C. Hall
2-5-85

CLINICAL IMPEDANCE AUDIOMETRY

SECOND EDITION

James Jerger, Ph. D.

Professor and Head
Division of Audiology and Speech Pathology
Department of Otorhinolaryngology
and Communicative Sciences
Baylor College of Medicine
Houston, Texas

Jerry L. Northern, Ph. D.

Professor and Head
Audiology Division
Department of Otolaryngology
University of Colorado Medical Center
Denver, Colorado

Educational Services Division
american
ELECTROMEDICS CORPORATION
"the impedance people"

American Electromedics Corporation: 533 Main Street
P.O. Box 317
Acton, Massachusetts 01720

Clinical Impedance Audiometry Second Edition ISBN 0-913258-66-0

Last digit is the print number: 9 8 7 6 5 4 3 2 1

PUBLISHER'S FOREWORD

As a college student I remember asking a professor, "What will tomorrow's test cover?" His cool reply was simple: "Everything since birth . . ." and I had learned another lesson. If one were to ask a clinician what knowledge will be applied in solving a particularly difficult clinical problem the same reply would be appropriate. Thus we present this second edition of *Clinical Impedance Audiometry* in hopes of extending the clinical acumen of practicing audiologists and otologists performing or interpreting impedance tests. American Electromedics strives to accomplish this purpose by various intellectual pursuits. Sponsoring the publication of this state-of-the-art textbook on the subject is another way to continue to support ongoing professional education as we have done for the past six years or, "since birth."

This work was published in association with Brian C. Decker, Publisher who orchestrated the editors, typesetters, printers, and binders in matching the book's physical appearance to the excellence of its content.

Irwin Klar
American Electromedics
September, 1979

Preface to the Second Edition

Almost five years have passed since the publication of the first edition of this handbook, years that have seen continuing growth in the clinical applications of impedance audiometry. Progess has been particularly noteworthy in three areas: 1) The use of impedance measures in the mass screening of children for hearing disorders 2) Refinement of acoustic reflex measures to predict degree of sensori-neural loss 3) Exploitation of ipsi-contralateral relations in exploring disorders of the central reflex arc.

The first area, use of impedance measures in mass screening, has created considerable, and we believe, healthy controversy. Advocates of the concept point to the widespread prevalence of midddle ear disorder in children, to the sensitivity of impedance measures in detecting such disorders, to the shortcomings of conventional pure-tone screening in this regard, and to the documented effects of even minor sensitivity loss on the acquisition of language skills during critical periods of language learning. Critics, however, emphasize the typically high false positive rates associated with impedance screening procedures, the fluctuating nature of middle ear disorder in children, and the lack, in any event, of a rational treatment regimen for the problem. Whatever its ultimate outcome may be, this controversy has had a positive educational effect in areas beyond impedance audiometry, per se. All parties to the debate have learned a good deal about the concepts of *sensitivity* (how well does the test identify what it seeks to identify) and *specificity* (how well does it exclude what it does not seek to identify). They have also learned the hard lesson that you can't have one without the other. As sensitivity increases, specificity decreases and vice versa. The better the test works to identify a particular disorder, the more likely it is to give a false-positive result. Similarly, a test without false alarms is typically a test with poor sensitivity. Advocates of mass impedance screening who point to its remarkable sensitivity to middle ear disorder have had to learn a bitter lesson about the price one must, inevitably, pay to achieve this high degree of sensitivity. Critics and advocates alike, moreover, have learned a great deal about the general concept of screening. They have had to learn, from the hard lesson of over-referral, that failing a screening procedure means follow-up examination rather than immediate referral to a physician. They have learned the difficult lesson that, because of the inevitable false alarm problem encountered in any screening technique of adequate sensitivity, screening must always be a three-step procedure. If the child fails the screen, he must be subjected to careful follow-up examination. Only if he fails the latter should he be referred for medical evaluation.

In summary, the controversy surrounding mass impedance screening will probably continue for several years. In the meantime, advocates and critics alike are, of necessity, learning some valuable lessons about cost-effectiveness in screening the hearing of large populations of children.

Interest in the use of acoustic reflex measures to predict degree of sensori-neural loss has expanded so rapidly during the past five years that we devote a separate chapter to the topic. The early promise of this technique has been only partially realized. It seems clear, at this writing, that prediction can be quite accurate in children, but encounters serious problems in adults, especially the elderly. At least two problems have been clearly identified: 1) The confounding effects of even very mild middle ear disorder on relations among reflex thresholds; and 2) an age effect, itself, on acoustic reflex thresholds. Here, again, we find healthy controversy. Critics of the technique point to its lack of precision and to the possibility of substantial predictive error in individual cases. Supporters, on the other hand, emphasize its relative accuracy in children, where such prediction has more practical value than in the elderly, and emphasize that, in any event, such predictions can be useful as cross-checks on other predicions as part of a total pediatric battery.

This controversy, too, has had a positive educational effect. Critics of the technique have, in their discourse with clinicians, learned something of the real-life problems of pediatric evaluation and of the inevitable compromises with laboratory precision often involved in this challenging area of clinical evaluation. Proponents of the technique, on the other hand, have been encouraged (prodded?) to seek the underlying bases of predictive error, and to catalogue and scrutinize all possible variable relevant to the technique. In the process, we have all learned a good deal more about the acoustic reflex in normal and impaired ears.

The third area in which great strides have been made during the past five years is the diagnostic application of ipsilateral (uncrossed) versus contralateral (crossed) reflexes in the analysis of retrocochlear, and especially brain stem, disorders. Here, again, progress has been so great that we devote an entire chapter to developments in this rapidly unfolding area. Measuring and recording the ipsilateral acoustic reflex is still, to a certain extent, a technologic challenge. Interaction between the probe and reflex-eliciting signals in the external ear canal yields an omnipresent acoustic artifact of varying degree. Although this ipsilateral artifact is often disconcerting, it can always be differentiated from the true ipsilateral reflex activity on the basis of differences in temporal pattern. Evaluating the latter is greatly facilitated by computer averaging techniques, but a simple recording of the reflex on a strip chart, with synchronous signal markers, is usually sufficient for adequate analysis. With proper precaution for artifact analysis, the ipsilateral acoustic reflex adds immeasureably to the diagnostic significance of acoustic reflex measures.

The clinical exploitation of ipsilateral-contralateral reflex patterns, based on the neuroanatomy of the acoustic reflex pathways in the brainstem, is a vivid and dramatic example of the complementary roles that basic investigation and clinical evaluation play in furthering our understanding of the auditory system. The pioneering work of Eric Borg, in the rabbit, established the basic wiring diagram of the system; the clinical evaluation of reflex patterns in patient material has validated both its structural and functional accuracy. As we shall see in Chapter VIII, specific reflex abnormalities can sometimes provide quite precise localization of brain stem disorder.

Although progress in these three areas has been especially noteworthy during the past five years, of perhaps greater importance in the long run, has been the steady growth of impedance audiometry as an integral part of the basic audiometric examination, and the extension of the technique into other specialties. We have seen, for example, dramatic growth in the use of automatic tympanometers by pediatricians seeking to monitor middle ear disease more objectively in children. Finally, we have seen, in the past few years, preliminary evaluation of the value of impedance audiometry in veterinary medicine, a field with vast potential for impedance applications.

Our goal, in the preparation of this second edition of *Impedance Audiometry* has been three-fold: first, to continue to provide a basic manual of test administration and test interpretation for both new and experienced clinicians; second, to update readers to the important new developments of the past five years; and third, to impart some sense of the continuously expanding horizons for impedance audiometry in clinical auditory evaluation.

James Jerger
Jerry Northern

September, 1979

Preface to First Edition

During the past decade no new development has so profoundly affected the practice of clinical audiology as the advent of impedance audiometry. Within a very short span of years we have seen the measurement of impedance characteristics of the middle ear progress from a sophisticated research tool to a clinical procedure applicable to virtually every patient referred for audiologic evaluation. The purpose of this manual is to introduce the salient features of impedance audiometry to all audiologists who may benefit from its use.

Although several investigators have successfully studied characteristics of the middle ear by means of impedance audiometers for more than 50 years, the story of modern impedance audiometry begins in 1946 with the publication of the now-classic monograph by Metz on the clinical measurement of middle ear impedance. Metz constructed what was probably the first clinically practical impedance bridge. Using an electromechanical method for detecting relative changes in the acoustic impedance of the middle ear Metz showed that, in patients with sensori-neural hearing loss and loudness recruitment, contraction of the stapedius muscle could be elicited by acoustic signals at considerably lower sensation levels than in the normal ear.

During the decade of the 1950's the pioneering work of Metz was continued and expanded almost exclusively in the Scandinavian countries.

In Denmark, Terkildsen and his colleagues pioneered the development of a clinically practical impedance bridge based on an electro-acoustic rather than an electro-mechanical principle. Later Jepsen used this electro-acoustic method to explore details of the normal stapedius reflex, and Ewertsen extended Metz's original work on the relation between the stapedius reflex and loudness recruitment.

In Sweden Moeller studied characteristics of the normal reflex while Klockhoff mapped modifications imposed by various types of hearing disorder. During this same period Lidén, in Gothenburg, began his now classic studies of the dynamic characteristics of the tympanic membrane culminating in the modern technique of tympanometry.

This early work in the Scandinavian countries was characterized by an interest in the detection of relative changes in middle ear impedance, especially those changes elicited by the stapedius reflex, and an almost total commitment to the electro-acoustic principle of measurement.

Late in the 1950's however, Zwislocki, in the United States, returned to the electro-mechanical principle in order to design an impedance bridge capable of measuring the absolute impedance of the middle ear system in the resting state. Feldman used Zwislocki's bridge to study absolute impedance characteristics in a variety of aural pathologies, but the technique never received wide clinical exploration, probably because many clinicians who attempted to use this bridge found it cumbersome and unwieldy to apply in routine patient evaluation.

The ultimate expansion of true clinical impedance audiometry beyond its native Scandinavian soil was due principally to the excellent work of Brooks, in England, and Alberti, in Canada. Using electro-acoustic bridges based on Terkildsen's original work,these investigators showed that impedance audiometry could be a practical clinical tool, and an especially valuable tool in the evaluation of young children.

Modern impedance audiometry includes at least three separate types of measurement:

1. tympanometry
2. absolute or static compliance
3. stapedius reflex thresholds

TYMPANOMETRY

Tympanometry is a technique for determining how the compliance of the middle ear system changes in response to variation in the air pressure on the lateral surface of the tympanic membrane. The measurement is carried out by introducing controlled degrees of both positive and negative air pressure into the closed cavity of the external ear canal. As air pressure is varied, the change in compliance is noted. The resulting graphic plot of compliance versus air pressure is called a "tympanogram." Tympanograms may be either calculated manually in point-by-point fashion or recorded automatically on an X-Y plotter or other type of graphic recording device.

STATIC COMPLIANCE

Measurement of the compliance of the middle ear in its resting or static state is accomplished by determining the volume of air which has a compliance equivalent to the compliance of the middle ear system under test. The static compliance of the middle ear is then expressed as this equivalent air volume (in cm^3).

In order to carry out the measurement of static compliance, it is necessary to calculate two volumes; first, the actual volume of the closed cavity in the external ear canal; second, the total volume when the "equivalent" volume of the middle ear system is added. The difference between these two volumes (the total volume minus the volume of the external canal) is the compliance of the middle ear. This value may be expressed either in acoustic ohms or in cubic centimeters of an equivalent volume of air. In clinical practice the air volume notation is preferred for its simplicity.

There are actually two resting states at which the static compliance of the middle ear can be measured. One is the static compliance with atmospheric pressure at the lateral surface of the tympanic membrane. The other is the static compliance at the air pressure yielding maximum compliance on the tympanogram. Both measures of static compliance are useful and important. The former is relevant to the way in which the middle ear functions in the everyday world, while the latter is more valuable from the diagnostic standpoint. In order to preserve this distinction, compliance at atmospheric or ambient air pressure is denoted by the symbol C_A, whereas compliance at the maximum of the tympanogram is denoted by the symbol C_M.

STAPEDIUS REFLEX

The stapedius muscle contracts reflexively in response to sound of sufficient loudness. The reflex is bilateral. Sound in either ear causes both muscles to contract. This interesting property greatly facilitates the clinical measurement of stapedius reflex thresholds. The impedance bridge is coupled to one ear, and sound is presented to the opposite ear. If the sound is sufficiently loud, both stapedius muscles contract. The muscular contraction tenses and stiffens the ossicular chain, thereby increasing the impedance (i.e., decreasing the compliance) of the middle ear system. This decrease in compliance is detected by the impedance bridge in the ear to which it is coupled. The threshold of the stapedius reflex is the lowest sound level capable of eliciting a detectable change in compliance.

This arrangement of sound in one ear and bridge in the other ear effectively tests the entire reflex arc. The afferent or sensory portion of the arc translates sound intensity into the appropriate neural correlate of apparent loudness via the VIIIth cranial nerve. The central portion of the arc, in the brain stem, evaluates this neural signal, and if it exceeds a certain critical level, transmits a command signal to the efferent or motor portion of the arc. The latter conveys this command signal, via the VIIth cranial (facial) nerve to the stapedius muscle.

PURPOSE OF THIS MANUAL

The purpose of this manual is to show how these broad concepts can be applied in everyday clinical evaluation. We begin with an elementary exposition of the basic concepts underlying impedance measurement by Drs. Berlin and Cullen. In the next chapter Dr. Northern outlines the essential steps in the clinical examination. Then Drs. Harford, Dempsey, Djupesland, and Bluestone discuss, in detail, tympanometry, static impedance, reflex measures, and evaluation of Eustachian tube function. In the next chapter your obedient servant attempts to relate these findings to diagnostic interpretation. In the final chapter, Dr. McCandless, an impedance innovator in his own right, engages in some stimulating speculation about what the future may hold.

The appendix contains 15 illustrative cases selected to demonstrate the various concepts we have tried to convey in the body of the manual.

It is our modest hope that the reader will be inspired to share with us at least some of the excitement and satisfaction that impedance autiometry has brought to the professional life and work of each contributor.

James Jerger
Houston, Texas

August, 1974

Contributors

Charles I. Berlin, Ph.D.

Director, Kresge Hearing Research Laboratory of the South; Professor of Otorhinolaryngology and Physiology, Louisiana State University Medical Center, New Orleans, Louisiana
Physical Basis of Impedance Measurement

Charles D. Bluestone, M.D.

Professor of Otolaryngology, University of Pittsburgh School of Medicine; Pittsburgh, Pennsylvania; Director, Department of Otolaryngology, Children's Hospital of Pittsburgh
Assessment of Eustachian Tube Function

Denzil N. Brooks, M.Sc.

Manchester Audiology Clinic, Manchester, England
Impedance in Screening

John K. Cullen, Jr., Ph.D.

Assistant Director, Kresge Hearing Research Laboratory of the South; Associate Professor of Otorhinolaryngology and Physiology, Louisiana State University Medical Center, New Orleans, Louisiana
Physical Basis of Impedance Measurement

Gisle Djupesland, M.D.

Associate Professor, Ear, Nose and Throat Department, Riks-hospitalet, Oslo, Norway
The Acoustic Reflex

James W. Hall, Ph.D.

Director of Audiology, Department of Hearing and Speech Sciences, University of Maryland, College Park, Maryland
Predicting Hearing Loss from the Acoustic Reflex

Earl R. Harford, Ph.D.

Professor and Director of Audiology, Department of Otolaryngology, University of Minnesota Medical School, Minneapolis, Minnesota
Tympanometry

Deborah Hayes, Ph.D.

Associate Professor, Division of Audiology and Speech Pathology, Department of Otorhinolaryngology and Communicative Sciences, Baylor College of Medicine, Texas Medical Center, Houston, Texas
Diagnostic Applications of Impedance Audiometry: Middle Ear Disorder, Sensori-Neural Disorder

James F. Jerger, Ph.D.

Professor and Head, Division of Audiology and Speech Pathology, Department of Otorhinolaryngology and Communicative Sciences, Baylor College of Medicine, Texas Medical Center, Houston, Texas
Diagnostic Applications of Impedance Audiometry: Middle Ear Disorder, Sensori-Neural Disorder. Applications of Impedance Audiometry to Animal Research

Susan Jerger, M.S.

Research Associate, Division of Audiology and Speech Pathology, Department of Otorhinolaryngology and Communicative Sciences, Baylor College of Medicine, Texas Medical Center, Houston, Texas
Diagnostic Applications of Impedance Audiometry: Central Auditory Disorder

Robert W. Keith, Ph.D.

Director, Division of Audiology and Speech Pathology, Department of Otolaryngology and Maxillofacial Surgery, University of Cincinnati Medical Center, Cincinnati, Ohio
Use of Impedance Measurements in Hearing Aid Fitting

Larry W. Mauldin, B.A.

Research Assistant, Division of Audiology and Speech Pathology, Department of Otorhinolaryngology and Communicative Sciences, Baylor College of Medicine, Texas Medical Center, Houston, Texas
Applications of Impedance Audiometry to Animal Research

Geary A. McCandless, Ph.D.

Professor, Department of Communication; Head, Audiology Division of Otolaryngology, University of Utah Medical Center, Salt Lake City, Utah
Use of Impedance Measurements in Hearing Aid Fitting

Jerry L. Northern, Ph.D.

Professor and Head, Audiology Division, Department of Otolaryngology, University of Colorado Medical Center, Denver, Colorado
Clinical Measurement Procedures in Impedance Audiometry
Impedance Measurements with Distinctive Groups

Contents

Chapter One

THE PHYSICAL BASIS OF IMPEDANCE MEASUREMENT

CHARLES I. BERLIN, Ph.D.
JOHN K. CULLEN, Jr., Ph.D.

INTRODUCTION

This chapter has been written in a number of parts for readers with different backgrounds. The introductory material and programmed sections are designed for the reader who prefers to learn by verbal analogy rather than by mathematic equation. However, in the interests of accuracy and stimulating better understanding of the physics involved, we have included sections on the necessary physics and mathematics.

The measurement of the total impedance of the ear at all frequencies is, in fact, not presently performed with most commercially available devices. The chapter will clarify how only one of the many contributing variables is generally assessed. The reader will wish to keep uppermost in mind that a clinically evaluated "ear with high impedance" has generally been studied for one variable (stiffness) at one frequency (typically 220 Hz), or at most, at a few frequencies; however, the data obtained are nevertheless useful in understanding the mechanical state of the middle ear.

IMPEDANCE BY ANALOGY

Impedance simply is a measure of the acceptance or rejection of energy per unit time. A mechanical system with high impedance accepts energy less readily than a mechanical system with low impedance. Imagine a canoeist who moves his paddle through the air. It moves quickly and easily. Conversely, if he is to move the paddle through water at the same speed as through air, he must apply a much greater force.

Preparation of this document was supported in part by NIGMS Fellowship 1 FO3 GM 52343 to one of the authors, USPHS Training Grant NS-05531, and Clinical Research Center Grant USPHS NS-11647.

We thank our colleagues for their respective editorial efforts and criticisms, and Pamela Burrell for her assistance in preparing this manuscript.

Relatively speaking, air is a low-impedance medium and water is a high-impedance medium. Here you can see the relationship between applied force, resultant velocity, and impedance which will be amplified in a later section.

Systems that are properly impedance-matched permit energy to be passed from one system to another. A good analogy to appreciate impedance matching is as follows:

A. Hold a piece of paper by one corner in front of you. With your other hand, make a fist and try to tear the paper by punching it in the middle section. The paper will almost float away from your fist. It is clear that very little of the energy in your hand can be used to break this paper apart unless the paper can somehow be made to accept more energy.

B. If the paper were held stiffly in space, let's say by two colleagues each holding two corners, you could then easily punch through the paper. The impedance of that system has been adjusted so that a more efficient transmission of energy from your fist to the paper can take place.

C. Now, substitute a brick wall for the paper. Common sense tells us that if you hit the brick wall with as much force as you hit the paper, there would be so much reflectance of energy that most of it would be dissipated in your hand and the high impedance of the wall would be painfully obvious. However, energy transfer from your hand to the wall is possible if we have a more efficient way of impedance matching.

One of the more common ways to do this is to use a hammer and nail. In Figure 1-1 you see two ways of using a nail. The nail in Position "B" is a far better impedance-matching device than the nail used in Position "A." By bringing the force of the hammer to bear on only the point of the nail, you have reduced the area over which the force from the hammer is spread. You have, in fact, increased the force-per-unit area transmitted to the wall without actually increasing the total force from your arm. Thus, the nail and hammer arrangement is an impedance-matcher effectively transmitting energy from your arm to the wall.

The tympanic membrane and ossicular chain act as an impedance-matching device to bring sound from the air into the cochlea. Since the cochlea is made up of fluid resembling sea water, it presents a reflective barrier to airborne sound. This is similar to the barrier the wall presented to your fist. The impedance-matching capability of the middle ear is primarily related to the ratio of the area of the tympanic membrane to that of the stapes footplate. In Figure 1-2 you can see how similar this arrangement is to a carpenter's nail. However, there are three ossicles that also operate to increase slightly the mechanical advantage achieved by the favorable areal ratio of the tympanic membrane to the stapes. The combination of the mechanical lever advantage and the areal ratio in the human ear helps compensate for the sound-reflecting properties of the fluids of the inner ear.

The Effects of Frequency

One of the problems with the hammer and nail analogy is that it suggests sound energy has only one aspect, namely a simple forward motion. In fact, sound waves, as they impinge upon the tympanic membrane, have both inward and outward motions that exert forces on the middle ear structures. Accounting for this back-and-forth motion generates a complicated problem in which we have to consider not only the

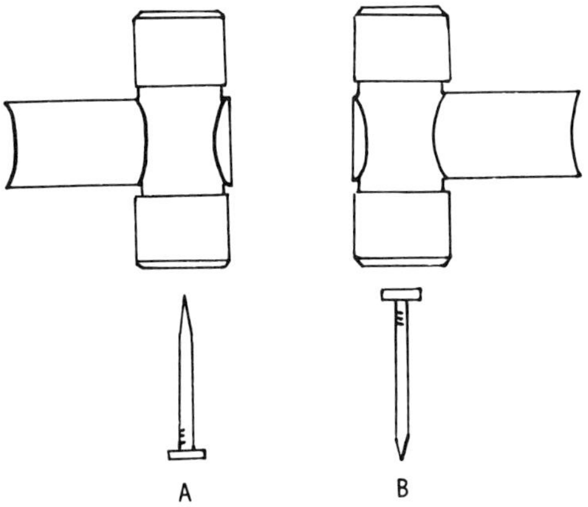

Figure 1-1 An analogy of impedance matching. The force of the hammer hitting the nail is the same in both diagrams A and B; however, the nail in position B will be driven into the wood more efficiently since the force from the hammer is concentrated over a very small unit of area.

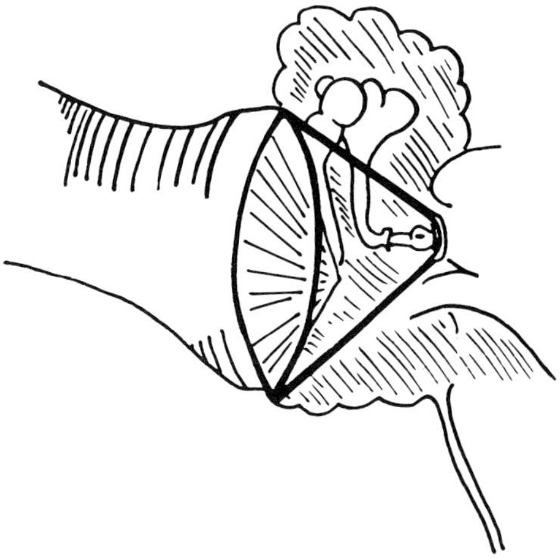

Figure 1-2 The "coning down" of area, typified by the hammer and nail analogy of Figure 1 is demonstrated in the ear.

incoming force in the positive direction but also the force in the negative direction, and all points in time between maximum positive and maximum negative deflection. In doing so, we find that the acceptance or reflection of energy in the middle ear is, to a great extent, frequency-dependent. The next section will show us how frequency enters into the picture.

The Impedance Equation

There are three factors that determine how much energy is accepted or reflected and in what frequency (f) ranges. The three factors are the *mass* (M) of the system, the *stiffness* (k) of the system, and its *resistance* (R). Mathematically speaking we express this as follows:

$$Z = \sqrt{R^2 + \underbrace{6.28\ fM}_{\substack{\text{mass}\\ \text{reactance}}} - \underbrace{\frac{k}{6.28f}}_{\substack{\text{elastic}\\ \text{reactance}}}{}^{2}}$$

Here reactance equals the contribution of either the mass term or the stiffness term to the total impedance.

The factor related to mass (6.28 x fM) is called the mass reactance. The factor dealing with stiffness is called the stiffness reactance, or more properly, the elastic reactance (k/6.28f). The resistance component, however, is simply resistance and is generally related to energy loss due to friction. Reactance differs from resistance in that resistance is not frequency-dependent.

The number 6.28 is a rough approximation of 2 x π, or 2 x pi. When 2 x π is multiplied by the frequency of the signal, we have what is called "angular frequency of the signal," designated later in this chapter as (ω).

Programmed Section

Let us now move into a partially programmed format to emphasize the points in this section. Cover the column to the left and fill in the blanks after the numbered statements. Check your response before you proceed to the next item.

mass	1. The three major factors that must be considered in analyzing the impedance of any mechanical system are its . . ., its stiffness, and its resistance.
stiffness	2. The three factors that interact in a complex fashion to account for the impedance of any mechanical system are the mass, the . . ., and the resistance.
resistance	3. The three major factors that are not strictly additive but interact in a complex fashion to generate the impedance of any mechanical system are the mass, the stiffness, and the . . . .
mass	4. The portion of the total impedance figure attributable to the . . . is called the mass reactance.
mass reactance	5. The portion of the impedance attributable to the mass is called the . . . .
stiffness	6. The portion of impedance attributable to . . . is called the elastic reactance.
elastic reactance	7. The portion of impedance attributable to stiffness is called . . . .
resistance	8. The portion of impedance attributable to . . . is called simple resistance.
mass reactance elastic reactance	9. Therefore, it is correct to say that the total impedance of the ear is composed of the complex interaction of . . ., . . ., and the resistance.
mass reactance elastic reactance resistance	10. Total impedance of the ear is not additive but, in fact, is the complex interaction of the . . ., the . . ., and the . . . .

D

11. Choose the correct statement. Impedance is the:

A. sum of mass, stiffness, and resistance;
B. product of mass, elasticity, and stiffness;
C. complex interaction of mass, resistance, and friction;
D. complex interaction of mass reactance, elastic reactance, and resistance.

One of the simplest ways to encode large amounts of verbal information precisely, but in small spaces, is with a mathematical equation. Notice that in question 11 the words "complex interaction" were easy to overlook. They are very important, as you will see.

Mathematically speaking, we express the complex interaction between mass, elasticity, and resistance as follows:

$$Z \text{ (the total impedance)} = \sqrt{R^2 + 2\pi fM \left(\frac{-k}{2\pi f}\right)^2}$$

Let us analyze this expression in parts: the expression that says $2\pi fM$ represents the mass reactance; and the expression that says $\frac{k}{2\pi f}$ is the elastic reactance.

mass reactance

12. Substitute the language equivalents for the part missing in the equation:
$Z = \sqrt{R^2 + \ldots \text{minus} \left(\frac{k}{2\pi f}\right)^2}$

elastic reactance or stiffness

13. Do the same for the missing parts here:

$$Z = \sqrt{R^2 + (2\pi fm \text{ minus } \ldots)^2}$$

total impedance, resistance (or R)

14. Try this expression:
$\ldots = \sqrt{\ldots^2 + 2\pi fM - \left(\frac{k}{2\pi f}\right)^2}$

resistance

15. As you can see, R stands for the third term in the impedance equation, ...

mass reactance, elastic reactance (or stiffness), and resistance

16. The three factors that interact in a complex fashion to generate the total impedance of any mechanical system are: . . ., . . ., and . . . .

$Z = \sqrt{R^2 + 2\pi fM - \left(\frac{k}{2\pi f}\right)^2}$

17. State the equation for the total impedance of any mechanical system: . . . .

For the sake of illustration, let us calculate a simple problem. If the mass of a given unit is "1" and the frequency of stimulation is 100 Hz, we might say that mass reactance of this system is "628 mass reactance units" (remember: mass reactance = $2\pi fM$ or 2 x 3.14 x 1 x 100 = 628). Now, there are two ways of increasing this mass reactance. One way is to increase the mass itself. In this case, if the frequency is held at 100 Hz and the mass doubled, the mass reactance will now go up to "1256 mass reactance units." However, if the mass remains the same and the *frequency* is doubled to 200 Hz, we will still have 1256 units of mass reactance. Mathematically, we would obtain $2\pi fM = 2 \times 3.14 \times 1 \times 200 = 1256$. *Thus, mass reactance increases in direct proportion to frequency.*

If we look at the elastic reactance (the expression related to stiffness) we see that if we have a stiffness value of 1 and a frequency of 100, we have an elastic reactance of 1/628 units. (Remember, elastic reactance $= \frac{k}{2\pi f} = \frac{1}{2 \times 3.14 \times 100}$ or $\frac{1}{6.28}$.)

If the stiffness increases, the value of that fraction increases and, therefore, the elastic reactance increases. However, if we hold the stiffness constant and increase the frequency of stimulation, we find that the elastic reactance *decreases* as frequency goes up. Thus, if $f = 200$, we would obtain $\frac{1}{2 \times 3.14 \times 200} = \frac{1}{1256}$ units.

As you can also see, resistance is *independent* of the frequency of stimulation. The units for mass reactance, elastic reactance, resistance, and total impedance are called *ohms*; the higher the ohm value, the greater the impedance.

A Clinical Auditory Application

Notice that if we increase the stiffness of a given system, the effect of the increased stiffness will be to weaken transmission in the low frequencies. If we increase the mass of the system, the effect will be to weaken transmission in the high frequencies. In the audiograms of Figure 1-3, pick the audiogram that represents a "tilt due to increased

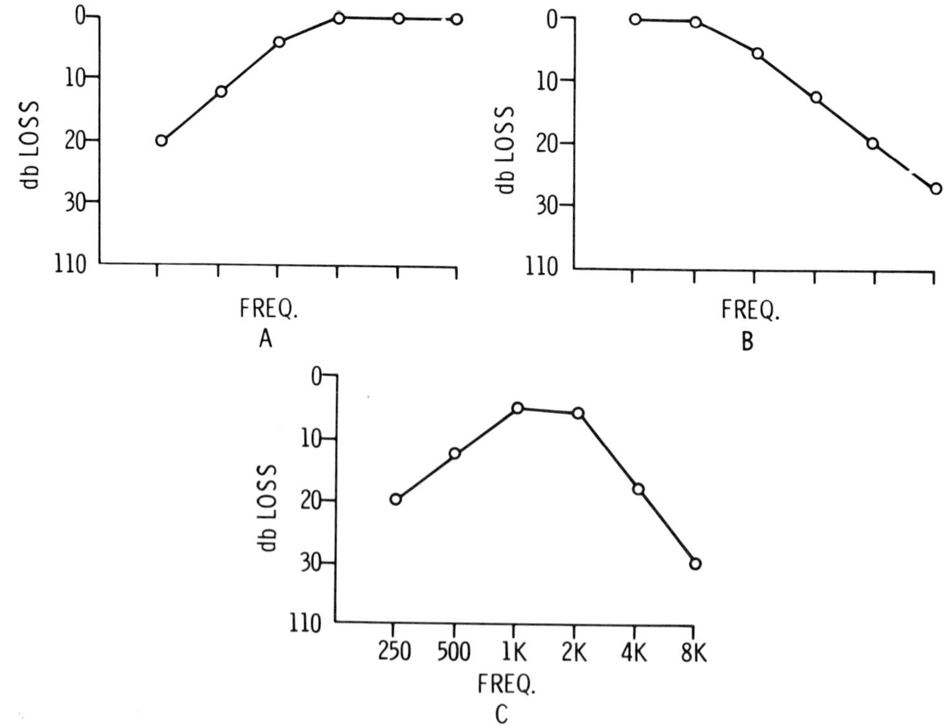

Figure 1-3 Audiograms representing a stiffness (a) to the mass (b) tilts, and mixtures of both (c).

stiffness." Audiogram A is the textbook audiogram often given for early otosclerosis, a lesion that causes a low-frequency hearing loss for pure tones.

In Figure 1-3, pick the audiogram that represents the "tilt due to increase in mass." In Audiogram B, a mild-to-moderate high-frequency pure-tone audiogram loss can be seen with an increase in the mass of the tympanic membrane and ossicular chain complex. (Cholesteatomas sometimes yield such a pattern.)

Note Audiogram C. It may represent an ear that has both mass and stiffness problems. It is "in resonance" around 1500 Hz, one of a number of resonance points in the human ear. Such an audiogram is often (but not always) associated with suppurative otitis media.

Notice also that total impedance is so frequency-dependent that we cannot express "the impedance of the ear" with one simple number. We need to express the frequency, as well as other information,[1] to get a complete picture of the ear's mechanical properties. For clinical convenience, the 220 Hz is typically used as a tone to infer the impedance of the ear. At that frequency, remember we are essentially measuring only the effects of elastic reactance, or *stiffness.*[2]

The Concept of Vectors

By way of review, there are three factors that interact to yield a measure of impedance. They are mass, stiffness, and resistance. This interaction is complex. That is, the expressions for resistance and reactance do not combine as simple additive factors; rather, they add to form a vector. You will notice the new term "vector"; some digression is required for the reader who may not be familiar with the concept of vectors. In Figure 1-4, you see a picture of a sailboat being driven by the wind in Direction A. The wind is driving the sailboat at 10 mph. However, the sailboat is also being subjected to a current at a 90° angle to the path of the wind. The current, marked "B," is a 10-mph current. At the end of one hour, the boat will have been driven 10 mph to the sailor's left. Where will the boat finish? At Position X,Y, or Z? You are correct if you chose Position Y.

Now let us further complicate this picture by introducing Vector C (Fig. 1-5, which will be the natural tendency of the sailboat to swing to the right side at about 2 mph. Two of the vectors here are additive, and therefore, one way to restate the problem is to subtract the 2-mph negative vector C from the 10-mph positive vector B and rewrite the problem as "A" (a 10 mph wind) interacting with "B" (an 8-mph current), in which case the craft would be at Point W.

Let us look at the next diagram (Fig 1-6), in which we substitute for A,B, and C as follows:

Resistance is substituted for A (the wind), stiffness is substituted for B (the current), and mass is substituted for C (the swing to the right). The resulting vector is analogous to the *position* of the sailboat and represents impedance of a system. As you can see, the contributing variables of mass, stiffness, and resistance are not directly additive, nor are they all three directly subtractive; they are combined in different values to give you a vector resultant.

---

[1]Phase angle, which will be discussed later.

[2]The term most often encountered in the current literature is "compliance." Compliance is simply the reciprocal of stiffness.

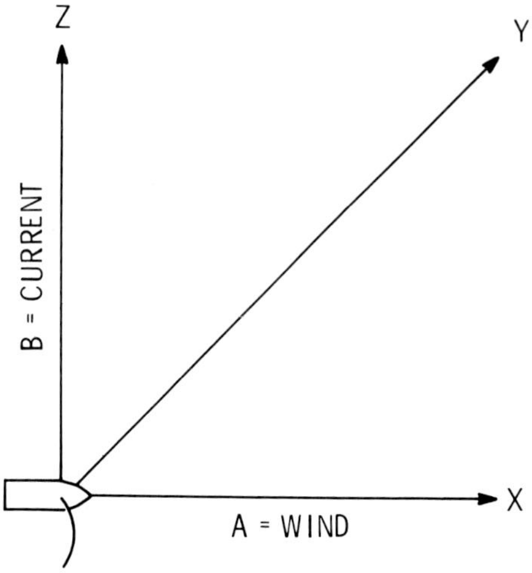

Figure 1-4 An example of vector notation in sailboat analogy.

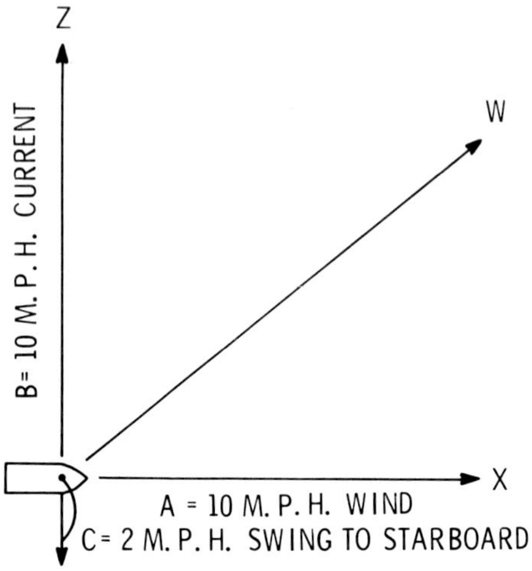

Figure 1-5 The same analogy with an additional 2 mile per hour swing to the starboard.

Most clinical measurements devices used in the ear ignore the contribution of each of the three factors independently, and present an approximation of the resultant vector as a total impedance measure. Most of the impedance changes in the human ear with pathologic findings are reflected as changes in stiffness; the changes of resistance due to pathologic factors in the ear have yet to be systematically demonstrated.[3] Changes due to mass are seen at such high frequencies that under conditions where most bridges are used, mass effects are negligible. Therefore, the elastic reactance (or stiffness) is essentially all we look at in making clinical measures of the ear's impedance.

Expressing Impedance in Equivalent Volumes of Air

In this section we will try to clarify the logic behind expressing impedance in terms

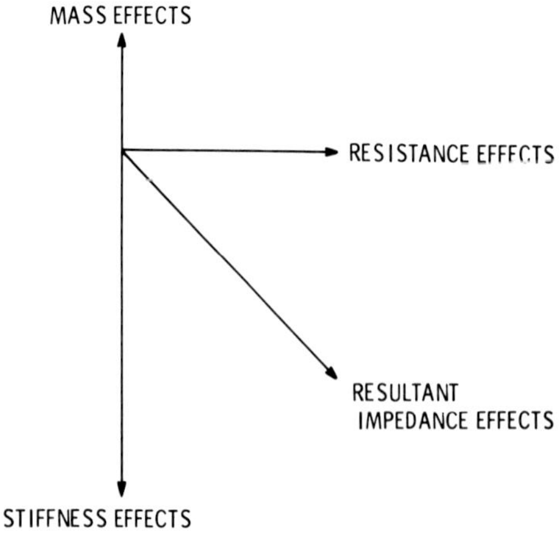

Figure 1-6 An impedance diagram showing the vector nature of resistance, mass, and stiffness components.

[3]Although lengthy test sessions may increase the resistance of the air trapped in the external meatus.

of an equivalent volume of air. In Figure 1-7 you see three cylinders of equal diameter but different total volumes. If you had to compress the air in those cylinders with a piston, which of the three air pockets do you think would accept the most energy from the piston, and which would be the "stiffest"? You are correct if you say that the air in the largest volume cylinder can accept the most energy from the piston, and the smallest volume would generate the greatest stiffness. It would also be correct to say that the larger volume of air has an impedance of fewer mechanical or acoustic ohms than the smaller cylinder. Thus, the stiffness of the ear measured with a bridge can be expressed in terms of a volume of air whose mechanical properties are equal to the ear in question. If we keep the air at a static pressure of 760 mm of mercury (e.g., at sea level pressure) we find that one cubic centimeter of air has about 1100 ohms of impedance to a 220-Hz signal.[4]

Review of the Verbal Section on Impedance

mass reactance elastic reactance (or stiffness) resistance or viscosity	1. The three factors that interact to account for the impedance of the ear are: A. . . . . . . B. . . . . . . C. . . . . . .
high	2. The effects of mass are seen at . . . (high or low) frequencies.
low	3. The effects of stiffness are seen at . . . (high or low) frequencies.
Stiffness or elastic reactance	4. Most clinical bridges, in fact, assess only one of the three factors related to impedance, namely . . ..
C	5. The three factors that interact to generate the total impedance of the ear (choose one): A. add linearly at all frequencies. B. are products of one another, especially at high frequencies.

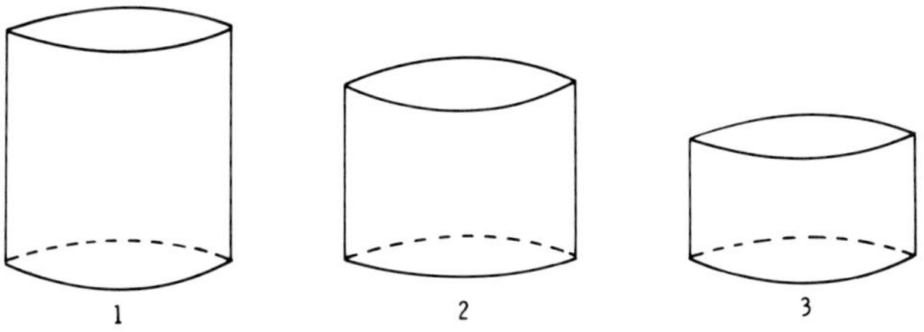

Figure 1-7 Volumes of air with different inherent impedances.

[4]Keep in mind that this "equivalent volume of air in cc" is subject to changes in atmospheric pressure and temperature. Therefore, the "normal impedance" of an ear would appear to be lower at high altitudes, like the city of Denver as compared with Brooklyn, New York.

If you missed this question, go on reading the next section.

C. interact in a complex fashion as a function of frequency.
D. can be added without attention to frequency.
E. are mostly accounted for by stiffness at all frequencies.

Skip this section if you got the last item correct.

If you chose A, or B, or D, remember: The factors that make up the impedance equation do not add or multiply; they interact in a complex fashion as a function of frequency. If you chose E, remember that the impedance audiometer, which uses a low-frequency probe tone, assesses primarily the stiffness of the ear. Stiffness effects are *not* uniform at all frequencies, and therefore C is the best answer.

The next section covers similar material but with the precision and accuracy inherent in mathematic statements, which cannot be matched by words alone.

IMPEDANCE FOR THE PHYSICALLY ORIENTED READER

Introduction

As we said earlier, impedance may be roughly defined as a measure of a physical system's ability to transmit or accept energy per unit time (power). Under this definition, one would expect that a sound-conducting system characterized as having a high impedance situated between a loudspeaker and a microphone would allow less of the sound power generated at the speaker to arrive at the microphone than would a system characterized as having a low impedance. While this "feeling" for impedance is not wrong, it provides little information as to how the intensity of the acoustic signal picked up by the microphone will vary as a function of changes in frequency or of alterations in the dimensions of the sound-conducting system. To gain an appreciation of the factors making up the term impedance, it is necessary to review some basic physical principles.

Review of Physics

Force (F)[5] is a quantity with which most of us are familiar. For example, a wind blowing at 25 mph exerts more force on an open umbrella than does a light breeze. In the English system of units, force is measured in pounds, while the unit of force in the centimeter-grams-seconds (cgs) system often used in acoustic is the dyne.

Work has a specific meaning in physics which differs somewhat from its general connotation. We would feel that we had "worked" very hard if we spent several hours attempting to lift a very heavy box that would not move. Yet, in the physical sense, no work would have been accomplished, since, in spite of the large force we applied, the

[5]F is used to designate force in this section, and f is used to designate frequency.

box did not move. In physics, work (W) is force (F) operating through a distance (x), or W = Fx. In the cgs system, work is measured in dyne-centimeters. Power (P), measured in watts, is the rate of doing work, or work/unit time (t). We may write this as $\Delta W/\Delta t = P$, or $P = F\Delta x/\Delta t$, where Δ is used to indicate change. Since x is distance displaced, $\Delta x/\Delta t$ corresponds to change in displacement per interval of time, or velocity (v). We can now say P = Fv. Power is thus the product of force and velocity. Naturally, the force impressed on a system, and the subsequent velocity, are not independent in a mechanical system. Rather, they are related to one another by the physical characteristics of the system such that F = Zv. Z is termed impedance, and in cgs units, has the dimensions of dyne • sec/cm.[6] This is often called the mechanical ohm in honor of Georg Simon Ohm (1789-1854), who first used a similar concept to characterize voltage-current relationships in electrical circuits. If Z is small, the force needed to achieve a given velocity is small; if Z is large, F must also be large to obtain this same velocity.

In an acoustic system, the physical characteristics encompassed by the term Z are the mass of the medium, its compressibility, and resistance or viscosity. We now wish to examine how these various characteristics interact with force.

The relationship between force and the movement of a mass is given by Sir Isaac Newton's (1642-1727) second law: The product of mass (M) and acceleration (a) is equal to the applied force, or F = Ma.

Compressibility of a medium may be thought of as analogous to a spring that can be streched or compressed. Common experience tells us that a compressed spring "pushes" back while a streched spring "pulls" back, the degree of "push" or "pull" being predicted on the size and material of the spring. The suspension spring of an automobile might be characterized as being "stiffer" than a screen door spring, since a larger force is needed to stretch the car spring one inch than is required to stretch the door spring a comparable distance. This relation can be stated mathematically as F = kx, where k is the stiffness coefficient; the larger k, the more force must be applied in order to stretch or compress the spring a distance (x).

The resistive, or viscous, qualities of a medium result from molecules bumping into one another and sliding along the walls that make up the boundaries of the system. This bumping and sliding results in the production of heat in a manner similar to the heating of a drill while boring wood at high speed. Heat produced in this way is a loss of power, and the force (F) necessary to overcome this loss is proportional to velocity (v). Formally, F = Rv, where R is a quantity representing the viscous characteristics of the medium; the larger R is, the larger must be the applied force to achieve a given velocity.

Incorporating these principles, we may picture an acoustic system as in Figure 1-8. Here the spring represents the compressibility or elasticlike characteristics of the medium, M its mass, and the piston device to the right, its viscous nature. We may now examine how this system behaves when a force is applied at, say, Point A, using the force relations given above. When the system is subjected to an applied force, the mass will accelerate in accordance with the relation F = Ma; the spring will compress (or stretch) in agreement with the relation F = kx, and the piston will move with a velocity determined by the relation F = Rv. Since the elements of the system are connected, they will act as a unit. That is, the elements acting together will produce a force that is

[6] The dimensions of the cgs mechanical ohm are often given as grams/sec. These are equivalent to the above dimensions, since dynes = grams • cm/sec². Substituting this relation yields grams/sec.

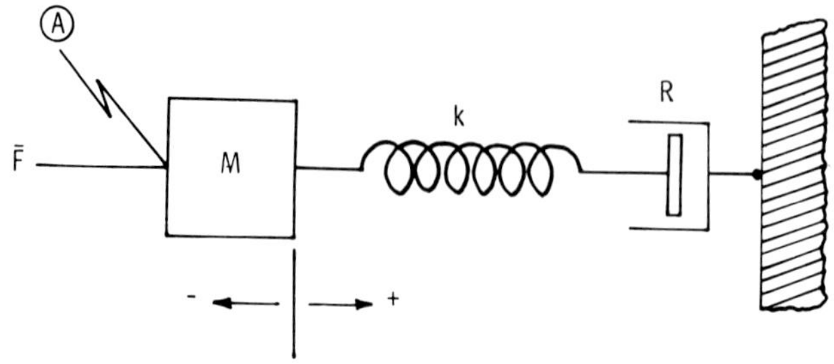

Figure 1-8 A mechanical analog of an acoustic system.

opposed, but equal to, the applied force. Therefore, $F = kx + MA + Rv$.

Consider now the situation in which the magnitude of the applied force varies periodically, as would be the case if the force were a pure tone. F could then be written as $F = F^* \sin\theta$, where F^* is the maximum value of the force and θ is a function of time. We may then diagram (Fig 1-9) the displacement (x), velocity (v), and acceleration (a) of the elements for one complete cycle of the applied force. Relating these diagrams to Figure 1-8, we can see that when the spring is maximally compressed (maximum positive displacement), the velocity must be zero, since the system is about to reverse its

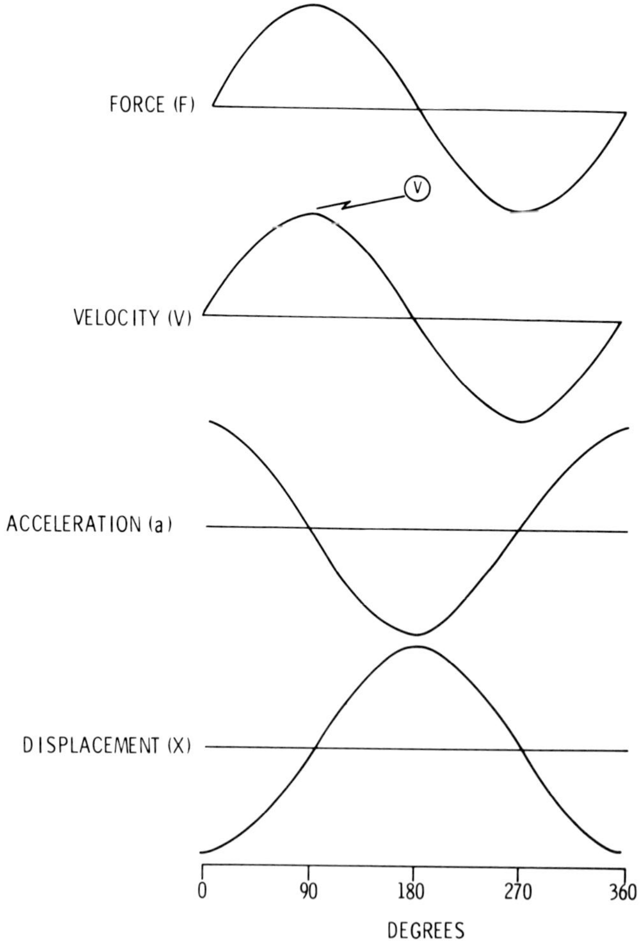

Figure 1-9 The phase-angle relationship between force, velocity, acceleration and displacement.

direction of motion and the acceleration must be at its largest negative value to bring the system to a stop to allow for the reversal. Similarly, when the spring is fully stretched, the velocity must again be zero and the acceleration must have its largest positive value.

The velocity curve is in phase with the force curve. That is, maxima and minima for the two curves occur at the same times in the cycle. The acceleration curve, on the other hand, has its maximum and minimum displaced a quarter of a cycle (90°) ahead of those for the force and velocity curves. The displacement curve is exactly out of phase (180°) with the acceleration, so that when displacement is at a maximum, acceleration is at a minimum, and vice versa. If we stand on the maximum of the velocity curve (Point V, Fig 1-9) and observe the relative positions of the maxima for acceleration and displacement, we see that the acceleration maximum occurs a quarter of a cycle (90°) before the velocity maximum, while the displacement maximum occurs a quarter of a cycle later. We may plot these phase relations on a graph, as in Figure 1-10.

So far we have been able to formulate a relation between an applied force and the mass, stiffness, and resistance linked, respectively, to acceleration, displacement, and velocity. Recall that, in accordance with our earlier definition, the impedance relation we seek must be the ratio between the applied force (F) and the velocity (v), or $Z = F/v$. Therefore, we want to express displacement and acceleration in terms of velocity. Because we are dealing with harmonic motion, the displacement can be expressed as v/ω and the acceleration as ωv, where $\omega = 2\pi f$, or angular frequency as defined previously in the section on Impedance by Analogy. This allows us to write our formula for force as $F = [(\omega M < +90) + (k/\omega < -90) + R]v$. Here, the $< +90$ symbol is used to designate the phase relations shown in Figures 1-9 and 1-10. Dividing both sides of the equation by v and rearranging terms gives us $F/v = Z = [R + (\omega M < +90) + (k/\omega < -90)]$. This relation for impedance can again be plotted in polar coordinates where the length of the arrows, or vectors, represents the magnitude of the various terms (Fig 1-11). These vectors can be considered as projections of another vector Z on the coordinates of a Cartesian coordinate system. The magnitude of Z (i.e., its length in Figure 1-12) can be obtained by use of the Pythagorean theorem of geometry: The

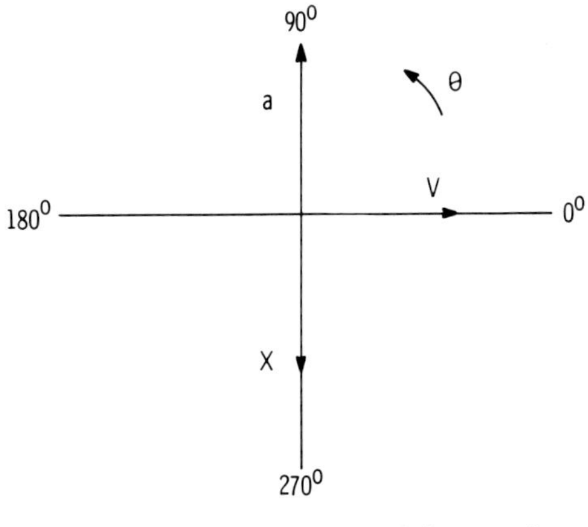

Figure 1-10 The relationship of force, velocity, acceleration, and displacement in polar coordinates.

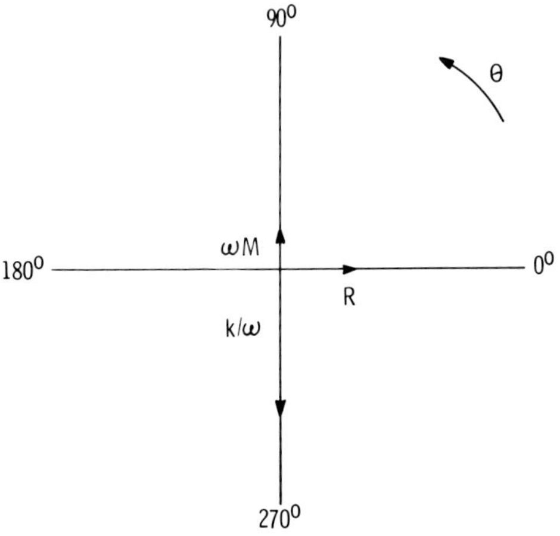

Figure 1-11 Polar representation of impedance components.

square of the hypotenuse of a right triangle is equal to the sum of the sides squared (as shown in Figure 1-13). Applying this theorem, the magnitude of Z is given by:

$$Z^2 = R^2 + (\omega M - k/\omega)^2$$

or

$$Z = \sqrt{R^2 + (\omega M - k/\omega)^2}$$

This is the relation for the impedance magnitude given previously and most often seen in textbooks. Note that there can be many values of R and (ωM - k/ω) which give a magnitude Z. Therefore, to specify Z unambiguously, we must know the angle of Z relative to the positive x-axis. This is given by θ = arctan [(ωM - k/ω)/R]. In writing Z, we often specify it as Z = /Z/<θ, where it is understood that /Z/ represents the magnitude and <θ, the angle of Z relative to the coordinate system.

The components of Z along the positive x-axis are commonly called mechanical resistance, while those along the y-axes are called reactance. In either case, they have the value of mechanical ohms (dyne • sec/cm).

Examining the equation for Z, one can see that the magnitude of the mass reactance component increases directly with frequency (=2πfM),[7] while elastic reactance decreases directly with frequency (= k/2πf). At some value of frequency, these two components will be equal and will combine to be zero. This value of frequency is often termed the "resonant frequency" of the system. Note that the resistive (viscous) component along the x-axis is invariant with frequency.

We have developed our concepts of impedance in mechanical terms for clarity. However, the conversion to acoustic quantities is not difficult when it is realized that pressure (p) is actually force divided by area, and the velocity in which we are interested is the velocity of a cross-sectional area of gas (u). Thus, acoustic impedance equals p/u and has the dimensions of dyne • sec/cm^5 or gram/cm^4 • sec. That is, the

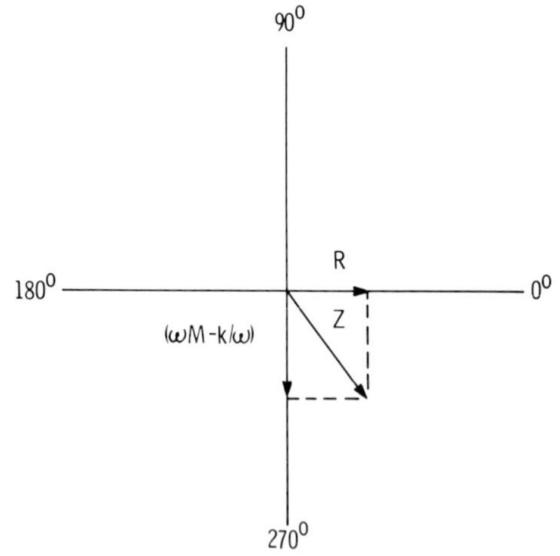

Figure 1-12 The equivalent impedance vector (and its components) in Cartesian form.

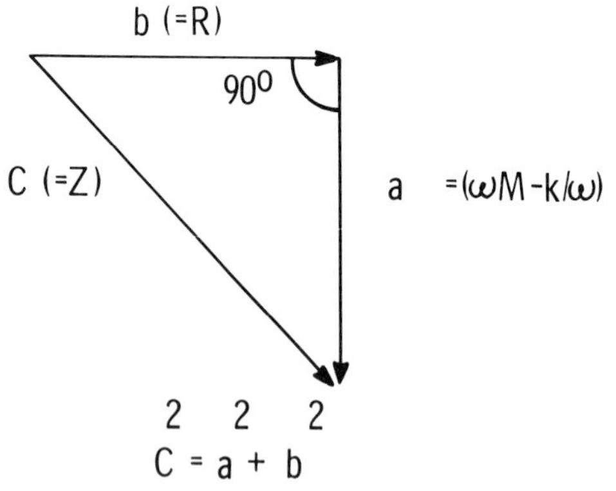

Figure 1-13 The application of the Pythagorean theorem of geometry to the relation of overall impedance to the contributing components.

[7]Recall that $\omega = 2\pi f$.

acoustic impedance of a sound-conducting system is equal to its *mechanical impedance*, scaled by a factor of 1 divided by the square of the cross-sectional area.

Impedance Principles in Clinical Use

In the previous sections, we have developed the physical basis for impedance. We now wish to apply this to obtain a better understanding of clinical impedance determinations.

Currently available electroacoustic bridges employ an ear insert containing a small acoustic generator and microphone which are sealed into the external meatus by inflatable cuffs, soft rubber seals, or other means. This traps a small volume of air between the seal and the tympanic membrane. This volume may be treated, for practical purposes, as being confined to a rigid walled tube. Since the dimensions of the cylinder of air are small relative to the wave length of the sound used to measure the impedance,[8] the motion of the cylinder is the same as a mechanical system having the properties of mass, stiffness, and resistance. The air will move as a unit, providing the mass of the system; the compression and expansion of the air provide the stiffness. The resistance component arises from the viscous nature of the entrapped air. We may, therefore, write the impedance of this volume as $Z = R + (\omega M < +90) + (k/\omega < -90)$, as in the previous section.

Because of the small volume of the air cylinder, the mass (calculated as density times volume) will be small. Since the measuring frequency is low, the value of the mass reactance (ωM) in the impedance expression will also be small. Viscosity is negligible, since the volume of air is moving as a unit. The elastic reactance[9] (k/ω), on the other hand, is large at these low frequencies. Using a diagram similar to Figure 1-12, we can represent the impedance components of the air volume qualitatively (Fig. 1-14). Since R and ωM are small, the resulting vector Z is approximately equal to k/ω at an angle of -90° (Fig. 1-15). Because of this, we may consider the impedance of the entrapped air as solely a stiffness reactance without appreciable error.

Experimental measurements taken of the middle ear components at these frequencies, when corrected for the volume of air in the external meatus, show that these structures also appear as an elastic reactance. That is, the mass of the tympanic membrane and ossicles, and the viscous forces associated with their movement, are small relative to their stiffness. Therefore, we may consider the measurement of the ear impedance, including the air entrapped in the external meatus, as equivalent to measuring a large volume of air composed of two compartments: the volume of air in the external meatus and an *equivalent* volume of air which would have a stiffness equal to that of the middle ear mechanisms. This is shown diagramatically in Figure 1-16.

To make static measures of middle ear impedance clinically, we obtain a measure of the stiffness of Block C or, alternatively, its *equivalent* volume. This is accomplished by introducing an increased pressure into the external meatus sufficient to prohibit movement of the tympanic membrane and ossicular chain. This then yields a measure

---

[8]The frequency used in most clinical measurements is 220 Hz. This yields a wavelength of approximately 161 cm for this low frequency at a temperature of 37°C.

[9]Generally, this is expressed in terms of acoustic compliance (c) where $k = 1/c$; the larger the value of c, the smaller the value of k.

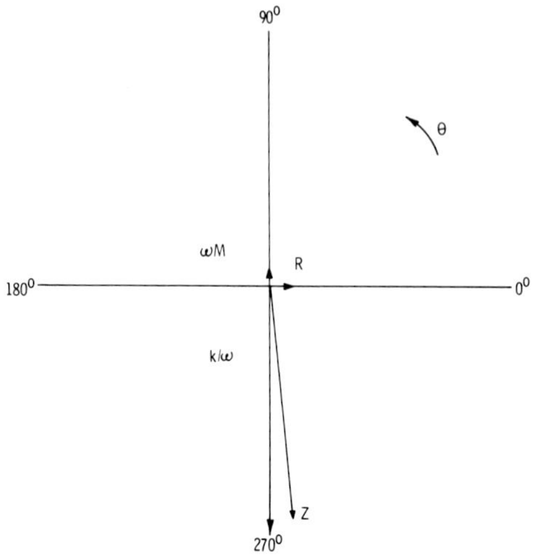

Figure 1-14 The impedance components of a small air volume at low frequencies.

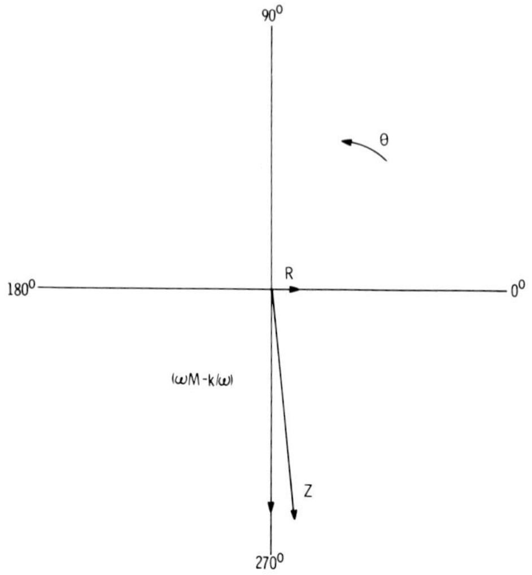

Figure 1-15 The practical results of having small mass reactances and resistances in the ear.

of the air volume in the external meatus (Block B). If the increased pressure is then bled off, we can obtain a measure of the larger volume (Block A). The *equivalent volume* representing the impedance of the middle ear can be deducted by subtraction: Vol. C (equiv.) = Vol. A - Vol. B.

In making tympanograms, we are observing the changes in the *equivalent volume* representing the stiffness of the middle ear components as the pressure in the external ear is varied. Here we can assume that the volume of air in the external meatus does not vary. The changes in impedance measured as the pressure is varied thus represent changes of stiffness for the middle ear. These changes as a function of pressure provide the curves that correlate with specific middle ear disorders. Likewise, middle ear muscle reflexes produce changes in the stiffness of the middle ear components without affecting the volume of air within the external meatus. The impedance changes measured during a reflex directly reflect the alteration of middle ear impedance produced by contraction of the middle ear muscles.

The Electroacoustic Bridge

The previous sections have dealt with the physical basis of impedance and the

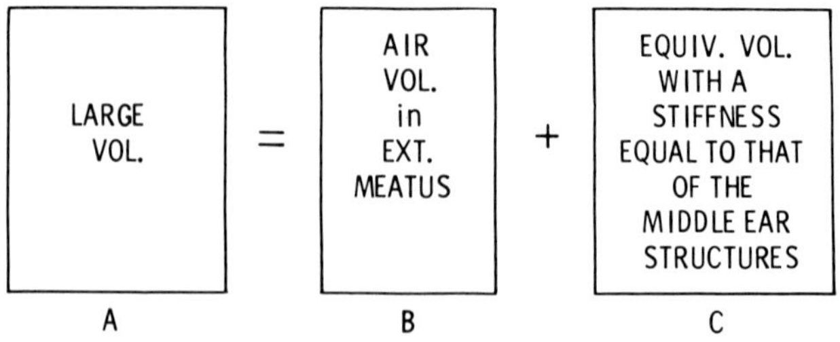

Figure 1-16 An analysis of the use of "equivalent volumes of air" as an index of the stiffness equal to that of the middle ear mechanism alone.

principles behind the clinical measurement of ear impedance. Here, we wish to treat briefly the theory of the electroacoustic bridge or impedance audiometer.

The ear insert of the bridge consists of an acoustic generator and measuring microphone which may be sealed into the external meatus. The generator is made to function through a small tube of high acoustic impedance. In this acoustic system, the volume velocity u will equal p/Z_t where p is the sound pressure at the generator and Z_t equals the sum of the acoustic impedance of the tube (Z_x) and the combined impedance of the entrapped air volume (Z_a) and the middle ear (Z_b). Since Z_x is much larger than Z_a or Z_b, Z_t is approximately equal to Z_x, and u will be approximately equal to p/Z_x. That is, volume velocity will depend on Z_x, not Z_a or Z_b (Fig. 1-17).

The measuring microphone is also specially constructed to operate through a small tube of high impedance. This permits measurements of pressure at the ear insert-external meatus interface to be made without being affected by the presence of the microphone.

Recall that, for all conditions, u will be a relative constant. Thus, the pressure value will be proportional to the magnitude of the combined impedances Z_a and Z_b. This value can be read on an appropriate meter or, as is most commonly done, read on a meter that can be nulled to zero. After initial closure of the meatus with the insert, the volume of the entrapped air will not change and Z_a is constant. Therefore, changes in the measured sound pressure (or, equivalently, deflections of the meter) represent changes in the impedance of the middle ear component, Z_b.

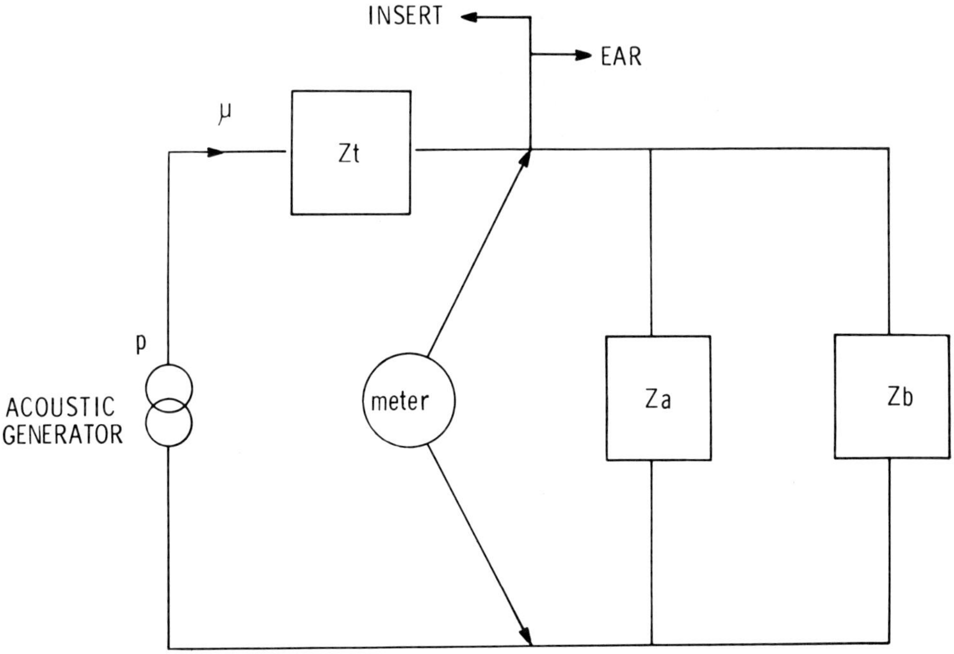

Figure 1-17 A block diagram clarifying why the volume velocity depends more on the acoustic impedance of the insert tube rather than on the smaller values generated by the sum of the impedances of the entrapped air volume plus the middle-ear impedance.

RECOMMENDED ADDITIONAL READING

Beranek, L.L.: *Acoustics.* New York, McGraw-Hill, 1954.

Kinsler, L.E. and Frey, A.R.: *Fundamentals of Acoustics.* New York, Wiley, 1962.

Lilly, D.J.: Acoustic impedance at the tympanic membrane. In Katz, J. (Ed.): *Handbook of Clinical Audiology* (Chap. 23). Baltimore, Williams & Wilkins Co., 1972.

Metz, O.: The acoustic impedance measured on normal and pathological ears. *Acta Otolaryng. (Suppl.)* 63: 1, 1946.

Møller, A.R.: Network model of the middle ear. *J.A.S.A.* 33: 168, 1961.

Terkildsen, K. and Scott-Nielsen, S.: An electroacoustic impedance bridge for clinical use. *Arch. Otolaryng.* 72: 339, 1960.

Zwislocki, J.: Analysis of the middle-ear function. I. Input impedance. *J.A.S.A.* 34: 1514, 1962.

Chapter Two

CLINICAL MEASUREMENT PROCEDURES IN IMPEDANCE AUDIOMETRY

JERRY L. NORTHERN, Ph. D.

INTRODUCTION

The operational principles underlying the electroacoustic impedance audiometer are relatively simple, and the technical manipulations of the test procedures are also not particularly complex. The clinician should thoroughly understand the operation of the instrument to facilitate development of skills in performing the clinical tests. The clinician should practice these test procedures on a number of subjects before attempting to test patients. The clinician who must refer to notes to carry out the impedance test battery creates a considerable credibility gap for the patient; likewise, the difficult-to-test patient may not wish to cooperate while the novice clinician fumbles through the impedance test battery. In skillful and experienced hands, the impedance test battery can be easily completed in a minute or two per ear with little or no discomfort for the patient. The operational steps necessary to perform each test are described in the instruction manuals that accompany each impedance meter. The purpose of this chapter is to explain the principles of each test in the impedance test battery and to describe various applications of impedance audiometry in routine clinical use.

The impedance test battery consists of tympanometry, static compliance, acoustic reflex tests, and the physical volume test. Although each of these tests provides some information about the function and integrity of the auditory mechanism (Alberti and Kristensen, 1970), the technique becomes much more meaningful when relationships among the four procedures are considered. Diagnostic judgments can be made with greater authority and assurance when the overall configuration of the entire impedance battery is available. Jerger (1970) states that tympanometry alone is useful to only a limited degree, static compliance norms are too variable for accurate diagnosis, and absence of the acoustic reflex may be due to several possible factors. Although each individual test has limitations, when they are considered in combination, the battery yields patterns of great diagnostic value. Complete information and data regarding each of the elements in the impedance test battery are featured in later chapters in this text (Fig. 2-1).

PREPARING THE PATIENT

Because of the objective nature of the impedance test battery, little cooperative effort is required from the patient. The patient may be tested while seated wearing a comfortably fitted headset. The earphone is fitted over one ear and the transducer assembly is positioned on the patient's temple, forward of the opposite ear. If the transducer box is placed too close to the patient's ear, it is often difficult for the clinician to view the patient's ear canal clearly.

The patient is instructed that he is about to be given a type of hearing test in which a small plug will be inserted into his ear canal. It may help to show the patient the probe tip. The patient should be told that he is to sit still until the test is completed. Sometimes it may satisfy the patient's curiosity to inform him that the test is a measure of "how well his eardrum moves." The only additional patient instruction is offered prior to attempting to elicit the acoustic reflex. The patient is then warned that he may hear a very loud sound and not to be startled by the signal.

It is routinely necessary to fit a protective cuff onto the tip of the probe tip. This cuff is used to provide an airtight seal of the probe tip in the patient's ear canal. Because ear canals come in a variety of shapes and sizes, cuffs of different sizes and shapes must be available. Inflatable catheter tubes of varying diameters can be fitted to the probe tip. Adhesive tape can be wrapped around the probe tip until the desired diameter is achieved. Some clinicians prefer ear impression mixtures which they mix and set up around the probe tip in the ear canal. It makes no difference to the test procedure which type of cuff is selected, as long as an airtight seal can be achieved (Richards, 1973). Occasionally, when all else fails, a thin coating of Vaseline on the

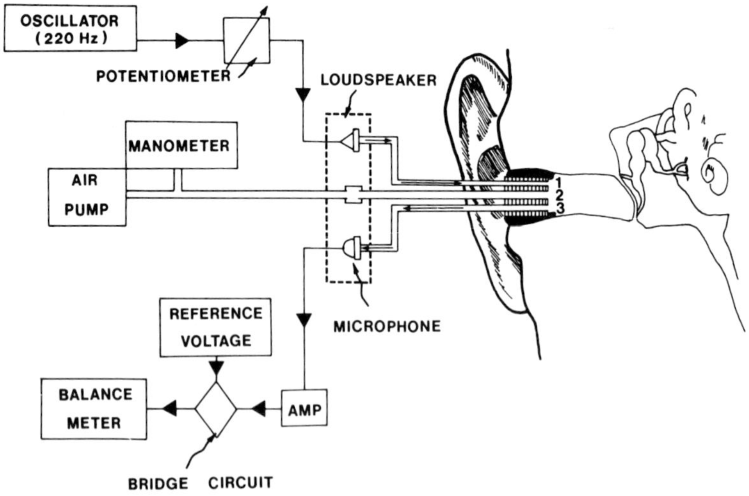

Figure 2-1 Diagrammatic representation of an electroacoustic impedance meter with probe tip inserted into the ear canal. The three operational systems include an oscillator to produce the probe tone, an air pressure manometer to control ear canal air pressure, and a microphone to compare SPL in the ear canal with a reference SPL.

outside of the cuff that fits the canal best will help produce a good airtight seal. Vaseline, however, may clog the probe tip holes if used too often, and tends to make the patient's ear canal quite slippery.

Proper placement of the cuff on the probe tip is important. The cuff must be fitted tightly enough so that it will not slip off and remain in the patient's ear canal when the probe tip is removed. However, the cuff should be seated on the probe tip in such a way that it extends slightly over the tip, so that ear canal debris and wax will be pushed ahead of the probe tip by the cuff, thereby reducing the possibility of plugging the tiny holes in the tip of the probe.

The cuffs should, of course, be cleaned after each use. The use of alcohol as a cleaning agent tends to make the rubber cuffs very hard and ultimately uncomfortable for the patient. Zephrin (benzalkonium chloride) is a good substitute for alcohol and cleans the cuff quite well. Liquid surgical soap may be rubbed vigorously on the cuffs, which are then rinsed with hot water and set aside to drain and dry. High-frequency sonic cleansers such as hearing aid dealers often use to clean earmolds are not very successful in the cleaning of the probe tip cuffs.

Obtaining the airtight seal of the probe tip in the patient's ear canal often poses the most serious problem to the novice in the performance of impedance audiometry. There is no substitute for experience. Every clinician should expect to encounter some difficulty in obtaining the seal while conducting initial impedance tests. Skilled clinicians may occasionally meet a patient in whom a seal simply cannot be obtained. Such patients are rare, however, and probably comprise less than 2 percent of the clinical population.

A cursory physical examination of the patient's external ear must be done before attempting to select a probe cuff. It is usually quicker to select the largest size cuff and work toward smaller sizes than to begin with the small cuffs. The pinna of the patient is then raised and pulled posteriorly. This will expose and straighten the ear canal. Care should be taken to insert the probe and cuff into the ear canal so that it is not being forced directly into the wall of the ear canal. Slight rotation of the probe and cuff helps to slip the tip into the canal comfortably. The cuff should fit into the canal fairly tightly even with the pinna distended. When the probe and cuff are settled securely in the ear canal, the pinna is released and the canal is allowed to collapse around the probe cuff.

The hermetic seal of the probe tip is quickly checked by increasing the air pressure in the external canal to plus 200 mm H_20, while the clinician observes the air pressure meter to see if the positive air pressure can be maintained. A slow leak can be tolerated, and impedance audiometry can be accomplished by experienced clinicians under less-than-airtight conditions.

TYMPANOMETRY

Tympanometry is the measurement of eardrum compliance change as air pressure is varied in the external canal. Using the impedance bridge it is possible to determine middle ear pressure and quantitate Eustachian tube function behind an intact tympanic membrane. Compliance of the tympanic membrane is measured as the relative change in the sound pressure level (SPL) in the entrapped ear canal cavity as the air pressure is increased and decreased. When sound waves strike the tympanic membrane, some energy is reflected back, identical in frequency to the probe tone frequency but differing in phase and amplitude. The amount of difference in phase and amplitude between the probe frequency and the reflected wave depends upon the impedance characteristics of the tympanic membrane and the middle ear system. Acoustic impedance purists worry about measurements of the phase difference, but knowledge of the phase offers little, if any, clinical information. The resultant graph or tympanogram (pressure-compliance function) shows the compliance change of the tympanic membrane as a function of air pressure variations by measuring the relative sound pressure level change (Figs. 2-2 and 2-3).

The point of maximum compliance (measured as the point of lowest sound pressure level in the external cavity) occurs when the pressure in the middle ear is balanced by the introduced pressure in the closed external ear cavity. Thus, tympanometry provides an indirect measure of existing middle ear pressure by identifying the air pressure in the external canal at which the eardrum shows a peak of maximum compliance.

The mechanical aspects of tympanometry begin by pushing or "clamping" the tympanic membrane into a position of poor compliance with air pressure equal to plus 200 mm H_20. At this point the stiffened eardrum reflects most of the probe tone energy, creating a high SPL measurement at the probe pick-up microphone. Air pressure is then reduced in the ear canal cavity, permitting the compliance of the tympanic membrane to increase; the impedance meter now measures a decrease in reflected SPL. The lowest SPL is achieved at the maximum compliance of the tympanic membrane, and as negative air pressures are created in the external auditory canal, compliance decreases and is noted by an increase in the SPL meter. Clinicians tend to conceptualize the tympanogram as "the way the eardrum moves." Actually, the tympanogram is a graphic recording of changes in SPL in the external ear as air pressure is varied by the clinician.

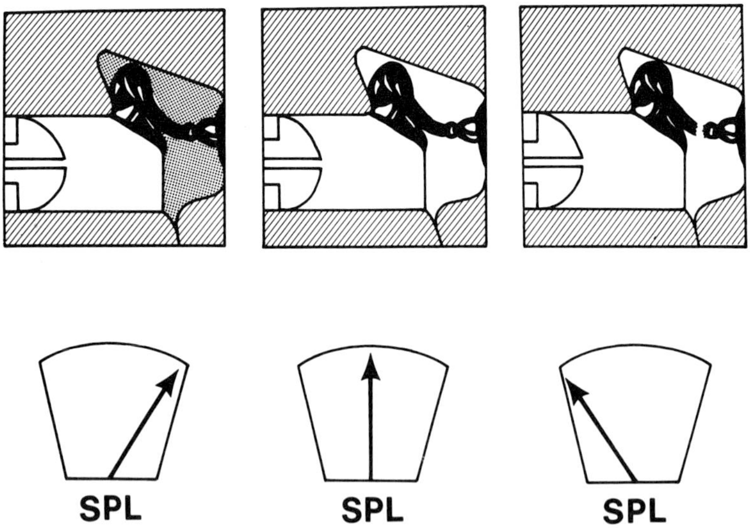

Figure 2-2 The impedance meter measures reflected sound pressure level in the external auditory canal. The middle diagram represents a normal middle ear and an "average" sound pressure level reflection; the diagram on the left represents a high level of reflected probe tone energy due to middle ear effusion; the diagram on the right represents a low reflected sound pressure level due to a highly compliant tympanic membrane with an ossicular discontinuity (from Katz, J.: *Handbook of Clinical Audiology*, 2nd Ed. Baltimore, Williams & Wilkins Co. 1978.)

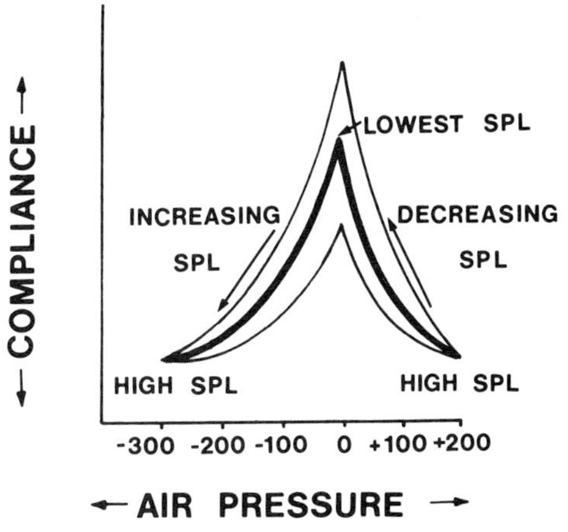

Figure 2-3 The tympanogram is a graphic record of change in sound pressure level (SPL) in the external ear canal as air pressure is varied. (From Katz, J.: *Handbook of Clinical Audiology*, 2nd Ed. Baltimore, Williams & Wilkins Co. 1978.)

By displaying the tympanograms in terms of the relative change in compliance from a standard arbitrary reference compliance at plus 200 mm H_20, the amplitude of the tympanogram is independent of the size of the ear canal. In this way a "standard range" of normal tympanograms is available for most impedance meters independent of patient, age, and individual variance in anatomy. Utilization of that tympanogram "norm" pattern is an important guide for clinical interpretation. Pathologic conditions that render the tympanic membrane nonmobile simply show no SPL change as a function of varied air pressure. "Tympanograms" from ears with perforations or with ventilation tubes in place have a constant SPL in the external auditory canal and middle ear cavity. Alteration of air pressure has no influence on the entrapped SPL. Tympanic membranes retracted from serous otitis media may not be influenced by pressure equal to plus 200 mm H_20. Ear canals occluded with cerumen demonstrate a constant small volume size with no change in "compliance" as air pressure is varied (Northern and Grimes, 1978).

STATIC COMPLIANCE

Static compliance is also a measure of middle ear mobility. The factors of compliance include mass, friction, and stiffness, which work together in a complex manner to facilitate or impede motion of the middle ear system. Historically, this test procedure is referred to as acoustic impedance. Currently, however, compliance seems to be a more appropriate term than impedance. Considerable controversy exists in the United States concerning the clinical contribution of static compliance to otologic and audiologic diagnosis. Unfortunately, because a wide range of compliance values exists for various otologic pathologic factors that overlap with normal middle ear mechanisms, diagnosis of ear problems based only on the static compliance measure must be considered with extreme caution.

Static compliance is measured in terms of equivalent volume in cubic centimeters based on two volume measurements. The first volume measurement (C_1) is made with the tympanic membrane clamped in a position of poor compliance with plus 200 mm H_20 air pressure in the external ear canal. The second volume measurement (C_2) is made with the tympanic membrane at the maximum compliance pressure. Since sound is more easily transmitted by the tympanic membrane during the second volume measurement (C_2), the probe-sound pressure in the enclosed cavity of the external canal is lower than noted in the first volume measurement (C_1), and a larger "equivalent volume" will be indicated (Fig. 2-4).

The static compliance measure is contaminated by the compliance of the air in the external canal itself. Static compliance is calculated by subtracting C_1 from C_2, which cancels out the compliance due to the volume of air in the external ear canal. The remainder is the compliance due to the middle ear mechanism. Thus, $C_2 - C_1$ equals the static compliance of the middle ear in units of equivalent air volume in cubic centimeters. In general clinical use, static compliance is abnormally low when the value is smaller than 0.28 cc and abnormally high when the value is larger than 2.5 cc. The major clinical contribution of the static compliance measurement is to differentiate between the fixated middle ear and the middle ear with an ossicular discontinuity, but even here it is not always accurate. Only static compliance values that clearly exceed the 0.28 or 2.5 cc norms should be considered diagnostically significant.

Middle ear compliance is influenced by many variables including patient age, sex, and pathologic state. The static compliance measure is corroborative information following tympanometry, since both these tests measure "compliance." The static compliance measure is considered by many to be the least valuable test in the impedance battery, and many clinicians omit it in routine clinical assessment. Indeed, Feldman (1974) indicates that the static compliance measure is appropriate only when the patient's tympanic membrane is devoid of any abnormalities. Dempsey (1975) summarizes the current status of static compliance by pointing out the irony that this "impedance" measure—for which the meter is named—is of questionable usefulness.

ACOUSTIC REFLEX THRESHOLD

The stapedial muscle contracts reflexively when the ear is stimulated with a sufficiently loud sound. This contraction occurs bilaterally, even when only one ear is stimulated. Researchers have consistently documented that the necessary intensity

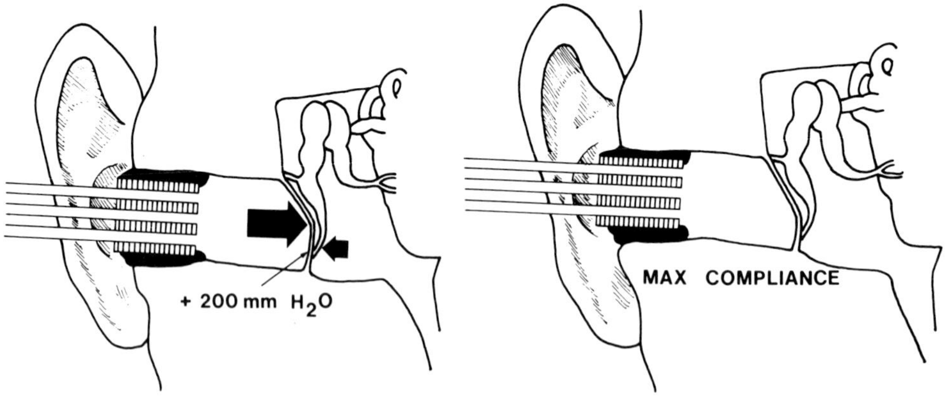

Figure 2-4 Static compliance is based on two volume measurements. The first measurement (A) represents the near-absolute volume between the probe-tip and the eardrum "clamped" with positive air pressure; the second volume measurement (B) is made with the tympanic membrane at the position of maximum compliance. (From Katz, J.: *Handbook of Clinical Audiology*, 2nd Ed. Williams & Wilkins Co. 1978.)

range is 70 to 100 dB hearing threshold level (HTL). The median threshold value for the stapedial reflex to pure-tone signals is approximately 85 dB HTL and approximately 65 dB HTL for white noise.

In the demonstration of the acoustic reflex, the electroacoustic impedance technique measures the sudden change in sound pressure caused by the decrease in compliance of the middle ear system as the muscles contract. The acoustic signal is introduced through an earphone attached to the impedance audiometer headset. If the signal to the earphone ear is sufficiently loud to elicit the bilateral acoustic reflex, the contraction of the stapedius muscle in the ear containing the probe tip will suddenly decrease the compliance of that eardrum (creating a sudden increase in the cavity sound pressure level) synchronously with the presentation of the stimulating earphone signal. The contralateral technique of eliciting the acoustic reflex is recorded as the acoustic reflex threshold for the stimulated ear. Under some circumstances the clinician is interested in the presence or absence of the acoustic reflex in the probe ear; on other occasions, the ear of interest is the earphone or stimulated ear. Regardless of which ear is under examination, it is standard clinical practice to record the acoustic reflex for the stimulated ear (Fig. 2-5).

PHYSICAL VOLUME TEST (PVT)

A most valuable application of impedance measurement is the Physical Volume Test (Northern and Downs, 1978). The electroacoustic impedance meters rely on the physical principle that intensity is a function of cavity size. A signal of fixed intensity introduced into a large cavity and a small cavity will produce two different sound pressure levels in the two cavities. The larger cavity will have a lower sound pressure level; a higher sound pressure level will exist in the smaller cavity. Thus, when the impedance probe emits the probe tone into an ear canal with an intact eardrum, the meter will balance at a cubic centimeter value of 1.0 to 1.5 in a normal adult; the PVT reading in normal children is approximately .7 cc to 1.0 cc (Fig. 2-6).

If the tympanic membrane is not totally intact, the physical volume measure will be quite large (three to four times greater than the normal volume values), often exceeding 5.0 cc. Thus, the physical volume test (PVT) can be used as a means to rule out nonobservable perforation behind an exaggerated anterior overhang or beneath an

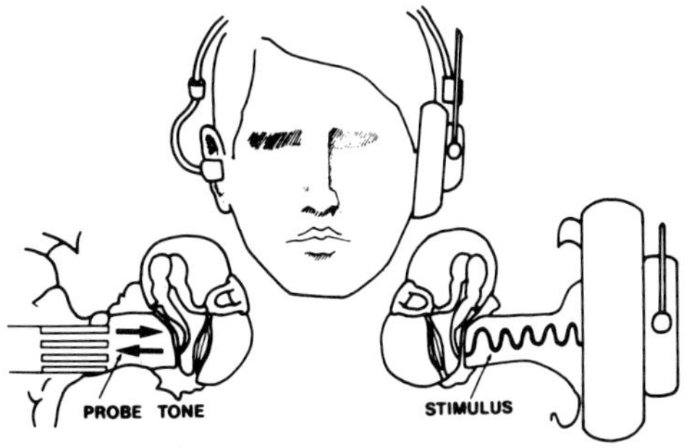

Figure 2-5 Diagrammatic view for measuring the contralateral acoustic reflex. When the earphone stimulus is loud enough to cause bilateral stapedial muscle contraction, the probe tone in the opposite ear measures an increase in reflected SPL due to reduced compliance of the eardrum and middle ear ossicular chain. (From Katz, J.: *Handbook of Clinical Audiology*, 2nd Ed. Williams & Wilkins Co. 1978.)

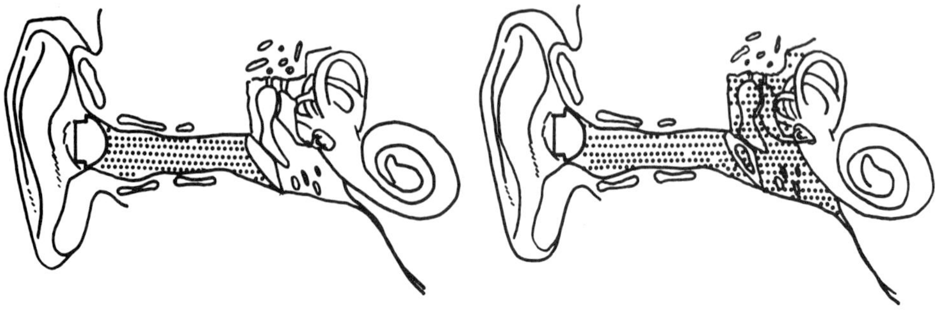

Figure 2-6 Diagrammatic representation of the measurement of near-absolute volume known as the Physical Volume Test (PVT). The PVT indicates intactness of the tympanic membrane, and cc volume values in eardrums with perforations or patent ventilation tubes are four or five times greater than when tympanic membrane is intact.

adherent crust. Or the PVT can identify obstruction of ventilating tubes, as well as possible blind attic retraction pocket perforations.

Knowledge of the physical volume in cubic centimeters will help clarify the etiologic factors responsible for B-type tympanograms. Nonmobile tympanic membranes with volmes larger than 2.5 cc (or 2.0 cc in children) are usually indicative of a perforation or patent ventilation tube; flat tympanograms with normal volume measurement are indicative of a nonmobile tympanic membrane. Abnormally small physical volumes may be related to cerumen occluding the external canal, or perhaps the probe tip is pressed against the canal wall.

MANAGEMENT OF IMPEDANCE AUDIOMETRY WITH CHILDREN

The main limitation of impedance measurements in young children is that the test battery cannot be completed while the youngster is vocalizing—speaking, crying, yelling, or any combination of these noises. Stapedial muscle reflex contraction and Eustachian tube changes during vocalization cause the compliance of the tympanic membrane to change rapidly, thereby making impedance measurements impossible. The clinician's most challenging task is to make the youngster stop vocalizing for just the necessary few moments to obtain impedance data. Each clinician must devise his or her own techniques for momentarily distracting the screaming child. Impedance skill with children requires the highest competency in manipulating both the equipment and the child.

The information presented below includes a number of practical suggestions pertinent to impedance measurements in children. Although these techniques are especially good with children under two years of age, we have also found them useful in working with other difficult-to-test pediatric patients, including the mentally retarded, the deaf-blind, the congenitally deaf, and other children with multiple handicaps (Northern, 1977a).

For children less than three years of age, it is also helpful and probably essential that a second or even a third person be utilized for obtaining impedance measures. Practice and coordination of these personnel are helpful, and they must be in constant

---

The author is indebted to Geary McCandless, Ph. D., University of Utah Medical Center, for permission to use material from his NIH-sponsored project, "Manual for Impedance Testing in Children," which describes some pediatric impedance techniques developed at the University of Colorado Medical Center.

communication during all aspects of the test to ensure rapid and reliable results. It is difficult for one person to manipulate the ear insert while at the same time operating the pressure pump and other dials on the impedance devices. It is preferable to have one person operate the impedance instrument while a second stabilizes the child's head and inserts the probe tip. This latter person either must be apprised at all times as to whether or not a seal has been obtained, or else the pressure manometer must be in a position to be observed directly. Sometimes it works well to hold the probe tip in place by hand after insertion and, with the help of the assistant, stabilize the head during the test to prevent a loss of pressure seal due to head movement.

A suggested technique in handling the headpiece is to remove the headphone and hold it over the contralateral ear. The headpiece itself can be placed over the wrist and the insert placed into the ear canal. In younger children, it is helpful to have a parent cradle the child with an arm, passively immobilizing him, then place the headpiece over the parent's shoulder and insert the earpiece into the child's ear while holding the headphone on the contralateral ear.

The age range between two months and twelve months presents one of the most difficult periods in which to obtain impedance tests. The children are not old enough to understand the test or to respond to verbal enticements, yet they are old enough to react (sometimes decisively!) both to the test situation and to the insertion of the probe tip in particular. We have found that it is most effective to employ a distractive technique to redirect the youngster's attention from the test. The form of distraction is relatively unimportant as long as it is sufficiently novel to compel the infant to disregard the insertion of the probe tip. The external stimuli can be visual, tactile, auditory, or any combination of the three. Before assuming a distractive procedure to be essential in impedance testing, one should first try to place the probe tip quickly, but gently, in the ear. Frequently, this takes the child by surprise, and further games are not necessary. Often the entire impedance battery can be completed before the child really has time to react or respond. However, at the first hint of a reaction from the child, the clinician should be prepared to present a distraction. If habituation to one mode of distraction occurs, instantly alter or introduce other diversionary tactics. If the diversions fail, it may be possible to apply passive restraint to the child's body, head, or hands to complete the test.

Distractive or diversionary tactics are most effective if the headset is not used. Instead, rely on an assistant to insert the probe tip while holding the headpiece over the wrist or over the parent's shoulder with the child in the parent's lap. When using visual distraction, keep the diversionary object well within the child's field of vision to prevent undue head movement which produces artifacts.

The following are examples of the many possible distractive techniques that can be used with children under the age of three years. The number and type of devices are limited only by the ingenuity of the examiner:

Flashlight. Direct the light toward the child or shine it on objects or people well within the child's visual field. Constantly change the rate of movement from slow to fast. If habituation occurs, take the child's hand and repeatedly place it over the light source.

Animated toys. Introduce animated toys only as required at critical times necessary to complete the test. Avoid movement artifacts by keeping the toy well out of the reach of the child.

Cotton swab. Gently brush the back of the child's hand, arm, or leg in a slow, even motion. Make the distraction visual as well as tactile by making oscillatory or exaggerated movements of the swab.

Pendulum. Using a bright and unusually shaped object, make a pendulum with an 18-inch string. This technique is highly effective if the examiner swings the pendulum about in various motions within various areas of the infant's vision. Swing the pendulum rather slowly in short excursions, permitting easy visual following. Frequently stop or alter the swinging motion to provide novelty to the pendular action.

Mirror. To an infant less than one year of age who is capable of reacting and attending to faces, a large mirror is sometimes irresistible, at least for a period sufficiently long to place a probe tip and to perform the impedance test battery.

Toys that produce sounds. Toys or other devices that emit intense sounds should be avoided if at all possible, since they may evoke an acoustic or other reflexive response from the child. Toys that produce softer sounds in no way interfere with the test and can therefore be used effectively, especially if the sound is somewhat novel.

Food. Although swallowing and sucking movements are notorious for producing artifacts in the tympanogram and reflex measures, food can still be used as a distractive technique. Flavored gelatin or soft-drink powder in water, honey, or sweetened lemon juice can be dropped into the child's mouth at intervals during the test. Avoid taking measures until the reflexive sucking action has subsided. Administering small amounts of liquid at well-spaced intervals can keep the child occupied for many minutes.

Watch. In front of the child, simply remove one's wristwatch, manipulate or wind it well out of reach of the child, or point to it.

Shoe. A simple yet effective technique is to lace and unlace a child's shoe, either on or off his foot. This should be carefully timed to coincide with the insertion of the probe tip into the ear. Move slowly and methodically and do not appear to have any object in mind except to lace and unlace the shoe.

Action toys. A variety of toys that perform repetitive actions are available, such as a monkey that climbs down a stick pole. Often these are not the best distractive devices because children one year and older often wish to handle or manipulate this type of toy.

Wad of cotton or tissue. A cotton ball can facilitate effective passive attention when balanced on the hand, arm, or knee of the child or on the hand of the assistant. It can be squeezed or otherwise manipulated; it can be blown or allowed to fall repeatedly from the hand. A tissue can also be used as a parachute, torn slowly into strips, rolled into small balls and placed in the child's hand, waved, punctured, and so forth.

Tape. A roll of adhesive or paper surgical tape has been found to be one of the most effective distractive devices. Bits of tape can be torn off or stuck on various parts of the child's or examiner's anatomy. The child can be allowed to pull the tape off, objects can be picked up with the adhesive side of the tape, fingers can be bound together, links can be made with small strips, rings can be formed, fingernails covered, and innumerable other manipulations can be performed. Tape works wonders for the few seconds necessary for obtaining impedance measures.

Lollipop. A lollipop can be utilized when the child is cradled and partially immobilized in the examiner's or parent's arm. The examiner can stroke the child's lips or tongue with the lollipop. Careful spacing of the lollipop permits completion of the entire impedance test battery.

Miscellaneous devices. Tongue blades, cotton swabs, colored yarn, or similar devices are all effective as distractive devices. They are best utilized when manipulated or "played with" by the examiner. If the child insists, he can be allowed to manipulate the device. But care must be taken to permit only passive action so as to reduce movement artifact while the test is proceeding.

There is no way to predict the behavior or reaction of children between one and three years of age. Their reaction to the test situation is influenced by past exposure to other tests and other clinicians and by their age, their personalities, and their general evaluation of what they see is about to happen to them. They are often most concerned about whether or not the procedure will be painful. For these reasons, some general rules apply when testing children in this age group. First, never ask a child for permission to perform impedance tests; calmly assume you are going to administer the test and proceed to do so. Second, avoid undue explanation regarding the test procedure. Instructions to the child contribute nothing to the test results unless they help reduce physical movement. Besides, the child would not understand explanations even if given. It is sufficient to say something like this, "Here, listen to this," or "Hold still," or "Listen to this radio," and then proceed with the test. Most often it is better to say nothing unless the child reacts to placement of the headset or insert. Explanations usually take longer than the test itself!

For most children older than three years of age, no special distraction is required when applying impedance measures unless the child is particularly apprehensive in an unfamiliar clinical situation. Only one or two of every hundred children in this age category will demonstrate adverse reactions to impedance testing. Where necessary, one can reduce anxiety by saying simply, "We are going to test your hearing, please hold still," or other uncomplicated statements of reassurance. Most three-year-olds can be tested with a single examiner.

Allowing the child to observe other children or adults being tested helps to allay any fears that pain will occur. With these children, as with the younger group, refrain from asking permission to perform the test. Distractive techniques are viewed with suspicion, so treat this age category essentially as you would adults except for mild and occasional words of instruction or encouragement.

Sedation

On occasion it may be necessary to consider the use of sedation to quiet a noncooperative youngster for acoustic impedance evaluation. Chloral hydrate and secobarbital are often used because of ease of administration and general effectiveness. The action of chloral hydrate and secobarbital is such that drowsiness, quieting, and sometimes deep sleep are achieved within an hour. Following the impedance evaluation, the youngster can be aroused and taken home. The major disadvantage of chloral hydrate and secobarbital is that both drugs are long-acting sedatives. Acoustic reflexes can be observed in patients sedated with chloral hydrate or secobarbital, but researchers have shown the acoustic reflex thresholds to be elevated (Borg and Møller, 1968; Gicomelli and Mozzo, 1965; Robinette et al., 1974).

Clinicians must be aware, however, that a child's reaction to such medication is not always as expected. Children vary considerably in their response sensitivity to sedatives, and the recommended dosages may not be sufficient to induce the desired effect. The same dosage in other children may actually increase activity and excitement levels so that the desired impedance study is still not possible.

Mentally retarded children are often maintained on medication for management of behavioral or convulsive disorders. Thus, the absence of acoustic reflexes in this population may be drug related. Richards and colleagues (1975) evaluated impedance findings in ten functionally retarded, normal-hearing children on phenobarbital. These authors reported that low-level amounts of phenobarbital have no effect on the acoustic reflex threshold.

Impedance evaluation under conditions of general anesthesia is not always successful. Results are influenced by the anesthesia technique and drug agent. Middle ear pressure is increased under inhalation of some gases, such as nitrous oxide, thereby decreasing the compliance of the tympanic membrane and obscuring the acoustic reflex (Thomsen et al., 1965). Researchers have shown that nitrous oxide collects in closed gas-filled body spaces (Eger and Saidman, 1965; Matz et al., 1967; Starr and Schwartzkroin, 1972). Middle ear pressure measurements taken during endotracheal inhalation anesthesia showed increased middle ear pressures as great as plus 450 mm H_20 with nitrous oxide, while no pressure elevation was noted with halothane or ethrane (Patterson and Bartlett, 1976).

An interesting study was recently reported on the effect of various anesthetic agents on normal and deseased middle ears (Mitchell and Richards, 1976). Thirty patients were intubated with one of six anesthetics while undergoing various surgical procedures. A summary of results indicates that preanesthetic medications (belladonna drugs and mild sedatives) had no effect on middle ear muscle thresholds. The acoustic reflexes, however, followed the same pattern demonstrated by other observable reflexes, such as deep tendon and pupillary reflexes, through the various anesthesia states. Acoustic reflex thresholds were elevated 20 to 25 dB at 1000 Hz during plane I; by the time plane III anesthesia maintenance was reached, the middle ear reflexes were completely abolished.

According to Borg (1976) barbiturates have varying influence on the stapedial reflex mechanism. Central depressant drugs have been evaluated with the stapedial reflex in man by Lidén and colleagues (1974). Research with pentobarbital in the rabbit shows that the acoustic reflex offset wave pattern is altered. The stimulus had to be increased 4 dB to match predrug reflex wave-form amplitude (Borg and Møller, 1975). Sedation with diazepam and meperidine in adults has been recently reported to have no significant effect on tympanometry, static compliance or acoustic reflex measurements. Oramas (1977)indicates that he routinely uses ketamine (a dissociative anesthestic) for acoustic impedance evaluation in conjunction with electrocochleography measurements in children. The acoustic reflexes are unaffected by ketamine, but at our facility the drug is reluctantly used by anesthesiologists because of possible umpleasant emergence reactions.

Often one must decide whether the impedance test results merit the problems and risks related to sedation. Any drug that alters central nervous system responses may have a dilatory or inhibitive effect on the acoustic reflex.

CLINICAL IMPLEMENTATION OF IMPEDANCE MEASURES

Impedance audiometry offers much to the practice of audiology and otology in the diagnosis of clinical problems. The impedance audiometer is an indispensable tool when fully utilized by an experienced clinician. This instrument was originally developed to evaluate conductive hearing impairment, but its utility has now been extended so that evaluations of the inner ear, and retrocochlear and brain stem problems are common practice. The impedance technique has proven valuable in predicting or confirming audiometric findings regarding the nature of conductive or sensorineural hearing loss, the differentiation of various types of conductive hearing impairment, the elucidation of sensorineural hearing loss into problems of the cochlear or eighth nerve, the quantification of degree of hearing loss, as well as the integrity of intact auditory reflex pathways in the brain stem.

Maximum diagnostic implementation of impedance audiometry requires careful consideration and caution. The powerful diagnostic implications of impedance audiometry may give naive clinicians an unwarranted sense of security. For example, absence of the acoustic reflex may be due not to a single simple cause, but rather to a complex combination of unsuspected conductive hearing impairment not identified in routine audiometry or otoscopy, a subtle peripheral facial nerve problem, or an undetected eighth nerve or brain stem problem.

Clinicians using impedance audiometry must follow several guidelines:

1. *Learn to recognize overall patterns in the impedance test battery.* Do not use any single test in the battery to reach diagnostic conclusions; avoid specific clinical interpretations based solely on one element of the impedance test battery. Impedance measurements are strongest when combined with other evaluation procedures including otoscopy, audiometry, and behavioral observations.

2. *Pay little attention to the absolute value of any of the impedance test battery results.* Little useful information is obtained from the absolute value of the amplitude or height of the tympanogram; static compliance should be regarded as being within normal limits, below normal limits, or above normal limits—exact knowledge of the static compliance is not important; and it is often sufficient to know that the acoustic reflex is present or absent, within normal limits, elevated, or at a reduced sensation level. Clinicians may overlook the total clinical impedance picture if they are too concerned with the absolute numbers involved in each element of the impedance battery.

3. *Beware of implicit diagnostic conclusions based only on the impedance test battery.* No test is infallible; few otologic problems have one, and only one, cause. The clinician must realize that several reasons may cause an abnormal tympanogram and that all these reasons may influence the measurement of the acoustic reflex threshold. The impedance test battery results from a patient with otosclerosis may be the same as the impedance results obtained for a patient with profound sensorineural hearing loss. The impedance technique is a strongly diagnostic tool, but the sophisticated clinician bases final decisions on the patients total presentation of complaint, history, audiometry, physical examination, and impedance test battery (Northern, 1976).

A common clinical protocol suggests initial pure-tone air conduction and speech audiometry followed by evaluation with the impedance test battery for *all* patients. Patients with sensorineural hearing loss and normal hearing have bone-conduction thresholds equal to their air-conduction thresholds. Thus, when the impedance battery indicates no conductive element to the hearing loss, bone-conduction tests are at the discretion of the clinician. Bone-conduction measurement is imperative only for those patients with conductive pathologic findings to determine the amount of the air-bone gap and to evaluate the cochlear reserve or hearing sensitivity of the inner ear. Deletion of bone-conduction measurement on patients with normal hearing and sensorineural hearing loss will result in significant time-saving for routine clinical practice. The lack of standardized bone-conduction testing techniques and the need for careful application of masking during bone-conduction measurements make the bone-conduction test one of the most difficult testing procedures. Audiologists disagree about many aspects of bone-conduction measurement, including placement of the bone oscillator on the mastoid or frontal bone, procedures for calibration of the bone oscillator, masked or nonmasked bone-conduction testing techniques, and recording of bone-conduction responses. In our practice, bone-conduction testing is performed on patients with known conductive hearing losses identified through abnormal tympanometry or abnormal static compliance measures, accompanied by the absence of the acoustic reflex. The clinician, however, must be aware of the otosclerotic patient whose impedance findings may look like a profound sensorineural hearing loss with a normal tympanogram, normal static compliance, and absent acoustic reflexes.

OTOLOGIC APPLICATIONS

The diagnostic implications of the acoustic reflex considerably outweigh the contributions of tympanometry and static compliance measurements. It is noteworthy that the impedance meter, which was originally used to identify conductive hearing loss, has now been extended so that evaluation of the inner ear and retrocochlear and brain stem problems is common clinical practice (Northern, 1977b).

Cochlear Hearing Loss

The acoustic reflex sensation level shows a "decibel-for-decibel" inverse relation to the degree of cochlear hearing loss (Jerger et al., 1972).The acoustic reflex sensation level decreases from approximately 70 dB for patients with a 20 dB cochlear hearing loss to approximately 25 dB for patients with an 85 dB cochlear hearing loss. Jerger concludes that as long as the cochlear hearing loss is less than 60 dB, there is a 90 percent likelihood that the acoustic reflex will be observed when the earphone is over the ear with the hearing loss, with a normal tympanogram in the opposite ear. As the sensorineural loss increases above 60 dB, chances of observing the acoustic reflex lessen. At 85 dB, the chances are only 50-50 of observing the acoustic reflex; if the loss is 100 dB HL, there exists only a 5 to 10 percent chance. Thus, the presence of acoustic reflex thresholds at a sensation level at 60 dB or less, in light of a hearing loss of 85 dB or less, provides a powerful indication for a cochlear site-of-lesion diagnosis. In patients with unilateral cochlear hearing loss less than 85 dB, the acoustic reflex should be easily observable bilaterally.

Conductive Hearing Loss

The acoustic reflex can be observed only in patients with mild unilateral conductive hearing loss. When the unilateral conductive hearing loss exceeds 30 dB HL, however, the acoustic reflex will be obscured bilaterally. When the stimulating sound is presented to the conductive-loss ear, the 30 dB + hearing loss is sufficient to prevent the signal from being perceived loudly enough to elicit the acoustic reflex. When the earphone is on the normal ear and the probe is in the unilateral conductive-loss ear, the mechanism causing the conductive loss prevents the eardrum from showing a change in compliance. Naturally, in a bilateral conductive loss, the acoustic reflexes will be absent bilaterally because the pathologic factor in each ear prohibits the probe from noting a compliance change when the opposite ear is stimulated with sound.

An example of the bilateral absence of the acoustic reflex in unilateral conductive loss can be appreciated in the classic example of ossicular discontinuity. Figure 2-7 shows an ossicular disarticulation at the incudostapedial joint which produces an audiogram and impedance study as shown in Figure 2-8. With a 60 dB hearing loss in the right ear, sufficient loudness cannot be appreciated by the patient when the earphone stimulates the conductive-loss ear; thus, no acoustic reflex will be noted. When the impedance headset is reversed and the probe is in the conductive-loss ear, no acoustic reflex will be seen because when the stapedial muscle contracts, the discontinuity prevents the ossicular chain from influencing the compliance of the tympanic membrane.

A unique exception to the bilateral absence of acoustic reflexes in unilateral conductive hearing loss occurs in the case of ossicular discontinuity in which the disarticulation lies medial to the attachment of the stapedial muscle, as seen in fractured crura of the stapes (Fig. 2-9). Although the audiogram and tympanogram findings are essentially similar to the traditional case of ossicular discontinuity, examination of acoustic reflexes will show unilateral presence, rather than bilateral absence (Fig. 2-10). When the probe is in the conductive-loss ear, contraction of the stapedial muscle will increase the impedance of the ossicular chain and decrease the compliance of the tympanic membrane. The unilateral presence of stapedial reflexes in ossicular discontinuity is pathognomonic of fractured stapedial crura (Northern, 1977b).

In general terms, the likelihood of absence of the acoustic reflex increases as the magnitude of the air-bone gap increases. When the earphone stimulates the conductive-loss ear, the reflex has little chance of being present as long as the hearing loss is in excess of 30 dB. Since conductive-type pathologic findings preclude tympanic membrane compliance change, the acoustic reflex can be expected to be absent when the probe tip is in a conductive-loss ear, regardless of how small an air-bone gap exists.

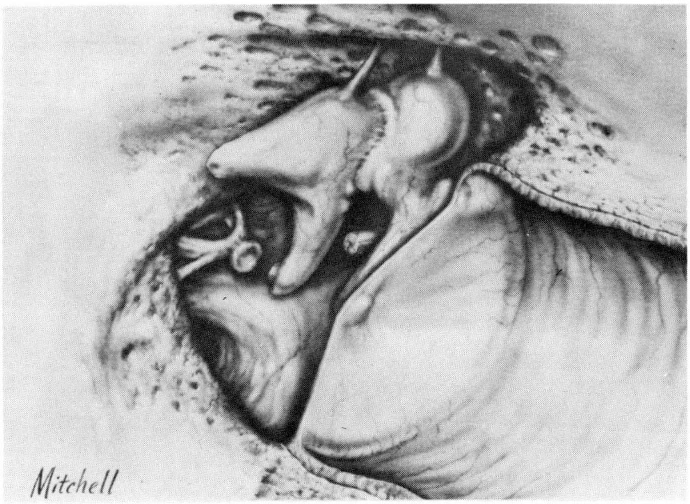

Figure 2-7 Discontinuity of the middle ear ossicular chain at the incudostapedial joint.

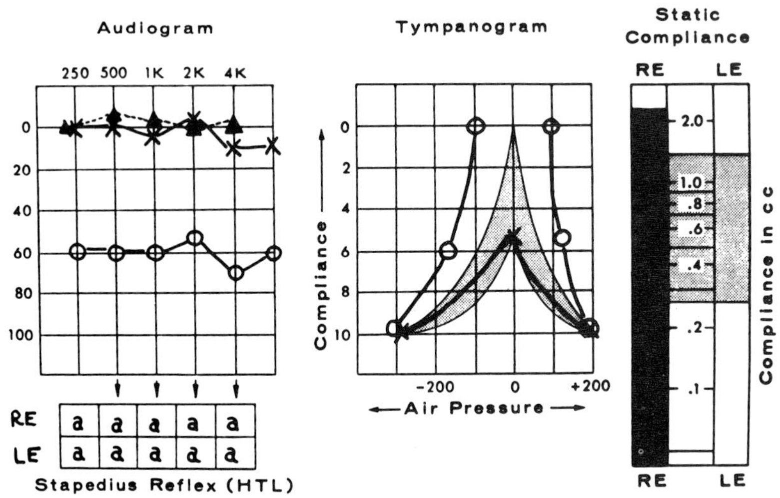

Figure 2–8 Audiogram and impedance results from unilateral ossicular discontinuity of the incudostapedial joint.

Jerger and colleagues (1974) reported that the presence of a small air-bone gap of only 10 dB is sufficient to obscure the reflex to the probe ear nearly 80 percent of the time. Conversely, if acoustic reflexes can be noted in the probe ear, it is virtually impossible for a significant conductive hearing loss to exist in that ear.

Eighth Nerve Pathologic Factors

Careful interpretation of the acoustic reflexes can also supply diagnostic information about the presence of acoustic nerve tumors. Anderson and colleagues (1970) suggested a test technique known as the Acoustic Reflex Decay Test. These researchers evaluated the acoustic reflex in seventeen patients with retrocochlear lesions. Of these patients, seven showed no acoustic reflexes. In the remaining ten

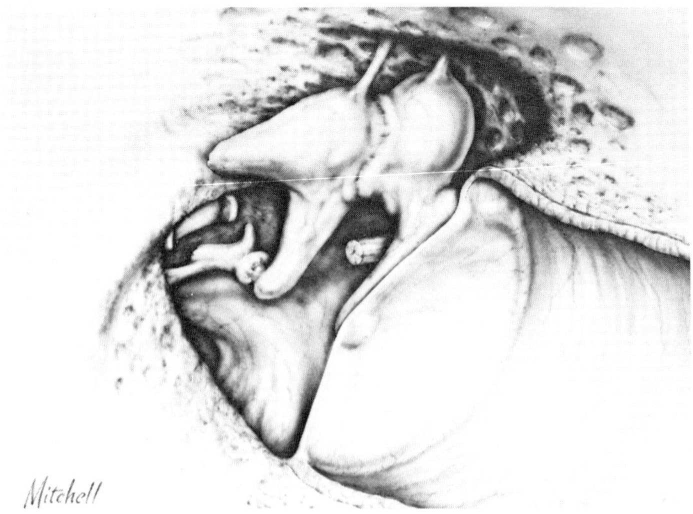

Figure 2–9 Discontinuity of the middle ear ossicular chain created by fracture of the stapes crura.

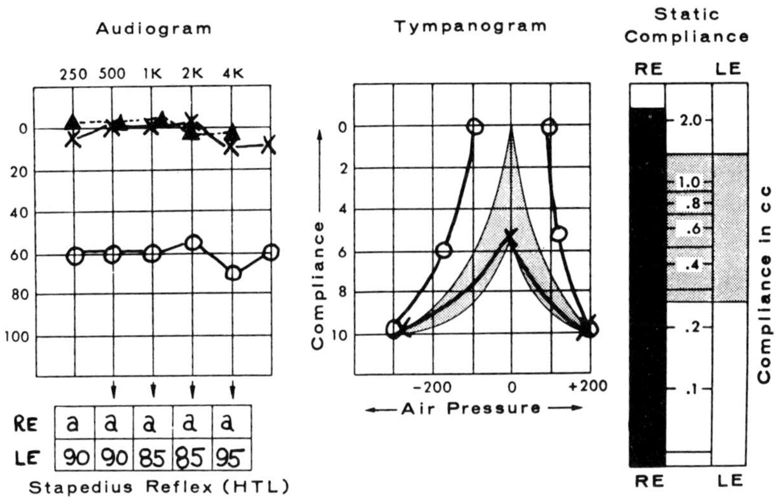

Figure 2-10 Audiogram and impedance results from unilateral ossicular discontinuity due to fracture of stapes crura.

patients, the acoustic reflex thresholds were elevated and could not be sustained at full magnitude for 10 seconds in the presence of an ongoing pure-tone stimulus. Accordingly, acoustic nerve tumors have two possible positive reflex findings: (1) the acoustic reflex is absent when one would expect it to be present, or (2) the acoustic reflex shows reflex decay under prolonged stimulation.

Researchers at Northwestern University and Baylor College of Medicine combined efforts to evaluate acoustic reflex findings in thirty patients with eighth nerve disorders. Acoustic reflexes were absent at all test frequencies in nineteen patients, present but elevated or with decay in four patients, and normally present in seven patients. Sheehy and Schlosser found similar acoustic reflex results in fiftysix cases of acoustic tumors. These researchers conclude that the acoustic reflex measurements are the single most powerful audiologic test in the diagnosis of eighth nerve tumors (Jerger et al., 1974b).

The most intriguing fact, evidenced from the Baylor-Northwestern data, is that the acoustic reflex is absent 30 percent of the time in patients with normal hearing who have eighth nerve lesions. The likelihood of absent reflexes quickly rises to 70 percent with a mild 30 dB hearing loss. The absence of the acoustic reflex, in light of normal or near-normal hearing levels, must be considered a suspicious finding until the presence of an acoustic tumor is ruled out. The conclusion in these studies was that acoustic reflex findings were more sensitive to the retrocochlear pathologic factors than Bekesy tracings, speech discrimination scores, tone decay test results, or the shape of the performance-intensity function for phonetically balanced monosyllables.

Postoperative Surgical Evaluation

Impedance audiometry may provide significant information concerning postoperative results in patients who have undergone ear surgery. Tympanometry can provide objective evidence concerning the healing and mobility of tympanoplasty grafts. Early tympanograms following tympanoplasty surgical procedures typically show the graft to be immobile. As the healing process thins the graft, the mobility of the tympanic membrane and middle ear pressure returns to normal. For staged middle ear surgical procedures, some surgeons see the stability of a normal tympanogram following the initial surgical operation as an objective time-lapse indication for the second surgical procedure. Postsurgical air-bone gaps that persist, or air-bone gaps that grow progressively greater with time may be evaluated with the impedance test battery. Interpretation of the tympanogram, the static compliance measure, and the presence or absence of the acoustic reflex can shed light on whether the postsurgical air-bone gap is caused by refixation of the middle ear system or by some discontinuity.

Patulous Eustachian Tube

At times the patulous Eustachian tube is difficult to document objectively. Patients with a Eustachian tube that is abnormally open complain of hearing their own breathing and their own vocalization and of the inability to converse at the dinner table while chewing. These are disturbing symptoms to many patients. The impedance meter can provide an objective diagnosis by establishing the presence of a normal tympanogram with normal middle ear pressure. Then the patient should inspire and expire through his mouth only, then breathe through his nose with his mouth closed, and finally stop breathing momentarily. Patients with a patulous Eustachian tube will show an increase in tympanic membrane compliance with each inspiration and a corresponding decrease in tympanic membrane compliance with expiration. Tympanic membrane compliance change will be greater during the period of nasal breathing than during the period of mouth breathing alone; momentarily stopping breathing dicontinues the abrupt changes in tympanic membrane compliance. When the impedance meter is in its most sensitive position it is often possible to observe compliance changes that are in synchrony with the patient's breathing, which verifies the presence of a patulous Eustachian tube even when the changes are so small as to be nonobservable by otoscopy.

Fistula Test

The principle of the fistula test is to apply direct positive pressure on the fluids of the inner ear. If a fistula exists, the positive pressure results in nystagmus and creates a sensation of vertigo in the patient. Utilization of the impedance audiometer air-pressure system allows a clinician to subtly and carefully create positive air pressure against the intact tympanic membrane, or through a perforated tympanic membrane, until the initial vertiges of dizziness are observed. In some clinics, the fistula test with the impedance audiometer is carried out with the patient hooked up to the electronystagmograph recorder to permit objective determination of nystagmus due to positive air pressure.

According to Swogger-Rosenberg and colleagues (1978) when using the tympanometric technique of sweeping ear canal air pressure changes between +400 mm H_20 and -400 mm H_20 and watching the patient's eye, one can observe nystagmus related to round or oval window fistula. She reports a series of eight patients in whom the fistula, subsequently confirmed by surgery, was initially identified during the tympanometric examination.

See Chapter Six for a more complete discussion of Eustachian tube function tests.

The Glomus Tumor

The glomus tumor is a vascular tumor of the middle ear which usually presents with symptoms of pulsatile tinnitus, possible hearing loss, and possible facial paralysis. This middle ear tumor is often difficult to observe otoscopically until it is of a relatively large size. The pulsations of blood through the tumor make earlier detection possible with the impedance technique. The air-pressure system is set at slight positive air pressure up to plus 150 mm H_20. The presence of a glomus tumor may be noted if the compliance change meter pulsates in synchrony with the patient's pulse. Confirmation of the diagnosis is provided when the pulsing of the compliance change meter decreases in amplitude as the carotid artery of the neck on the involved side of the patient is depressed by the clinician's thumb (Rock, 1974).

Lopes and colleagues (1972) described a case study of a woman with pulsatile tinnitus and low-frequency hearing loss in which the impedance fluctuations were ultimately related to a glomus tympanicum tumor. The patient was initially thought to have otosclerosis because of her symptoms, and the reddened tympanic membrane was thought to be due to Schwartze's sign. Balkany (1975) points out that pulsatile deflections noted during impedance audiometry may be related to problems other than the glomus jugulare tumor. He presents a case study of active chronic otitis media with pulsation of purulent fluid through a perforation, and a second case of pulsatile deflections related to objective tinnitus and spastic stapedial contractions from palatal myoclonus.

Facial Nerve Evaluation

Facial nerve testing is generally comprised of topographic (anatomic) and neurophysiologic (electric) techniques (Alford, 1974). The topographic approach relies on the anatomy of the facial nerve and its branches. Tests for tearing, stapedial reflex, taste dysfunction, and submandibular salivary flow establish facial nerve topographic function at several anatomic sites. Neurophysiologic test such as nerve excitability and electromyography indicate the status of nerve impulse condition. The major question of interest to the otolaryngologist is whether the facial nerve lesion is accessible through the transmastoid approach (below the geniculate ganglion) or whether the lesion must be reached through the middle fossa or translabyrinth approach at or above the geniculate ganglion (Luetje, 1977).

Since the stapedial muscle is intersected by a small branch of the seventh cranial nerve, the presence or absence of the stapedial reflex in a patient with facial paralysis may be used to help locate the site of lesion. If the patient has facial palsy and the stapedial reflex is present, it may be concluded that the site of lesion is distal to or at a lower level than the innervation of the stapedial muscle. With facial paralysis and no stapedial reflex present, the site of lesion may then be inferred to be proximal to, or at a higher level than the takeoff of the twig innervating the stapedial muscle. When using impedance audiometry to evaluate peripheral facial nerve function, the efferent nervous system is under investigation and the interpretation of test results is based on compliance changes in the probe ear. Regularly monitoring the presence or absence of the acoustic reflex, as well as its magnitude and briskness, may be a valuable technique in considering the necessity of surgical intervention in patients with active degeneration of the facial nerve. Observation of the return of the stapedial reflex in patients with degenerative facial nerve disease is often seen some ten days prior to the return of facial muscle function.

Citron and Adour (1978) evaluated forty eight consecutive patients with acute facial paralysis. Their results indicated that after nerve excitability testing, the acoustic reflex was the most efficient indicator of impending nerve degeneration and predictor of recovery. They reported a definite magnitude decrease of 50 percent one week after onset in the acoustic reflex of the affected side compared with the uninvolved side. These authors also suggested that topographic diagnosis cannot consistently predict the site of the lesion in acute facial paralysis, since a few patients who retained acoustic reflexes throughout the course of their palsy demonstrated decrease in lacrimal function.

REFERENCES

Alberti, P. and Kristensen, R.: The clinical application of impedance audiometry. *Laryngoscope* 80: 735, 1970.

Alberti, P.W. and Jerger, J.F.: Probe-tone frequency and the diagnostic value of tympanometry. *Arch. Otolaryngol.* 99: 206, 1974.

Alford, B.R. et al.: Diagnostic test of facial nerve function. *Otolaryngol. Clin. North Am.* 7: 331, 1974.

Anderson, H., Barr, B. and Wedenberg, E.: Early diagnosis of VIIIth nerve tumors by acoustic reflex tests. *Acta Otolaryngol. (Suppl.)* 263:232, 1970.

Balkany, T.J.: Pulsatile impedance tympanometry. *Impedance Newsletter*, Vol. 4, New York, American Electronics, 1974, 25

Borg, E.: Dynamic characteristics of the intra-aural muscle reflex. In Feldman, A. and Wilber, L. (Eds.): *Acoustic Impedance and Admittance—The Measurement of Middle Ear Function.* Baltimore, Williams & Wilkins, Co. 1976.

Borg, E. and Møller, A.R.: The effect of ethylalcohol and pentobarbital sodium on the acoustic reflex in man. *Acta Otolaryngol.* 64: 415, 1968.

Borg, E. and Møller, A.R.: Effect of central depressants on the acoustic middle ear reflex in the rabbit. A method for quantitative measurements of drug effect on the CNS. *Acta Physiol. Scand.* 94: 327, 1975.

Citron, D. and Adour, K.K.: Acoustic reflex and loudness discomfort in acute facial paralysis. *Arch. Otolaryngol.* 104: 303, 1978.

Dempsey, C.: Static compliance. In *Handbook of Clinical Impedance Audiometry.* New York, American Electromedics Corp., 71, 1975.

Eger, E.I. and Saidman, L.J.: Hazards of nitrous oxide anesthesia in bowel obstruction and pneumothorax. *Anesthesiology* 26: 61, 1965.

Feldman, A.: Eardrum abnormality and the measurement of middle ear function. *Arch. Otolaryngol.* 99: 211, 1974.

Gicomelli, F. and Mozzo, W.: An experimental and clinical study of the brainstem reticular formation on the stapedial reflex. *International Audiology* 4: 42, 1965.

Jerger, J.: Clinical experience with impedance audiometry. *Arch. Otolaryngol.* 93: 311, 1970.

Jerger, J., Jerger, S. and Mauldin, L.: Studies in impedance audiometry I Normal and sensorineural ears. *Arch. Otolaryngol.* 96: 513, 1972.

Jerger, J., Anthony, L., Jerger, S. and Mauldin, L.: Studies in impedance audiometry III. Middle ear disorders. *Arch. Otolaryngol.* 99: 165, 1974.

Jerger, J., Harford, E., Clemis, J. and Alford, B.: The acoustic reflex in VIIIth nerve disorders. *Arch. Otolaryngol.* 99: 409, 1974b.

Lidén, G., Peterson, J.L. and Bjorkman, G.: Tympanometry: a method for analysis of middle ear function. *Acta Otolaryngol. (Suppl.)* 263: 218, 1970.

Lidén, G., Nilsson, E., Laaskinen, O. et al.: The stapedius reflex and motor reaction time: a parallel investigation of the effect of drugs. *Scand. Audiol.* 3: 73, 1974.

Lopes, O., Granato, L. and Eligabestky, M.: The early diagnosis of a glomic tumor in the middle ear by means of acoustic impedance. *Impedance Newsletter*, Vol. 1 New York, American Electromedics, 1972.

Luetje, C.M.: Facial nerve dysfunction. *ENT Journal* 26, 1977.

Matz, G.J., Rattenborg, C.G. and Holaday, D.A.: Effects of nitrous oxide on middle ear pressure. *Anesthesiology*, 28: 948, 1967.

Mitchell, O.C. and Richards, G.B.: Effects of various anesthetic agents on normal and pathological middle ears. *ENT Journal* 55: 36, 1976.

Northern, J.: Clinical applications of impedance audiometry. In Northern, J. (Ed.): *Hearing Disorders*, Boston, Little, Brown & Co., 1976, 20-32.

Northern, J.: Acoustic Impedance in the Pediatric Population. In Bess, F. (Ed.): *Childhood Deafness, Causes, Assessment and Management* New York, Grune and Stratton, 1977a.

Northern, J.L.: Impedance Audiometry for Otologic Diagnosis. In Shambaugh, C. and Shea, J. (Ed.): *Proceedings of the Shambaugh Fifth International Workshop on Middle Ear Microsurgery and Fluctuant Hearing Loss.* Huntsville, Ala., Strode Publishers, p. 75, 1977b.

Northern, J.L. and Grimes, A.M.: Introduction to Acoustic Impedance. In Katz, J. (Ed.): *Handbook of Clinical Audiology*, 2nd Ed. Baltimore, Williams & Wilkins Co., 1978, 344.

Northern, J. and Downs, M.: *Hearing in Children*, 2nd Ed. Baltimore, Williams & Wilkins Co. 1978.

Oramas, R.: Personal communication (Caracas, Venezuela, 1977.).

Patterson, M.E. and Bartlett, P.C.: Hearing impairment caused by intratympanic pressure changes during general anesthesia. *Laryngoscope* 86: 3, 399, 1976.

Richards, G.B. and Kartye, J.P.: Comparison of three types of ear tips used for impedance audiometry. *Arch. Otolaryngol.* 97: 437, 1973.

Richards, G.B., Mitchell, O.C. and Speights, I.L.: Effects of phenobarbital on intra-aural muscle reflexes in retarded children. *EENT Monthly* 54: 69, 1975.

Robinette, M.S., Rhodes, D.P. and Marion, M.W.: Effects of secobarbital on impedance audiometry. *Arch. Otolaryngol.* 100: 351, 1974.

Rock, E.H.: Practical otologic applications and considerations in impedance audiometry. *Impedance Newsletter*, Vol. 3. New York, American Electromedics, 1974.

Starr, A. and Schwartzkroin, P.: Cochlear microphonic and middle-ear pressure changes during nitrous oxide anesthesia in cats. *J. Acoust. Soc. Amer.* 51 (Part II): 1367, 1972.

Swogger-Rosenberg, J., Brenman, A.K. and Rosenberg, P.: A changed concept of screening. In Harford, E., Bess, F., Bluestone, C. and Klein, J.O. (Eds.): *Impedance Screening for Middle Ear Disease in Children.* New York, Grune & Stratton, 1978.

Thomsen, K.A., Terkildsen, K. and Arnfred, I.: Middle ear pressure during anesthesia. *Arch. Otolaryngol.* 82: 609, 1965.

Chapter Three

TYMPANOMETRY

EARL R. HARFORD, Ph.D.

INTRODUCTION

Tympanometry measures the mobility of the tympanic membrane, or some acoustic quantity in the ear canal, during variation of air pressure in a hermetically sealed ear canal. Tympanograms (charts used for recording tympanometric measures) have been plotted in units of acoustic impedance and its components, acoustic resistance and reactance, and in acoustic admittance (the reciprocal of acoustic impedance) and its components, acoustic conductance and susceptance. Also, tympanograms have been plotted in probe sound pressure level, acoustic compliance, phase angle, and arbitrary compliance units (Margolis, 1978). Regardless of the unit of measure, tympanometry provides the simultaneous assessment of the mobility of the tympanic membrane, the status of the ossicular chain, and the air cushion of the middle ear, including the static air pressure in the middle ear space. As a clinical test, tympanometry has been found to be useful for the detection of an abnormal conductive mechanism, the delineation of various types of conductive lesions, and the evaluation of the sufficiency of function of the Eustachian tube.

HISTORICAL BACKGROUND

During the decade that followed the early work of Metz (1946), Thomsen (1958),and Terkildsen and Thomsen (1959) of Denmark explored the utility of tympanometry as a differential diagnostic technique for middle ear abnormalities. Much of the early work concentrated on the development of effective instrumentation and clinical methodology. This early work demonstrated the principles of tympanometry. That is, these researchers determined that it was possible to assess middle ear pressure by changing the air pressure in the ear canal until minimal impedance was obtained. Today this is done as a matter of course, but at that time it was a real feat. They used a mechanical bridge, and it was very difficult to obtain an airtight seal of the ear canal with this crude device. Thomsen therefore used a pressure chamber to conduct his early investigations. The term *tympanometry* was used by Anderson and colleagues (1956) to describe a clinical test, but the technique was not intended to measure middle ear pressure.

Except for limited isolated reports on clinical application, virtually no research was reported in the American literature on the subject of tympanometry until 1970, when Lidén, and colleagues (1970) Peterson and Lidén (1970), and Jerger (1970) published three successive articles in the *Archives of Otolarynology*. These articles prompted a surge of interest in tympanometry in the United States. In the months that followed there were numerous articles on this subject. In fact, within two years tympanometry had become an extremely popular clinical technique.

Tympanometry applies an objective measurement to the principle of Van Dishoeck's (1939) subjective pneumophone test and the early laboratory studies of Bekesy (1932). Van Dishoeck's technique was based on the principle that a sound delivered to the ear canal will be heard most distinctly when air pressure is equal on both surfaces of the eardrum. Modern automatic tympanometry utilizes an electroacoustic impedance unit incorporating a microphone to monitor changes in sound pressure and phase of the probe tone in the ear canal which correspond to changes in the compliance of the tympanic membrane. This monitoring takes place while the air pressure is simultaneously varied with a manometer in the sealed canal of the same ear. Thus, the probe tone is monitored while the air pressure in the ear canal is changing.

METHODOLOGY

The basic equipment for tympanometry consists of an indicating meter, a manometer, a headset with earphone and probe unit, and optionally, a strip chart recorder or xy plotter. The probe unit is inserted into the test ear and a hermetic seal is obtained. The meter is then adjusted to a reference level with the eardrum clamped by + 200 mm H_20 pressure. Ordinarily, the meter adjustment of the impedance unit is set to the maximum reading to utilize its full range when measuring the compliance of the eardrum.

The stylus on the recorder is also set for a position at the extreme edge of the recorder channel, again to allow for maximum use of the recorder range to measure an increase in compliance.

The air pressure in the sealed canal is then gradually decreased through zero into the negative range to a pressure of at least -200 mm H_20, or more. Pressure of -400 mm H_20 or more is often used today, especially in cases where a maximum compliance point is not obtained before reaching -200 mm H_20. This is accomplished either manually—by controlling the manometer by hand—or, preferably, by activating a motor that changes the air pressure automatically. The result of this change from positive to negative (or negative to positive) air pressure is a tympanogram or a graph relating compliance change of the eardrum to air pressure variation in the ear canal. Thus, a tympanogram is a pressure-compliance function. Stated differently, the observed or recorded change of the sound pressure level of the probe tone in the ear canal is an expression of the relative change of the compliance of the tympanic membrane as a result of varying the air pressure that is imposed on the eardrum. The impedance of the conductive mechanism can be inferred from the tympanogram. That is, the greater the compliance, the lower the impedance, and vice versa. Figure 3-1 illustrates a typical tympanogram or pressure-compliance function for a normal ear according to the American method of recording and displaying the function. Figure 3-2 is the same information as shown in Figure 3-1 but represents the method of

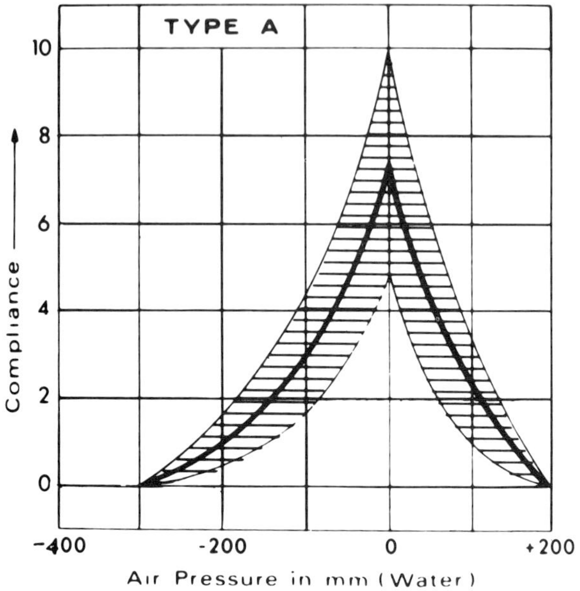

Figure 3-1 Typical normal pressure/compliance curve obtained by varying air pressure in sealed ear canal from positive through normal atmospheric pressure to negative pressure.

recording that was first introduced by the Scandinavian researchers.

As stated earlier, tympanometry can also be performed manually; i.e., without the use of a motor that automatically changes air pressure. This is accomplished by measuring compliance at several negative and positive pressure points, including zero atmospheric pressure, and plotting the compliance on a chart. The plots are connected by a smooth line curve and a tympanogram is displayed. The result from this manual method is presumed to be essentially the same as when the pressure is varied automatically and the compliance simultaneously plotted on a recorder. Both procedures yield a qualitative image of the compliance of the eardrum. Therefore, a tympanogram can be thought of as a qualitative counterpart of a static compliance measure. However, a tympanogram is likely to yield more information than a static

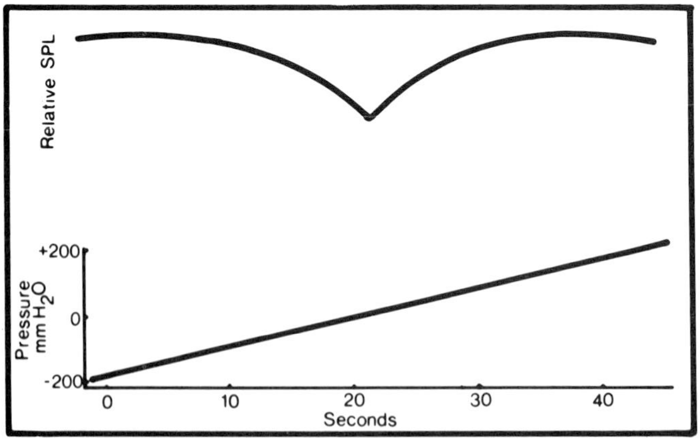

Figure 3-2 Type A, normal, tympanogram showing pressure/compliance function of normal ear drum and middle ear structure. This form of displaying tympanograms is popular in Scandinavia.

compliance measure because it has the capability of assessing the air pressure present in the middle ear. From the standpoint of clinical efficiency, it requires no more time to obtain a tympanogram than it does to establish static compliance measurements at three or four pressure points. Further, general classification (high, low, normal, etc.) of static compliance can be predicted from a tympanogram. Thus, tympanometry has gained wide clinical popularity, while static compliance measures are rarely used, especially since the quantitative results of the latter are subject to considerable variation and overlap among different middle ear abnormalities. Jerger (1970) reported that acoustic impedance, per se, which is computed from a static compliance measure, is simply too variable for accurate diagnosis. He found, in a large sample, about a 20 percent overlap between persons with normal hearing and those with a conductive hearing loss.

INTERPRETATION

As stated earlier, Lidén, Peterson, and Bjorkman (1970) stimulated much interest in tympanometry in the United States. A segment of their work involved the quantification of tympanograms. Figure 3-3 shows a normal tracing with various parameters which they suggest could be used for pruposes of quantification. Brooks (1969), another pioneer of impedance audiometry, advocated a method by which the gradient of a tympanogram could be calculated, as illustrated in Figure 3-4.

For the past several years, many clinicians have been using a fairly simple classification of tympanometric configurations. This classification involves three basic types of tympanograms: type A depicts a normal conductive mechanism and stapes fixation, type B is found in the presence of a fluid-filled ear or one with massive ossicular fixation, and type C depicts negative middle ear pressure resulting from insufficient Eustachian tube function and possibly accompanied by effusion in the middle ear. These three basic types are illustrated in Figure 3-5. Since there is an obvious difference between these three types of tympanometric tracings, a more

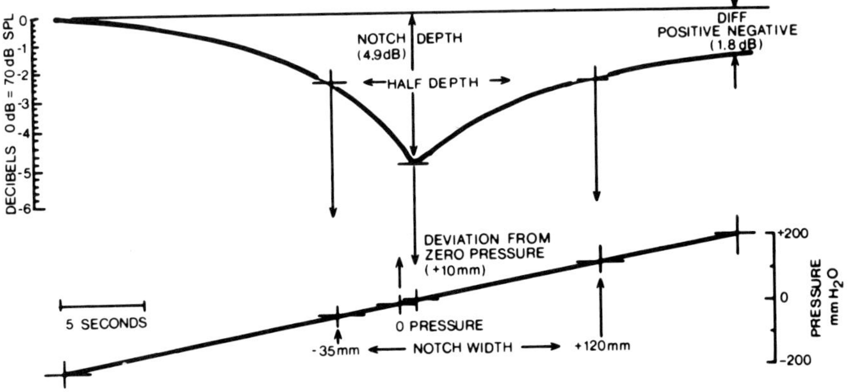

Figure 3-3 Tympanometric characteristics of 25-year-old woman with normal hearing and normal eardrum and middle ear. "V"-shaped curve shows tympanogram. Diagonal line is recording of air pressure change from −200 to + 200 mm H_2O. (Reprinted by permission of AMA *Arch. Otolaryngol.* from "Tympanometry," Lidén, G., Peterson, J. and Bjorkman, G., Vol. 92, pages 248–257, 1970.)

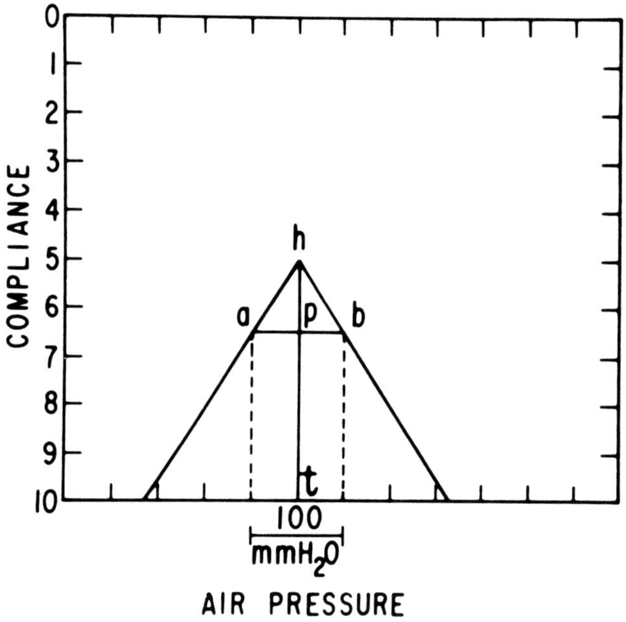

Figure 3-4 The gradient of a tympanogram is defined as ratio $\frac{hp}{ht}$, where ht equals overall height of tympanogram and hp equals vertical distance from peak to a horizontal line intersecting tympanogram, so that its width between points of intersection (a,b) is 100 mm H_2O. The higher the ratio $\frac{hp}{ht}$, the steeper the gradient. (After Brooks, 1969.)

precise analytic quantification of tympanograms, as proposed by Lidén and colleagues and Brooks seems to have limited value.

A rationale for adopting a more precise classification system for defining tympanograms is presented by Paradise, Smith, and Bluestone (1976) and is illustrated in Figure 3-6. Their system is based on correlations between the shape of tympanograms and the presence or absence of middle ear effusion, either as found at myringotomy or as diagnosed on pneumatic otoscopy. It is clear from this figure that one can obtain a variety of tympanometric curves that deviate from the simple A,B,C configurations. It is possible that more research on this issue will result in a method of classifying tympanograms that will yield a more definitive description of the status of the middle ear. Such a method is one of the highest priorities in tympanometry at this time. In the meantime, it appears that many clinicians continue to use the A,B,Cs in describing tympanograms.

Interpretation of tympanographic recordings is rather straightforward. A normal (type A) tympanogram is as easy to recognize as a normal audiogram. The peak represents the air-pressure point of greatest compliance of the eardrum. As expected in the case of a normal middle ear mechanism, this point of greatest compliance occurs at or near normal atmospheric pressure. It is not unusual to find this point of greatest compliance somewhat less or slightly more than 0 mm H_20. As much as -100 mm H_20, in the absence of any other indications of middle ear pathologic factors, represents the limit of a "normal" range; i.e., from 0 to -100 mm H_20. However, I should hasten to

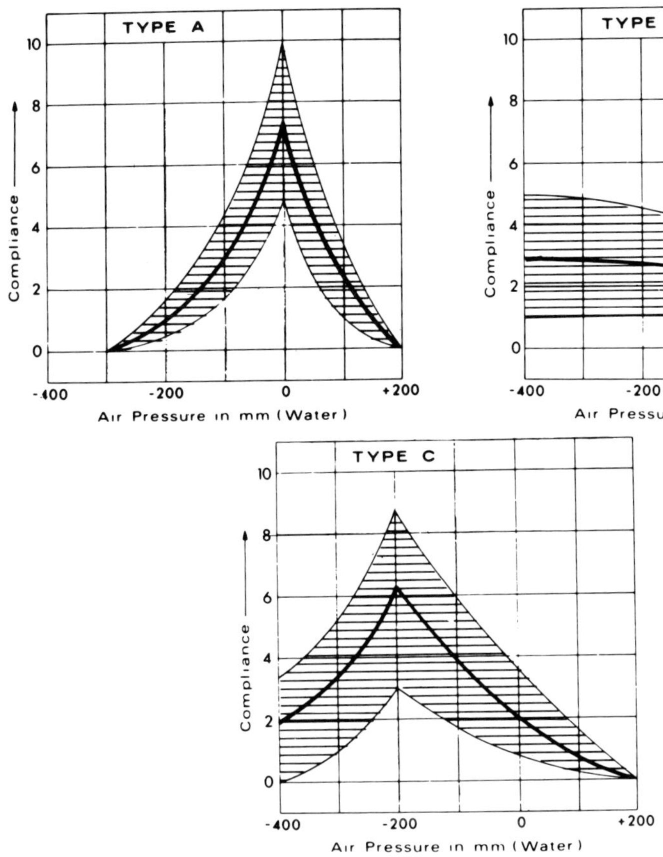

Figure 3-5 Three tympanograms, according to the American method of recording. Type A shows compliance of eardrum is greatest when air pressure in middle ear and in ear canal is equal to atmospheric pressure. Type B shows little change in compliance of eardrum with change in air pressure. Type C is indicative of underpressure in middle ear.

add that this question remains somewhat debatable and warrants further investigation.

Occasionally one will obtain a maximum compliance-pressure point above 0 mm H_2O. This finding also warrants further investigation and explanation, but it definitely occurs. Feldman (1976) claims that a positive pressure point for maximum compliance is suggestive of ensuing acute otitis media. It also suggests that the patient blew his nose, rose quickly in an elevator, or was crying just prior to the tympanogram.

We expect to find a normal tympanogram in persons with normal hearing and in those with a pure sensorineural hearing loss with normal middle ear pressure. However, the converse is not always true. That is, persons with normal hearing or a pure sensorineural hearing loss do not always manifest normal tympanometry. Some reports (McCandless and Thomas, 1974; Bluestone et al., 1973; and Brooks, 1971) suggest that a person's hearing thresholds for conventional pure-tone audiometry can be within the normal range (0 to 25 dB HL) and yet the person may have a mild conductive disorder that will be manifested by an abnormal tympanogram.

Lidén and colleagues (1970) reported a normal tympanogram in cases of stapedial otosclerosis (Fig. 3-7). This can also occur in other conditions leading to stapedial fixation. Thus, one can expect to obtain a normal tympanogram in cases of stapedial

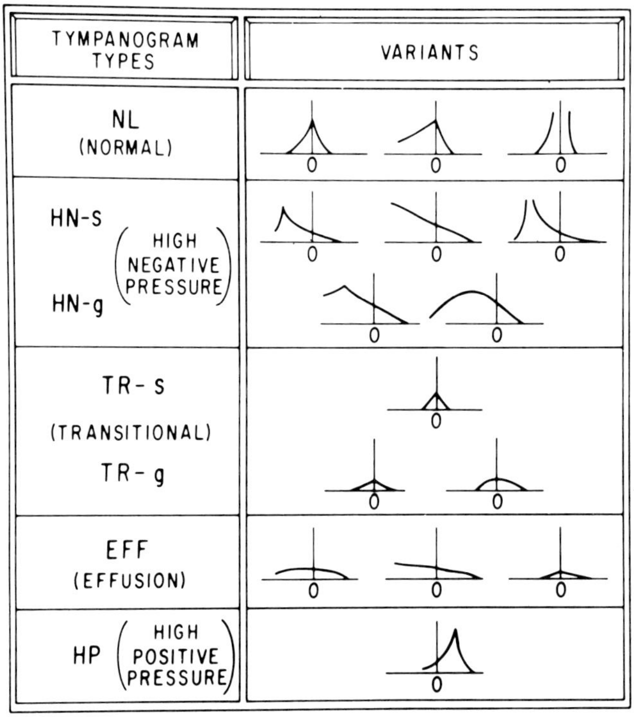

Figure 3-6 This figure illustrates examples of tympanometric configurations that can be obtained in a variety of ears in a typical clinical population. It is clear that these curves represent a continuum ranging from an essentially flat tracing to one that exceeds the limits of range of the recorder. (Reprinted by permission of *Pediatrics* from "Tympanometric detection of middle ear effusion in infants and young children," Paradise, J.L., Smith, C.C. and Bluestone, C.D., 58, pages 198–210, 1976.)

fixation or a tympanogram with a somewhat shallow peak, indicating a modest decrease in compliance. Fixation of the footplate of the stapes seems to have, at most, a minimal effect on the mobility of the eardrum under the stress of variation in air pressure.

It is important to keep in mind that tympanometry should be interpreted in conjuction with routine pure-tone audiometry, acoustic reflex measures, and an

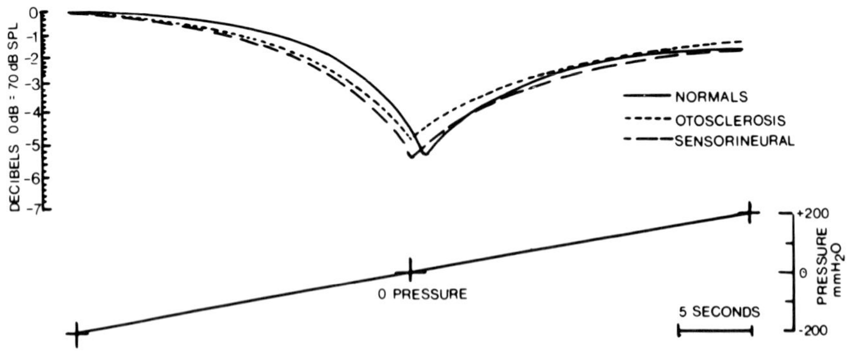

Figure 3-7 Mean tympanometric curves for 100 normal ears, 29 otosclerotic ears, and 27 sensorineural ears. (Reprinted by permission of AMA. *Arch.Otolaryngol.* from "Tympanometry," Lidén, G., Peterson, J. and Bjorkman, G., Vol. 92, pages 248–257, 1970.)

otologic examination. Thus, at the present state of the art, when a conductive hearing loss is in evidence, a normal tympanogram suggest the presence of stapedial fixation.

Once the interpretation of a normal (type A) tympanogram is understood, it is reasonably simple to predict the shape of a tympanogram for common abnormal middle ear conditions. For example, if a patient has a fluid-filled middle ear or massive ossicular fixation, the eardrum would not be expected to move much at all during variations in air pressure. Thus, there will be evidence of very little change in compliance, which suggests a high impedance. The result is a relatively flat (type B) or very shallow tympanogram indicating an immobile eardrum. A note of caution is warranted here. If a patient has a perforated eardrum, often a "seal" cannot be obtained. However, in some cases, it may be possible to obtain a seal with the probe. That is, the manometric gauge on the electroacoustic impedance unit does not show an air pressure leak. If this occurs, then the resultant tympanogram will be exceedingly flat. Obviously, this is because the compliance of the eardrum is not being assessed. Such an assessment requires an intact eardrum. Instead the air pressure is being changed in a large noncompliant cavity and the sound pressure level of the probe tone remains constant. In short, it is impossible to apply tympanometry for its intended purpose if the patient has a perforated eardrum. An absolutely flat tympanogram or rapid air pressure leakage at a positive pressure point is a good indication of a perforated eardrum. A rapid leak in the air pressure can occur if the Eustachian tube is forced open monentarily by an increase in air pressure. This measurement can have a useful purpose if the clinician wishes to determine if a ventilation tube in an eardrum is unobstructed.

Also, it is possible for the small hole in the probe, designed to deliver air pressure, to become occluded by residue or cerumen in an ear canal, while the other two holes remain open. This situation could cause a very flat tympanogram also; the reason is obvious. The air pressure may appear to be changing from an indication on the manometric gauge, but, in fact, the pressure is changing only to the place of occlusion in the probe and not actually in the ear canal. Thus, the sound pressure level of the probe tone will not change because there is no variation of air pressure on the eardrum. In short, be wary of the absolutely flat tympanogram; it may mean the presence of a perforated eardrum or a fault in the testing apparatus. A large amount of cerumen or impacted cerumen in an ear canal will usually prevent a tympanometric measure until it is removed. Also, if the tip of the probe is against the wall of the ear canal, especially in the case of a hand-held probe, a valid tympanogram cannot be obtained. This condition also results in a flat tympanogram.

If the middle ear is at negative air pressure relative to normal atmospheric pressure, maximum compliance will occur when the induced air pressure in the external ear canal approximates the negative air pressure in the middle ear cavity. Such a tracing is often referred to as a type C tympanogram. It is worthwhile to designate, as closely as possible, the amount of pressure where the maximum compliance occurs. It is important to be explicit for at least three reasons: (1) Further investigations will doubtless provide valuable data to allow for a correlation between the amount of negative (or positive) pressure and the nature or extent of causative factors; (2) if a patient is under treatment or is being monitored over time, or both, for an upper respiratory or middle ear condition, changes in middle ear pressure could provide valuable clues to the course of the abnormality; and (3) negative middle ear pressure can attenuate a stapedial reflex measure, and it is wise to compensate for such a condition by equalizing the air pressure in the ear canal with that in the middle ear when measuring the reflex. In brief, simply to state there is negative middle ear pressure without designating the extent yields an incomplete picture.

The presence of more than -100 mm H_20 negative middle ear pressure does not necessarily mean the patient has a middle ear abnormality. However, Bluestone (1973) cautions that children found to have middle ear pressure values of -100 mm H_20 or below should be considered to be at risk of developing otitis media, even if they are asymptomatic. He also states on the basis of considerable clinical experience, that it is possible that some children may be able to equilibrate high negative pressure intermittently and thus remain free of effusion.

It is presumptuous to assume that negative middle ear pressure signifies the presence of serous otitis media or a *nonfunctioning* eustachian tube or both. On the other hand, it appears that a more justifiable interpretation is an *insufficient* eustachian tube. Again, the results of tympanometry should be interpreted in conjunction with an otologic evaluation including a history and physical examination and with routine hearing tests, if possible. In young children and other difficult-to-test cases, the results of hearing tests may be inconclusive. However, when such inconclusive results are interpreted in conjunction with tympanometry and acoustic reflex measures, the nature of the problem may be greatly clarified. Jerger and colleagues (1974) have described this application of impedance audiometry very clearly. It will be delineated in some detail later in this chapter.

At this time, most commercially available impedance instruments, utilize a low-frequency probe tone; e.g., 220 Hz or 275 Hz. One unit offers both a 220 Hz and 660 Hz probe frequency. Of course, there are some "custom-made" units in use, and these may employ any number of different probe frequencies. Lidén's (1972) custom unit contains an 800 Hz probe tone, and it was Lidén and his associates (1974a) who called attention to two other types of tympanographic tracings not mentioned previously in this chapter. Lidén refers to them as a type D or "W" pattern, and Type E or undulating pattern. There is reasonably good evidence (Alberti and Jerger, 1974) today that these two patterns are directly associated with the frequency of the probe tone. Let us first discuss the type D.

This pattern appears in the shape of a sharp "W" as shown in Figure 3-8. This tympanometric pattern can be found in persons with absolutely normal hearing or a pure sensorineural hearing loss. In fact, Lidén and colleagues (1974b) report a high correspondence between the "W" pattern and simple scarred eardrum and in cases

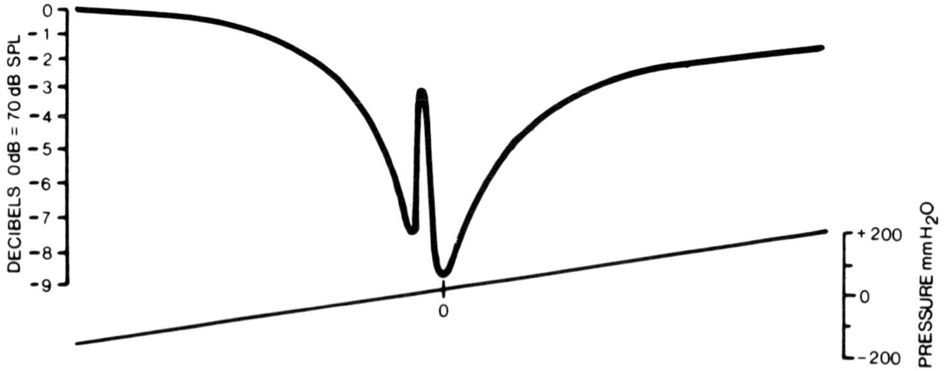

Figure 3–8 Type D tympanogram from 27-year-old normally hearing female on left ear. Tympanic membrane was thin and hypermobile. Probe tone frequency was 800 Hz. (Reprinted by permission of *Audiology* from "Automatic tympanometry in clinical practice," Lidén, G., Harford, E. and Hallen, O., Vol. 13, pages 126–139, 1974.)

with an atrophic or flaccid drum. They found that 8 percent of 182 subjects with perfectly normal hearing manifested a "W" or type D tympanogram. The reason for this tympanographic configuration can only be speculated at this time. Possibly these persons have a loosely coupled incudostapedial joint. Changes in the air pressure in the canal around barometric pressure may give rise to a partial decoupling of the cochlea. It is also possible that a small atrophic scar, even nonvisible, on the tympanic membrane may cause a "W" of type D tympanogram; many of these 182 subjects manifested visible scars. To explore this theory, Lidén coated the tympanic membrane with castor oil and, on a later occasion, with a thin plastic material (Nobercutane spray). Figure 3-9 illustrates the results of this experiment in one patient. It is obvious that the tympanographic configuration was virtually unchanged when the eardrum was treated with castor oil or plastic. This result tends to give some support to the hypothesis that partial decoupling of the incudostapedial joint may be one cause for a type D pattern in subjects with normal-appearing tympanic membranes. Margolis (1978) offers a detailed analysis of this type of tympanometric pattern based on the research of Vanhuyse, Creten, and Van Camp (1975). Their explanation is based on the arithmetic interaction between acoustic resistance and reactance. Further investigation and a clearer understanding of the W-shaped tympanogram is warranted, because it appears to be characteristic of normal neonate ears (Keith, 1973 and 1975; Cannon et al., 1974; Newman et al., 1974; Shurin et al., 1976; and Zarnoch and Balkany, 1978).

At this time, a type D tympanogram does not seem to have any significant diagnostic value. It appears to be a byproduct of a normal population when a probe tone frequency of 800 Hz or one slightly lower or higher is used. To avoid obtaining a "W" tympanogram in a usual clinical population, a lower probe frequency should be employed, such as 220 Hz, except in neonates, where the "W" appears even when a low-frequency probe tone is used.

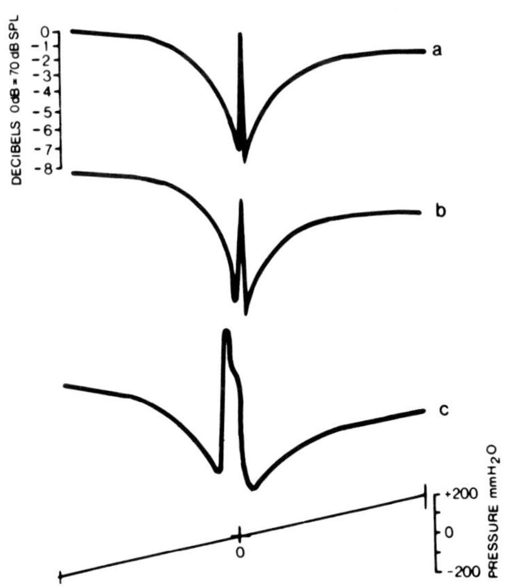

Figure 3-9 Tympanograms from 47-year-old male with hypermobile but otherwise normal tympanic membrane. (a.) Tympanic membrane uncoated; (b.) tympanic membrane coated with castor oil; (c.) tympanic membrane coated with a layer of plastic. (Reprinted by permission of *Audiology* from "Automatic tympanometry in clinical practice," Lidén, G., Harford E. and Hallen, O., Vol. 13, pages 126–139, 1974.)

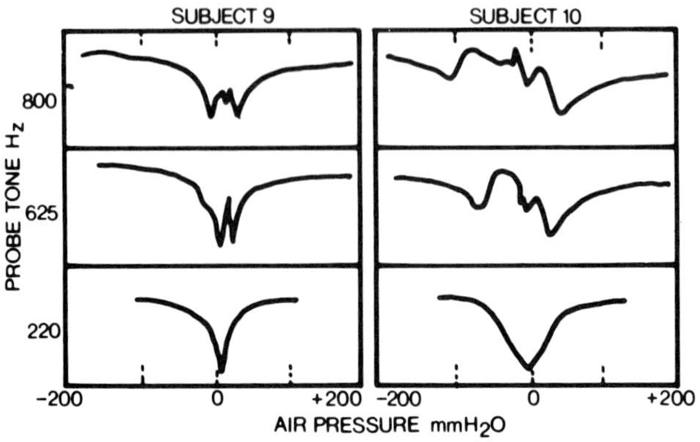

Figure 3-10 Three tympanograms for each of two subjects with confirmed ossicular discontinuity. Subject 9 is a 40-year-old man with cloudy tympanic membrane and scar in posterior quadrant. Subsequent tympanotomy revealed dislocation of both malleus and incus with discontinuity between incus and stapes. Subject 10 is 60-year-old woman who had stapedectomy in 1966. Present examination revealed thin scar in posterior superior quadrant of eardrum. Subsequent tympanotomy established that polytef piston had slipped from place, causing discontinuity. (Reprinted by permission of AMA *Arch. Otolaryngol.* from "Tympanometry for the diagnosis of ossicular disruption," Lidén, G., Harford, E. and Hallen O., Vol. 99, pages 23–29, 1974.)

The apparent significance of a type E or undulating tympanogram presents a conflict when selecting a probe tone frequency. Lidén and colleagues (1970) were the first to report this rather unusual tympanographic recording. They (1974b) claim that an undulating tympanographic pattern signifies the presence of an ossicular chain discontinuity. In support of this contention, they obtained three tympanograms on each of ten patients who had disruption of the ossicular chain which was subsequently surgically confirmed. A different probe tone frequency (220, 625, and 800 Hz) was utilized for each of the three tympanograms. Figure 3-10 illustrates the results from two cases with known disruption of the ossicular chain. Note that when a probe frequency of 220 Hz is used to generate a tympanogram, a rather deep type A pattern results. When a higher probe frequency (625 or 800 Hz) is used on the same ear, a different pattern emerges. True, in Subject 9, the 625 Hz probe frequency produced a pattern not unlike a type D, which could cause some confusion when interpreting results. However, when such a pattern occurs in a patient with an obvious conductive component, it is likely that the cause is a disruption of the ossicular chain. When a low probe frequency such as 220 Hz is used for tympanometry, the resultant tympanogram in a patient with ossicular disarticulation is expected to show a very high peak, or an incomplete tracing, like that illustrated in Figure 3-11. This tracing is often labeled A_D by those who use the alphabetic method for classifying tympanograms.

The shortcoming of Lidén, Harford and Hallen's 1974 report is that they used a sample of cases selected on the basis of a suspected ossicular disarticulation diagnosed by an otologist. They did not report tympanographic results on a variety of patients with a conductive hearing loss to explore the incidence of type E patterns in a cross section of the population with conductive type losses. Alberti and Jerger (1974) published an article detailing how this approach was taken by obtaining tympanograms on a cross section of the clinical population. Their sample included persons with normal hearing as well as those with a conductive- and sensorineural-type loss. In brief, they obtained tympanograms using probe frequencies of 220 Hz and 800 Hz on 1143 ears manifesting normal hearing and varying degrees and types of hearing

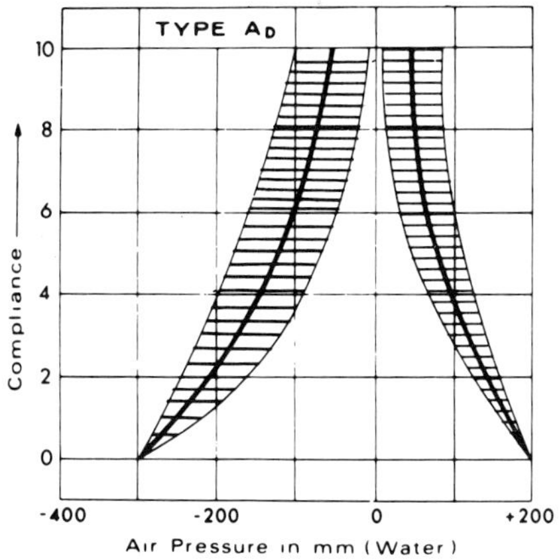

Figure 3-11 Typical tympanogram using 220 Hz probe tone, obtained from patient with ossicular chain disruption depicting very high compliance. Impedance meter and recorder go "off scale" around atmospheric zero.

impairment. The segment of their results pertinent to this issue is summarized below.

What appears to be their most significant finding was a "W" pattern for an 800 Hz probe frequency in ears with almost every type of middle ear disorder. In 969 ears (85 percent of the cases) the two different probe frequencies yielded the same pattern. However, in 174 ears (15 percent of the total group) there was a difference between the 220 Hz and 800 Hz tympanograms. In 141 ears they obtained a type A with the 220 Hz probe and a "W" shape (type D) with the 800 Hz probe tone. Forty of these ears manifested normal hearing and forty-five a sensorineural loss. The remaining fifty-six ears presented a variety of conductive type loss, eight with ossicular discontinuity, fourteen with otosclerosis, twenty-eight with otitis media, and six with a variety of miscellaneous causes.

In about half of the 141 ears the tympanic membrane was normal in appearance. In the other half, some type and degree of eardrum abnormality was observed—scarred, abnormally thin, hypermobile, post-tympanoplasty, and so on. Alberti and Jerger concluded that the most significant determinant of the "W" pattern was some degree of tympanic membrane disease. They went on to state that in general, the greater the degree of eardrum abnormality, the more complex the "W" pattern.

Alberti and Jerger's investigation highlights the fact that a higher probe tone frequency is likely to yield a "W" pattern in a variety of hearing disorders. Unfortunately, they do not really draw a clear distinction between a "W" (type D) and an undulating (type E) pattern. They tend to combine these two types into one group and call them a "W" pattern. It would be interesting to reexamine their data and separate tympanograms with a sharp "W" from those reflecting broad undulations. Recall that Lidén does separate these two patterns into type D and type E categories. He does not claim that the type D pattern has diagnostic significance but says that a type E does have diagnostic importance.

In any case, there seems to be some evidence that the frequency of the probe tone has a direct effect on the type of tympanographic pattern obtained on a variety of ears. Figure 3-12, for example, shows tympanograms at four probe tone frequencies in a patient with a grossly abnormal eardrum involving scarring and monomeric membrane. The "W" configuration is very much in evidence for 800 and 900 Hz tones, barely discernible for 660 Hz, and absent for the 240Hz probe tone. This

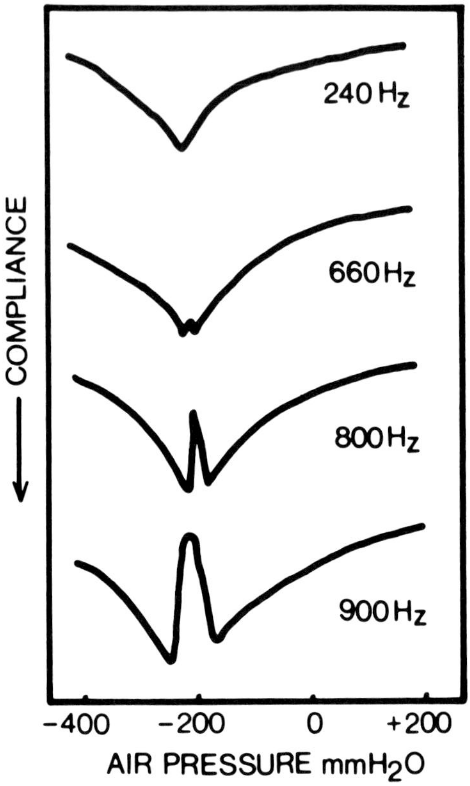

Figure 3-12 Effect of probe frequency on tympanogram in patient with grossly abnormal tympanic membrane. Note that "W" shape is obvious at 800 and 900 Hz, but only barely discernible at 600 Hz. (Reprinted by permission of AMA *Arch. Otolaryngol.* from "Probe-tone frequency and the diagnostic value of tympanometry," Alberti, P. and Jerger, J., Vol. 99, pages 206–210, 1974.)

supports Lidén's results cited earlier. Alberti and Jerger conclude that the "W" pattern either indicates some slight tympanic membrane abnormality or is simply a normal variant occurring in a small percentage of normal ears. Since the "W" pattern appears in most normal ears for probe frequencies above 900 Hz, it seems reasonable that the distribution of the normal "W" extends, with a small but definite probability, below 800 Hz.

Lidén and his associates (1974a, p. 29): launch into a more detailed speculation for the difference in patterns as they relate to the frequency of the probe tone. They make the following statements:

"The 800 Hz tone is closer to the resonant frequency of the middle ear than the 220 Hz tone. Interaction between the changes in resonance characteristics of the middle ear and the frequency of the probe tone due to changes of the air pressure in the ear canal will be greater and more pronounced at 800 Hz than at 220 Hz. Apparently, the lower, 220 Hz tone is virtually unaffected by changes in resonance.

"The impedance of the middle ear consists of a real or resistive part and an imaginary or reactive part. The resistance comes mainly from the cochlea. The reactive part includes the mass and the stiffness of the middle ear. Below the resonant frequency the middle ear system is stiffness-controlled and changes in resistance will pass nearly unnoticed at 220 Hz. Interruption of the incudostapedial joint implies disconnection of the cochlea and lowered resistance. Møller (1965) measured the impedance of the middle ear in cats with disruption of the ossicular chain and showed that the greatest change in resistance was found in the vicinity of the resonant frequency. In man, the resonant frequency of the middle ear is close to 800 Hz. Stated differently, the 220 Hz probe tone depicts mainly changes in the stiffness component of the reactance, while 800 Hz depicts changes in both resistance and reactance in the configuration of the curve.

"Changes of the air pressure in the ear canal have a strong effect on the impedance of the normal middle ear. The changes are more pronounced for negative than for positive pressure. Møller has shown in cats that the reactive part of the impedance has its lowest value when there is no pressure difference between the two sides of the eardrum and increases when the pressure is increased as well as decreased. The resistive part, however, is very low for negative pressure, indicating partial decoupling of the cochlea, but resistance increases with increased positive pressure. In cases with discontinuity of the chain, changes of the air pressure will exaggerate the changes in resistance and give rise to a tympanogram with undulations especially pronounced on the negative side."

Recall that a type D tympanogram has been observed in some (8 percent) normal subjects with very mobile but otherwise perfectly normal tympanic membranes. The cause for this configuration is still not clearly understood. However, it is possible that these subjects may also have a loosely coupled incudostapedial joint. Changes of the air pressure in the canal around barometric pressure may give rise to a partial decoupling of the cochlea.

Alberti and Jerger are not impressed with the value of a higher probe tone frequency for tympanometry. They report that they found that the 800 Hz tympanogram yielded no additional information of diagnostic value over and above the information yielded by the 220 Hz tympanogram.

Finally, Lidén and colleagues (1974a), in their article on tympanometry for the diagnosis for ossicular disruption, conclude:

"There is no doubt that tympanometry can offer valuable information for the differential diagnosis of conductive lesions. Before its full potential can be realized, we must reconcile some of the fundamental discrepancies in test results and interpretation that currently exist. In our judgment, the frequency of the probe tone has a major effect on the type of tympanographic recording obtained on cases of ossicular disruption. In our judgment, a probe tone frequency of 800 Hz is the one of choice."

Thus, there is a potential conflict concerning the value of a probe tone frequency higher than 220 or 275 Hz. The prospective user of impedance audiometry must judge what probe frequency to use for tympamometry. It appears that the higher the probe frequency, the more sensitive tympanometry is for the detection of abnormalities of the conductive portion of the hearing mechanism. At the same time, when a higher probe frequency is used (e.g., 660 Hz or 800 Hz), the clinician must be prepared to yield a greater percentage of false positive cases—that is, ears that appear to have an abnormality but actually do not have one of any particular consequence. This error can be reduced if other audiologic and otologic data are taken into consideration when interpreting the tympanometric results.

VARIABLES AND STANDARDIZATION

As we move well into the era of impedance audiometry in the United States, it seems appropriate to direct some attention to the matter of standardization in order to foster uniformity in procedures and reporting. The importance of standardization can best be appreciated by emphasizing the variables that can have an effect on the actual results or apparent results obtained from any clinical measurement. Although this principle is of supreme importance in inferential measurements, it is also significant in objective measures, such as tympanometry.

When reasonable care is exercised by the clinician, tympanometry is a reliable tool. During the formative period of impedance audiometry, concerns were expressed about the need for standards and uniformity of procedures so as to foster optimal communication for interpretation of impedance audiometry. A set of standards for instrumentation, as well as for terminology, has not yet been developed. A need still exists for standards of measurement of the commercial instruments, calibration procedures, reporting of specifications by the manufacturers, and the recording and reporting of tests used by clinicians. There is currently an ANSI (S-3 60) writing group in the process of developing some standards for impedance instruments. A report from this committee should be published in the near future. In the meantime, it seems that some attention should be given to the subject of reliability and stability of tympanometry. Feldman (1976) discusses some concerns relative to variables which may have an influence on the results obtained from tympanometry. He focuses primarily on the effect of speed and direction of change in air pressure on the peak location, amplitude, and shape of the tympanogram.

Lidén, Peterson, and Bjorkman (1970) reported the results of 20 consecutive tympanograms on the same person over a period of 10 hours. The probe was removed from the subject's ear after each tympanogram. Following a brief rest period, another tympanogram was obtained. Figure 3-13 shows the results of five of the twenty tympanograms on this subject. It is evident that they obtained essentially the same tracing with each test. We have obtained two or three tympanograms on the same ear during one sitting from numerous patients and obtained virtually identical results.

There are several impedance instruments on the market today. All of them purport to provide similar data on the status of the conductive auditory mechanism. There has been concern that one can obtain different results from the same ear on different instruments. We decided to explore this concern with a very simple procedure. We obtained a tympanogram on the same person on five different instruments (four manufacturers) within a period of twenty minutes. Figures 3-14 through 3-18 show the results. Clearly, each instrument provided nearly the identical result; a slight + 18 to 35 mm H_20 maximum pressure peak. At least on this one normal ear we were unable to demonstrate any real difference in the type of tympanogram obtained from these five different instruments. In fact, the range of peak pressure recorded on the five instruments was only 17 mm H_20 .

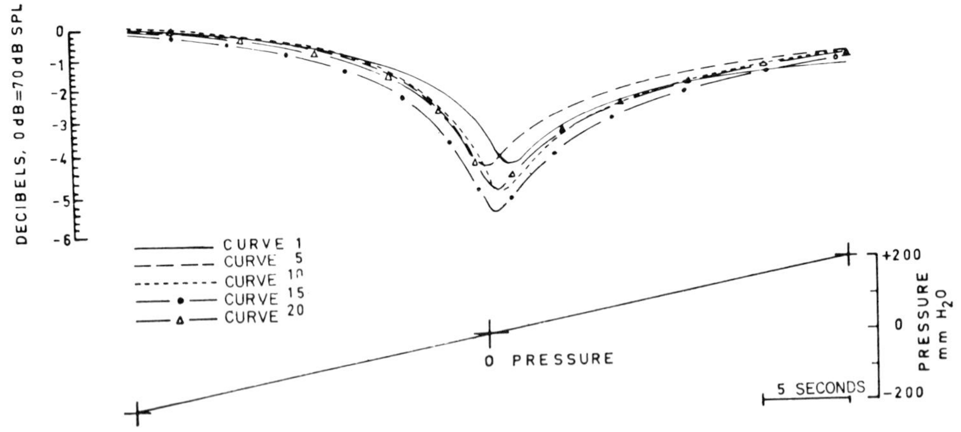

Figure 3-13 Test-retest comparison of five tympanograms for one ear with normal hearing and normal eardrum and middle ear, obtained over a consecutive ten-hour period. (Reprinted by permission of AMA *Arch. Otolaryngol.* from "Tympanometry," Lidén, G., Peterson, J.L. and Bjorkman, G., Vol. 92, page 253, 1970.)

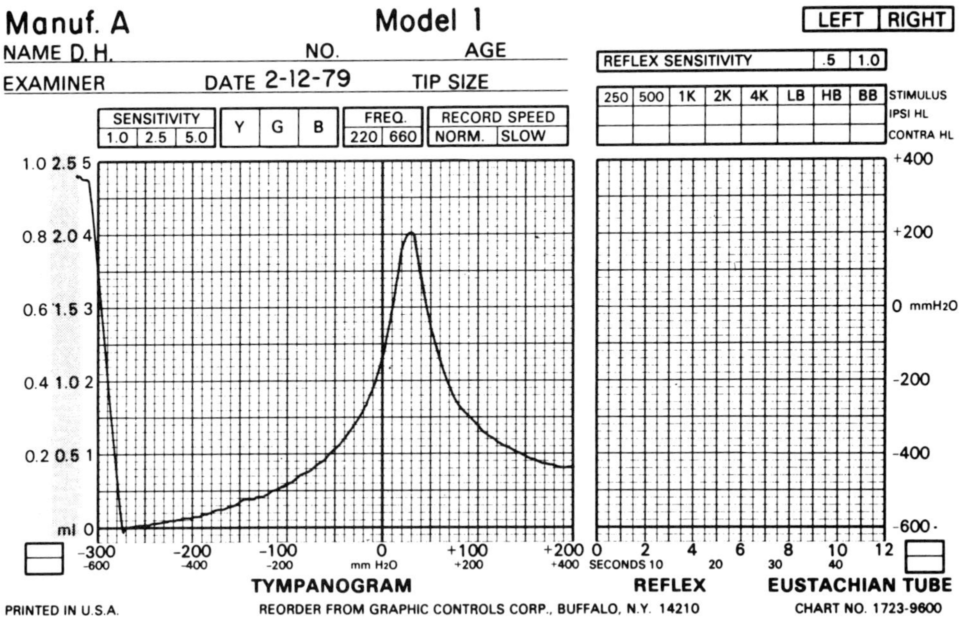

Figure 3-14

Figures 3-14 —3-18 Five tympanograms obtained on the same person within a period of 20 minutes using five different tympanometers manufactured by four different companies. There is essentially no difference in pattern or peak pressure with any of these instruments.

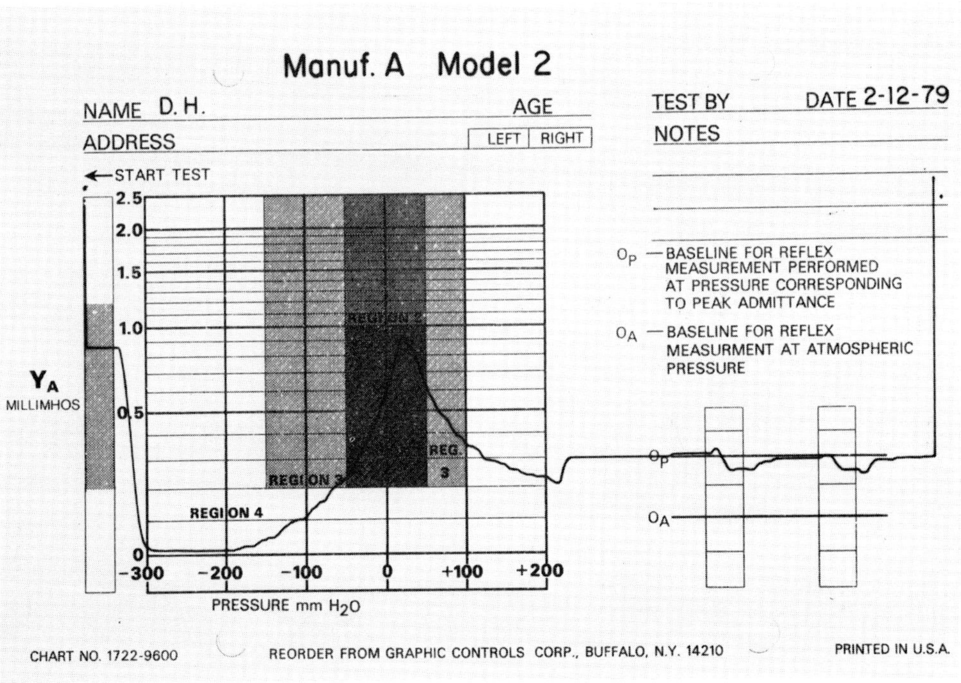

Figure 3-15

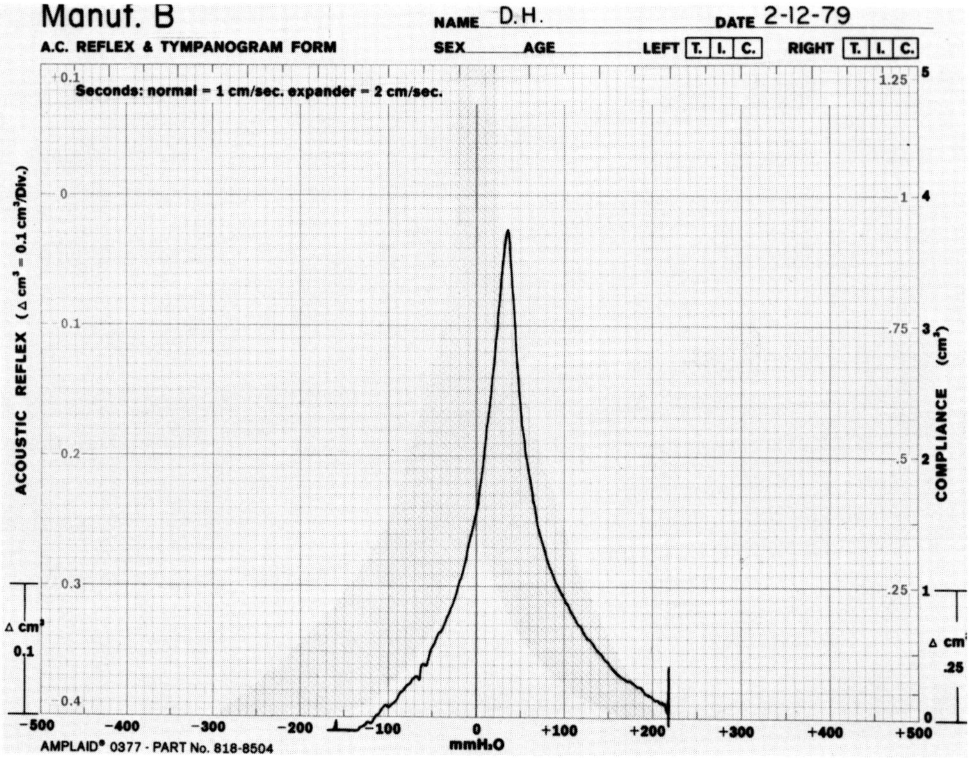

Figure 3-16

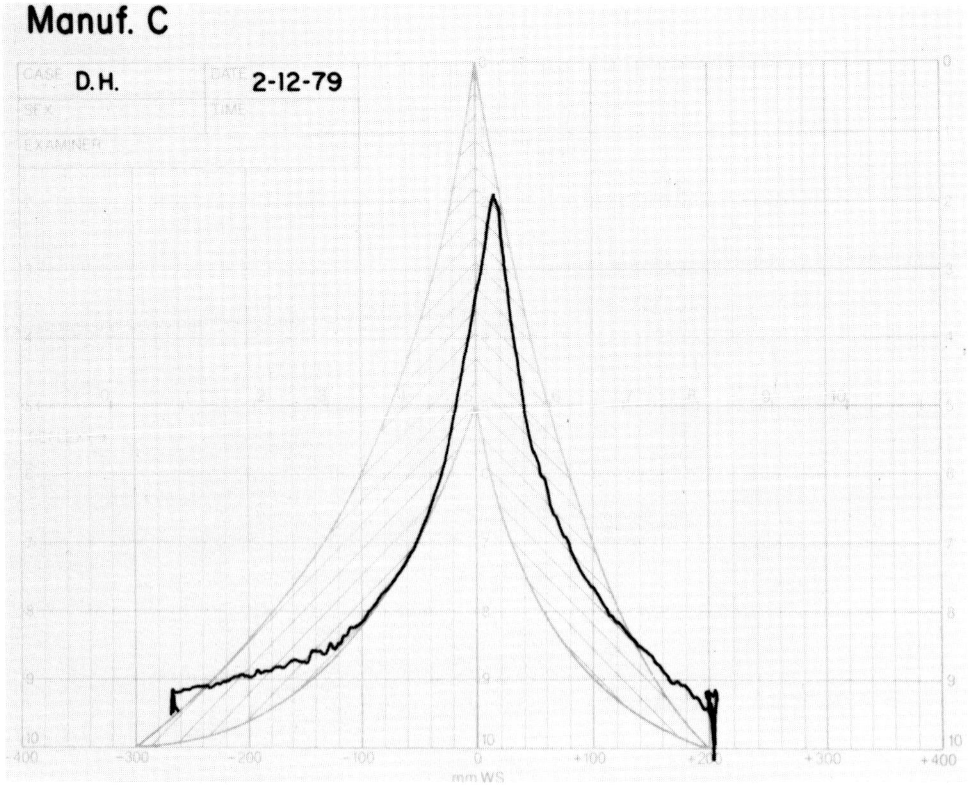

Figure 3-17

Manuf. D

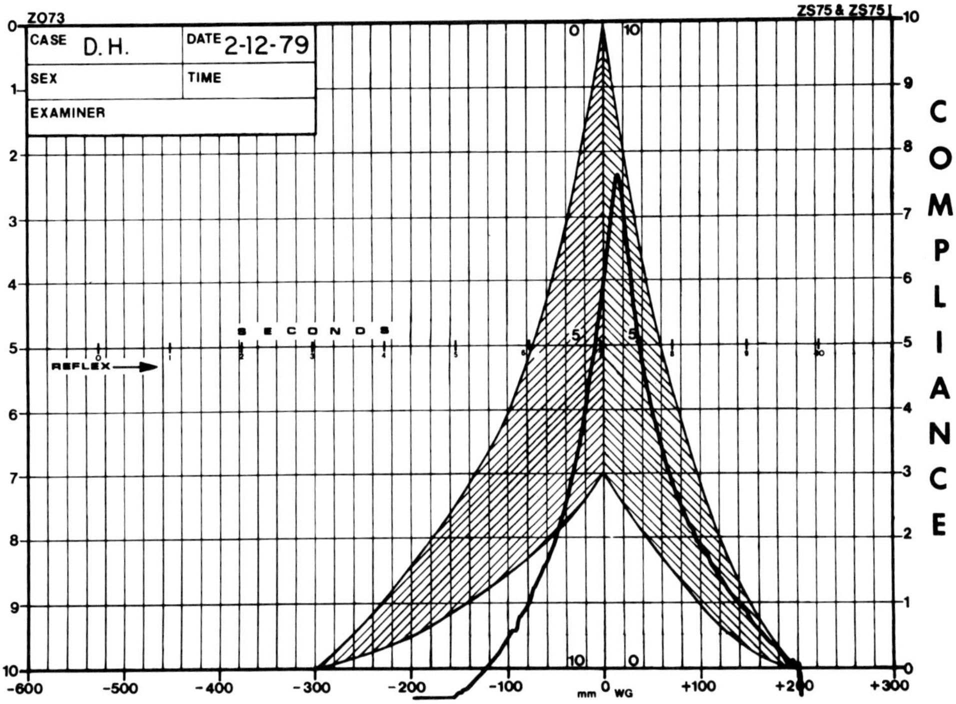

Figure 3-18

Figures 3-19 A and B and 3-20 illustrate the result of the direction of pressure change. The difference in the pressure peak apparently is a consequence of hysteresis. Note that when the air pressure is not equalized (Fig. 3-19 A,B), the change from positive to negative and negative to positive affects both the point of peak pressure and the amplitude of the tracing. On the other hand, when the air pressure is equalized following the positive to negative tracing, the peak is displaced but maintains the same amplitude during the negative to positive pressure change (Figure 3-20). Clinicians should choose one procedure for obtaining a tympanogram and use it consistently.

More research is needed on the subject of instrumentation and procedural variables. In the meantime, it is wise for the clinician to appreciate the possibility that the interpretation of tympanograms may be influenced by certain variables. Examples of some of these variables are listed below:

1. Frequency of the probe tone
2. Rate of air pressure change
3. Direction of air pressure change
4. Range of air pressure
5. Sensitivity of the recorder
6. Chart speed of the recorder
7. Unit of measure
8. Adherence to manufacturer's calibration procedure

Clearly, the formative period of automatic tympanometry is the appropriate time to develop standardization to avoid confusion in publications, verbal exchange of our mutual experiences, and clinical case reports. It is not the intention here to recommend

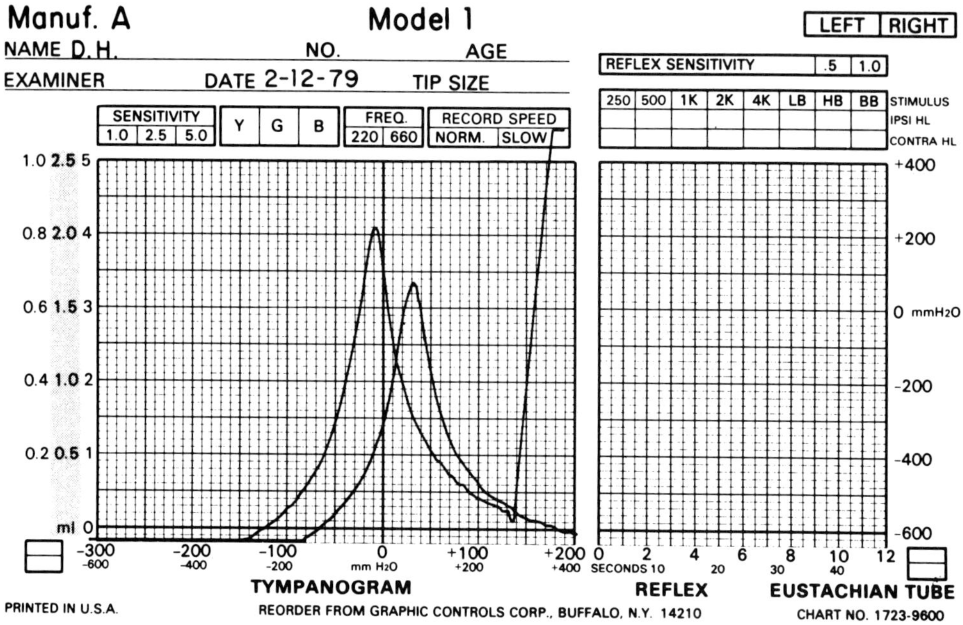

Figure 3-19 (A)Two tympanograms on same ear, obtained a few seconds apart. One tympanogram was obtained while changing air pressure from + 200 mm H_2O to negative pressure. The other was obtained while changing pressure from -200 mm H_2O to positive pressure. Note change in peak pressure *and* amplitude.

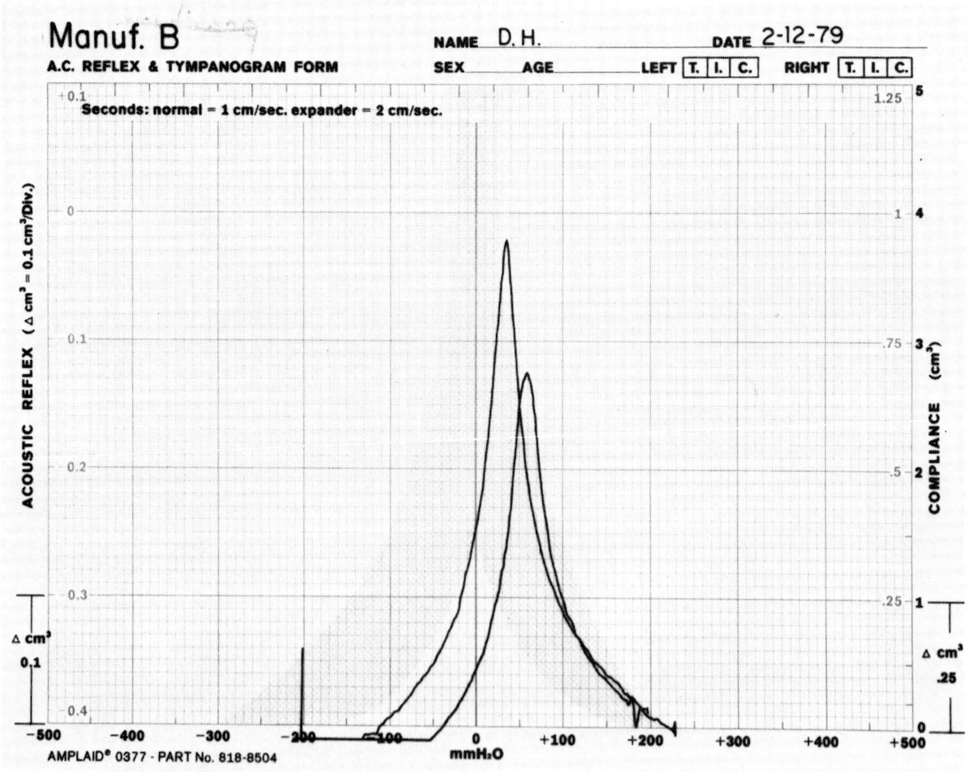

Figure 3-19 (B)Two tympanograms obtained as shown in (A), but with a different tympanometer.

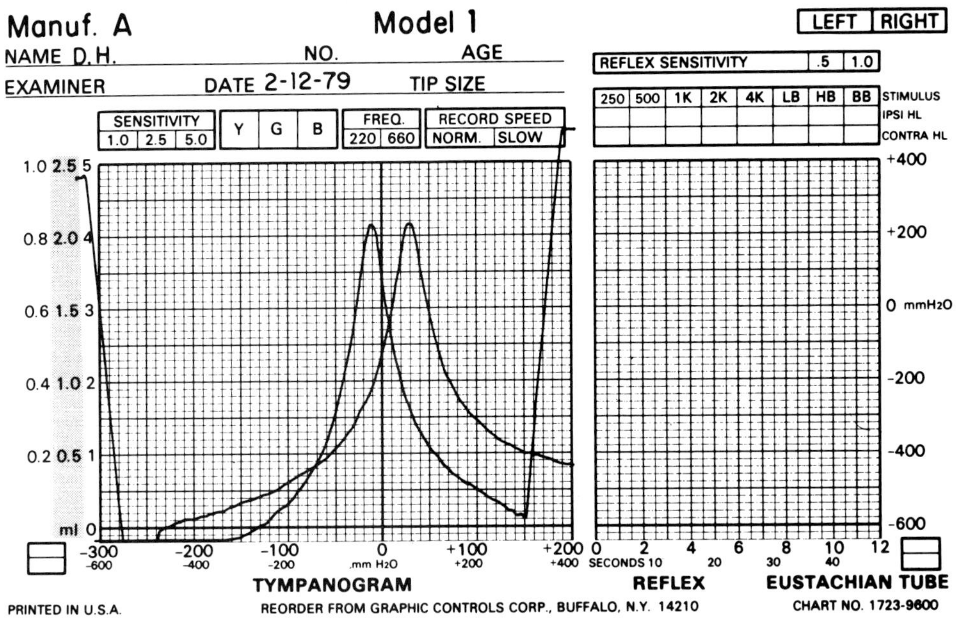

Figure 3–20 These two tympanograms were obtained the same way as those illustrated in Figure 3–19; however, between the two tympanograms, the air pressure in the ear canal was equalized to atmospheric pressure. Note the change in peak pressure; but the amplitude is the same.

the specifics for standardization, since this problem can be more appropriately dealt with by a body that represents a cross section of those who utilize information provided by automatic tympanometry. Instead, we will simply alert the clinician to the majority of factors that are likely to yield different results if they are varied from one test to another on the same patient during the same period of time.

CLINICAL APPLICATION

The intent of this section is to emphasize the clinical application of tympanometry. As stated at the outset of this chapter, tympanometry has become a popular technique for the differential diagnosis of middle ear disorders. It has become popular because it is an objective test, rather than inferential, as in the case of bone conduction audiometry, tuning fork tests, SAL (sensorineural acuity level), Bekesy audiometry, and other tests that require judgments by the patient. In addition to its objectivity, it is an easy test to administer, it is not time consuming, and the results are usually easy to interpret. As one gains more experience with tympanometry and more investigations appear in print, interpretation should be even more definitive.

Like many other tests, tympanometry should not be interpreted in isolation. Only by comparing the results of a tympanogram with other data can one expect to reap full benefit from this clinical measurement. At least an otoscopic inspection of the ear canal, and preferably a complete otologic examination should always precede or accompany tympanometry. It is essential that the ear canal be as free from residue as possible to have successful and meaningful tympanometry. It can be frustrating for the examiner if the probe tip becomes occluded each time it is inserted into the ear canal. This not only lengthens the time involved in this measurement, but may actually render it impossible if the residue is not cleaned out. Also, it is important to know if there is a perforation of the tympanic membrane for reasons cited earlier under the section on interpretation. If an otologist is not available at the time of the test, the examiner should inspect the patient's ear canal to ensure the absence of significant residue and perforation.

Although it is not essential, it is helpful to have some clue to the status of the patient's hearing disorder. The examiner should at least have some clue as to the differential diagnostic problem. For example, is there a conductive component or is this a pure sensorineural loss? Is this conductive loss due to stapedial otosclerosis or disruption of the ossicular chain? Are the ventilation tubes in the ear canals patent? Without such specific questions, the interpretation of results could have reduced significance. For example, in the presence of a hearing loss a normal tympanogram can signify either a pure sensorineural impairment, stapedial otosclerosis, or a mixed-type loss due to otosclerosis.

Further, tympanometry has considerably more significance when it is applied in conjunction with stapedial reflex measures. The reverse is also true. That is, an explanation for an absent stapedial reflex is often based on the presence of an abnormal tympanogram signifying conductive pathologic factors. Thus, tympanometry should always precede a stapedial reflex measurement. If the tympanogram reveals a negative middle ear pressure, the examiner will want to compensate for this negative pressure when attempting to elicit the stapedial reflex. This maneuver becomes important in those cases where a reflex is absent or elevated. If the stapedial reflex is in the normal range when negative air pressure is not compensated for, it is not likely that such an equilibration is necessary. Figure 3-21 simply illustrates in one selected case how only -100 mm H_2O of pressure in the middle ear can suppress a stapedial reflex. From our clinical experience, this suppression does not always occur, but it is important to be on the alert for it.

A few examples of the application of tympanometry coupled with stapedial reflex measures are included here to illustrate the significance of this technique. Jerger and colleagues (1974) have presented some excellent applications for the pediatric clinical population, particularly under the age of six years, but these could also pertain to the mentally retarded population with a much higher chronologic age. Some of these examples could also apply to perplexing differential diagnostic problems sometimes encountered in adults. The following is taken directly from Jerger's article (1974, p. 9):

"1. The behavioral audiogram suggests a unilateral loss by air conduction. Here impedance audiometry easily differentiates between a conductive and a sensorineural loss without the need for bone conduction thresholds. If tympanograms are Type A and reflexes are present in both ears or at least in the good ear, the loss is sensorineural. If, on the other hand, the tympanogram is A in the good ear, but B or C on the bad ear, and reflexes are absent from both ears, then the loss must be conductive. In very young children, the capacity to make this distinction without recourse to masked bone-conduction audiometry can be of some value.

"2. Behavioral results suggest a severe bilateral loss. The child seems to respond only to very intense signals. Here impedance audiometry confirms the picture if tympanograms are A and reflexes are bilaterally absent.

"3. Behavioral results suggest normal or near-normal hearing. The child seems to respond to familiar sounds at 20-30 dB HL. Here impedance audiometry confirms the picture if tympanograms are Type A and reflexes are present bilaterally. If, however, tympanograms are B or C on at least one ear, and reflexes are absent at all test frequencies from one or both ears, then a mild conductive loss must be considered likely.

"4. Behavioral results suggest reasonably good levels (20-30 db HL) but the parents report a great deal of fluctuation in sensitivity. Here Type B or C tympanograms and absent reflexes confirm the picture of recurrent otitis media.

"5. Behavioral results suggest reasonably good sensitivity to familiar environmental sounds (20-30db HL) but the parents report that the child seems to hear some sounds more consistently than

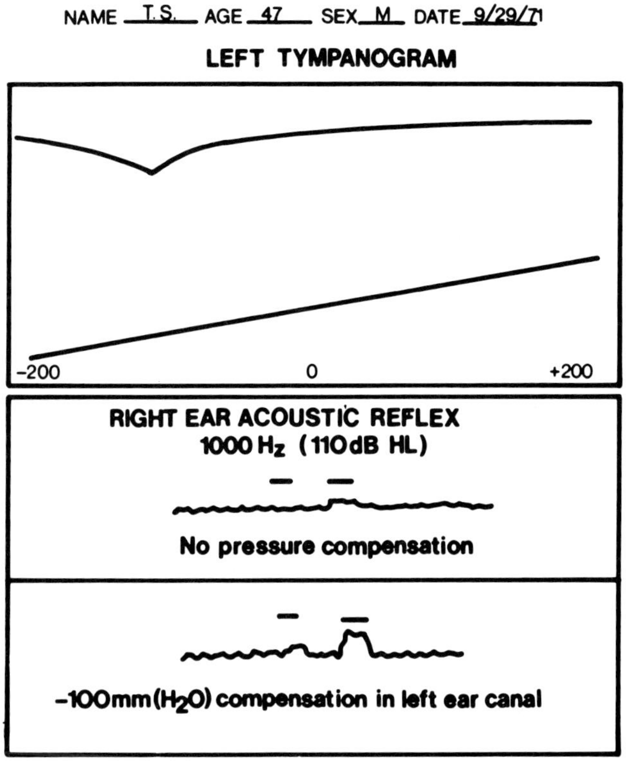

Figure 3-21 A tympanogram and acoustic reflexes for 47-year-old male with pure sensorineural hearing loss suspected as result of an eighth nerve tumor. Routine tympanometry revealed −100 mm H_2O pressure in left middle ear. Acoustic reflex threshold was reduced 5 dB without compensation for this negative middle ear pressure, and magnitude of reflex is also reduced. When −100 mm pressure is introduced into probe ear, acoustic reflex threshold is more obvious, as shown in lower tracing of acoustic reflexes. In this example, left ear is "probe ear" and right ear is "test ear."

others. Some parents may phrase this as, "He hears what he wants to hear. Sometimes he doesn't seem to hear us at all." Here Type A tympanograms combined with reflexes at 500 Hz and possibly 1000 Hz, but absent reflexes at 2000 and 4000 Hz confirm the picture of a steeply sloping high-frequency loss.

"6. Behavioral results suggest a total loss. The child fails to respond to sound at any level. If tympanograms are Type A and reflexes are absent, the impression of total deafness is confirmed. If, however, reflexes are present at normal levels, an alternative explanation for the behavioral observation must be sought (i.e., retardation, autism, etc.).

"7. The behavioral audiogram shows an air-bone gap of 15 dB but otologic examination is negative. Here Type A tympanograms and bilateral reflexes confirm the otologic examination and argue that the air-bone gap is invalid. On the other hand, abnormal tympanograms and absent reflexes support the audiogram and indicate that the otologic examination failed to detect a significant middle ear disorder."

Feldman (1976) approaches the clinical application of tympanometry somewhat differently, but in a very useful manner. Table 3-1 represents a chart that can be a guide to the clinician for the interpretation of tympanograms.

There appears to be a mounting interest in the application of impedance audiometry as a screening method for the detection of subtle middle ear impairment. This application of tympanometry is discussed in considerable detail in Chapter 11, consequently it will be mentioned only briefly in this section. The technique is simple. A tympanometric recording is observed and then a single frequency pure tone is used

TABLE 3-1. ANALYSIS OF TYMPANOMETRIC CONFIGURATION OF SOME COMMON MIDDLE EAR PATHOLOGIES*

			Shape	
Middle ear disorder	**Pressure peak**	**Amplitude**	**High-frequency probe tone**	**Low-frequency probe tone**
Serous otitis acute	None—severe negative	None—shallow	Flat—slight rising	Flat—falling
			Converging	
Serous otitis resolving	Moderate—negative	Shallow—normal	Normal	Normal
"Glue" ear	Moderate—severe negative	Flat-shallow	Flat	Flat-falling
			Converging	
Cholesteatoma	Normal—negative to absent	Non—shallow	Flattened	Lower at negative pressure
			Converging	
Acute otitis media	Positive	Normal	Normal	Normal
Blocked Eustachian tube	Mild—moderate negative	Normal	Normal	Normal
Glomus tumor	Non—normal	Extremely shallow	Vascular perturbations	Vascular perturbations
Otosclcrosis	Normal	Shallow	Normal	Normal
Malleolar fixation	Normal	Shallow	Normal	Normal
Incudostapedial interruption	Normal	Large	Peaked—normal	Deep notches, peaked and undulating
Crural interruption	Normal	Large	Peaked—normal	Deep notches, peaked and undulating
Healed TM perforation	Normal	Large	Normal—peaked	Notch—peaked
Perforated TM	None	Elevated base line	Flat	Flat
Stapedectomy	Normal	Large	Normal	Notched and undulating

*Reprinted by permission of Williams & Wilkins and Feldman, A.S. and Wilber, L.A.: *Acoustic Impedance and Admittance—The Measurement of Middle Ear Function*, Baltimore, Williams & Wilkins Co., 1976.

to elicit a stapedial reflex. If the tympanogram is abnormal or the reflex is elevated or absent, the child fails the screen. Yet to be determined is a logical negative pressure that can be safely tolerated before classifying a tympanogram as abnormal. Some clinicians use −50 mm H_20, others use −100 mm H_20, while others use −150 mm H_20. This question warrants further investigation. Also, the presence or absence of the stapedial reflex may not be a sufficient criterion for pass-fail on this aspect of the screen. That is, an elevated reflex, perhaps 100 dB HL, is a safer criterion for identifying a greater percentage of early middle ear abnormality than only an absent reflex.

Finally, those who advocate the use of impedance audiometry for screening purposes point out that this technique should not replace traditional pure-tone discrete frequency screening. Tympanometry cannot detect sensorineural hearing impairment. Thus, pure-tone screening will continue to play a role in detecting abnormal hearing caused by impairment of the sensorineural mechanism. This is particularly critical in cases of high-frequency hearing loss in children, a condition that can escape detection until a child receives a pure-tone screening test at school.

SUMMARY

Automatic tympanometry is one of the three basic components of impedance audiometry that was conceived and developed by Scandinavian clinicians. It is gaining rapid popularity in the United States. It is useful for the delineation of various types of abnormalities affecting the conductive transmission mechanism of the ear, including the sufficiency of the Eustachian tube. It also has promise as a screening device for the early detection of middle ear fluid in preschool and elementary school-age children. Tympanometry is an easy technique to employ. It yields information quickly and it does not require judgments by the patient. The results are relatively easy to interpret, and it can be a valid and reliable measure, provided the clinician respects the procedural and instrumentational variables that can influence the results.

REFERENCES

Alberti, P. and Jerger, J.: Probe-tone frequency and the diagnostic value of tympanometry. *Arch. Otolaryngol.* 99:206, 1974.
Anderson, H. and Barr, B.: Conductive recruitment. *Arch Otolaryngol.* 62:171, 1966.
Anderson, H., Holgren, L. and Holst, H.E.: Experiments with an objective method of testing the middle ear function. *Acta. Otolaryngol.* 46:381, 1956.
Bluestone, C.D., Berry, Q.C. and Paradise, J.L.: Audiometry and tympanometry in relation to middle ear effusions in children. *Laryngoscope* 83: 594, 1973.
Brooks, D.N.: A new approach to identification audiometry. *Audiol.* 10:334, 1971.
Brooks, D.N.: The use of the electroacoustic impedance bridge in the assessment of middle ear function. *Int. Audiol.* 8:563, 1969.
Brooks, D.N.: An objective method of detecting fluid in the middle ear. *Int. Audiol.* 7:280, 1968.
Cannon, S., Smith, K., Reece, C. and Thebe, J.: Middle ear measurements in neonates: a normative study. *Asha* 16:564, 1974.
Feldman, A.S. and Wilber, L.A.: *Acoustic Impedance and Admittance—the Measurement of Middle Ear Function.* Baltimore, Williams & Wilkins Co., 1976.
Jerger, J.: Clinical experience with impedance audiometry. *Arch. Otolaryngol.* 92:311, 1970.
Jerger, S., Jerger J., Mauldin, L. and Segal, P.: Studies in impedance audiometry for children less than six years old. *Arch. Otolaryngol.* 99:1, 1974.
Keith, R.: Impedance audiometry with neonates. *Arch. Otolaryngol.* 97:464, 1973.
Keith, R.: Middle ear function in neonates. *Arch. Otolaryngol.* 101:376, 1975.
Lidén, G.: The scope and application of current audiometric tests. *J. Laryngol. Otol.* 83:507, 1969.
Lidén, G.: Tests for stapes fixation. *Arch. Otolaryngol.* 89:215, 1969.
Lidén, G., Bjorkman, G. and Peterson, J.: Clinical equipment for measurement of middle-ear reflexes and tympanometry. *J. Speech Hear. Dis.* 37:100, 1972.
Lidén, G., Harford, E. and Hallen, O.: Tympanometry for the diagnosis of ossicular disruption. *Arch. Otolaryngol.* 99:23, 1974a.
Lidén, G., Harford, E. and Hallen, O. Automatic tympanometry in clinical practice. *Audiol.* 13:126, 1974b.
Lidén, G., Peterson, J.L., and Bjorkman, G.: Tympanometry. *Arch. Otolaryngol.* 92:248, 1970.
Margolis, R.H.: Tympanometry in infants: state of the art. In Harford, E.R., et al. (Eds.): *Impedance Screening for Middle Ear Disease in Children.* New York, Grune & Stratton, 1978.
McCandless, G.A. and Thomas, G.K.: Impedance audiometry as a screening procedure for middle ear disease. *Trans. Am. Acad. Ophthalmol Otolaryngol.* 78:98, 1974.
Metz, O.: The acoustic impedance measured on normal and pathological ears. *Acta. Otolaryngol. (Suppl.)* 63:1, 1946.

Møller, A.: An experimental study of the acoustic impedance of the middle ear and its transmission properties. *Acta. Otolaryngol. (Stockh.)* 60:129, 1965.
Newman, R., Stream, R. and Chesnutt, B. Application of the Niemeyer method of predicting hearing loss in neonates and infants. *Asha* 16:564, 1974.
Paradise, J.L., Smith, C.G. and Bluestone, C.D. Tympanometric detection of middle-ear effusion in infants and young children. *Pediatrics* 58:198, 1976.
Peterson, J.L. and Lidén, G.: Tympanometry in human temporal bones. *Arch. Otolaryngol.* 92:258, 1970.
Shurin, P., Pelton, S. and Klein, J.: Otitis media in the newborn infant. *Ann. Otol. Rhinol. Laryngol.* 85 (Suppl 25):216, 1976.
Terkildsen, K. and Thomsen, K.A.: The influence of pressure variations on the impedance of the human ear drum. *J. Laryngol. Otol.* 73:409, 1959.
Thomsen, K.A.: Investigations on the tubal function and measurement of the middle-ear pressure in pressure chamber. *Acta. Otolaryngol. (Suppl.)* 140:269, 1958.
Van Dishoeck, H.A.E.: Theorie and praxis des pneumophons. *Arch. Ohren* 146:5, 1939.
Vanhuyse, V., Creten, W. and Van Camp, K.: On the W-notching of tympanograms. *Scand. Audiol.* 4:45, 1975.
Von Bekesy, G.: Zur theorie des horens bei der schallaufnahme durch Knochenleitung. *Ann. Physik.* 13: 111, 1932.
Zarnoch, J.M. and Balkany, T.J.: Tympanometric screening of normal and intensive care unit newborns: validity and reliability. In Harford, E.R., et al. (Eds.): *Impedance Screening for Middle Ear Disease in Children.* New York, Grune & Stratton, 1978.

Chapter Four

THE ACOUSTIC REFLEX

GISLE DJUPESLAND, M.D.

MECHANISM OF THE ACOUSTICALLY ELICITED IMPEDANCE CHANGES

It has long been known that pure tones with an intensity level of 60 to 105 dB above the threshold of hearing produce impedance changes in both ears (Metz, 1946, 1951, 1952; Jepsen, 1951, 1955; Thomsen, 1955a, 1955b; Ewertsen et al., 1958; Klockhoff, 1961; Møller, 1961, 1962; Terkildsen, 1960b, 1962; Dallos, 1964; Djupesland et al., 1966; Lidén, 1970; Jerger et al., 1972; Hung and Dallos, 1972; Borg, 1972; Peterson and Lidén, 1972; Borg and Zakrisson, 1974; Woodford et al., 1975; Fria et al., 1975; Yonovitz and Harris, 1972, 1976; and Brask, 1978). On the other hand, there has been some uncertainty as to whether the impedance changes recorded are due to isolated contraction of the stapedius muscle, or whether the tensor tympani muscle is also involved.

One method used to study the function of the tensor tympani muscle in man is to observe or measure movement of the tympanic membrane. It is suggested that contraction of this muscle pulls the malleus and the tympanic membrane in a medial direction.

Visible or measurable inward movement of the tympanic membrane in connection with acoustic stimulation has been demonstrated, and has been interpreted as the expression of an acoustically elicited tensor tympani reflex (Mach and Kessel, 1872; Fick, cit. Lucae, 1874; Ostmann, 1898; Koehler, 1910; Mangold, 1913; Mangold and Eckstein, 1913; Cemach, 1920; Terkildsen, 1957, 1960a, 1962; Mendelson, 1957; 1961; Kawata, 1958; Weiss et al., 1962; Holst et al., 1963; and Lidén et al., 1970). On the other hand Waar (1923), Lüscher (1931), and Kobrak (1953) were unable to produce consistent visible reflex movements of the tympanic membrane by acoustic stimulation. Using the same method, Lüscher (1931) investigated patients with facial nerve palsy and assumed stapedius muscle paralysis but did not find an acoustically released contraction of the tensor tympani muscle in any of his cases.

Observation of changes in the acoustic impedance of the ear in which the stapedius muscle is paralyzed has been used to determine whether acoustic stimuli of high intensity might cause reflex contraction of the tensor tympani muscle. Jepsen (1955) was the first to use this approach. He investigated seven patients with unilateral stapedius muscle paralysis. The contralateral ear was stimulated by pure tones (maximum intensity 75 to 115 dB above the threshold of hearing), and noise (Bárány's noise box and beats on a cymbal). Changes in the acoustic impedance of the ear attributable to reflex contraction of the tensor tympani muscle were not observed.

Similar investigations have since been conducted with the same result by Terkildsen (1960a, 1962), Klockhoff (1961), Møller (1961), Borg (1968), Borg and Zakrisson (1973), Zakrisson (1975), Zakrisson and colleagues (1975), and Brask (1978). Acoustic stimulation of ears in which the connection between the stapedius muscle and the tympanic membrane was interrupted owing to a defect in the ossicular chain also failed to produced a change in the acoustic impedance of the ear (Klockhoff, 1961; Djupesland, 1967).

Using electromyography, Salomon and Starr (1963) also examined the tensor tympani muscle in a patient one week before therapeutic labyrinthectomy. It appeared that the acoustic stimuli (pure tones or repetitive clicks, 100 dB re 20 μ Pa) were only occasionally accompanied by increased activity of the tensor tympani muscle. This activity was initiated between 90 and 300 ms after the onset of the sound. Because of the inconsistent occurrence and the long latent period, Salomon and Starr interpreted the activity in the tensor tympani muscle as representing one component of a general muscle contraction elicited by loud sound.

In 1962 Djupesland (1962, 1964b, 1965, 1967) observed that during surgical treatment for otosclerosis it was possible to inspect and record contractions of the human tensor tympani muscle by direct methods. In an attempt to solve the problem concerning a possible acoustic tensor tympani reflex in man, Djupesland (1965, 1967) carried out electromyography of the tympanic muscles during stapedectomy. Eight patients with unilateral otosclerosis were investigated. The hearing in the contralateral ear was normal. Unipolar electrodes were placed in the stapedius and tensor tympani muscles, and the normal ear was stimulated by means of a burst of "white noise" from a TDH 39 telephone receiver producing an intensity of 134 dB re 20 μ Pa. A microphone was used to mark the acoustic simuli on the electromyogram.

The following results were obtained: When the white noise was presented unexpectedly, all the subjects showed rapid contraction of numerous muscles of the head and neck. (There was probably also contraction of muscles of the trunk and extremities, but this could not be seen, as the patients were partly covered during the operation). The most striking feature was contraction of the periorbital muscles, indicating a cochleopalpebral reflex. Simultaneously there was an increased activity of the stapedius and tensor tympani muscles (Figure 4-1). The increase of activity in the stapedius muscle started earlier (latent period about 10 ms) and was considerably greater than that seen in the tensor tympani muscle. The latent period for contraction

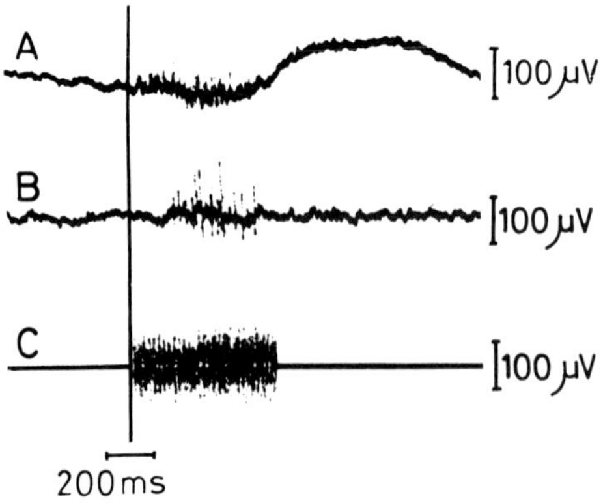

Figure 4-1. Electrical activity recorded in middle ear muscles during acoustic stimulation of contralateral ear (white noise, 134 dB re 20μ Pa) in patient with unilateral otosclerosis and normal hearing in contralateral ear. (A) Action potentials in stapedius muscle; (B) action potentials in tensor tympani muscle; (C) sound stimulus recorded. Microphone was placed just beside the earphone used. Vertical black line refers to onset of sound. (Djupesland, 1967.)

of the tensor tympani muscle elicited by acoustic stimuli varied between 80 and 290 ms, which is of about the same magnitude as that seen in skeletal muscles during a startle reaction elicited by loud sound (Davis, 1948). Repeated stimulation always caused increased activity of the stapedius muscle, while increased activity of the tensor tympani muscle was seen only in association with contraction of the muscles of the head and neck. Extensive muscle contractions of this type were seen when the test subject grimaced, signifying that the sound was disagreeably loud (defensive reaction). Similar experiments have been carried out by Salomon and Starr (1963) using electromyography, and by Brask (1978) using extratympanic manometry, and the results obtained correspond to those reported by Djupesland (1965, 1967).

On the basis of the results of electromyography (Salomon and Starr, 1963; Djupesland, 1965, 1967) and extratympanic manometry (Brask, 1978), it seems justifiable to conclude that loud acoustic stimuli usually lead to reflex contraction of the stapedius muscle alone, while the tensor tympani muscle contracts only when the sound is of such intensity or presented in such a way that it gives rise to a startle or a defensive reaction. In other words, a consistent acoustically elicited reflex contraction of the tensor tympani muscle does not seem to occur in man.

PATHWAYS OF THE ACOUSTIC STAPEDIUS REFLEX

The neural network involved in the reflex activation of the stapedius muscle during acoustic stimulation is not known in detail. Experimental studies in animals have shown that the pathways of the acoustic stapedius reflex are located in the lower part of the brain stem (Hammerschlag, 1899, 1902; Cajal, 1909; Lorente De Nó, 1933a, 1933b; Tsukamoto, 1934; Rasmussen, 1946; and Borg, 1973). A rough outline of the most direct pathways, based mainly on physiologic and experimental anatomic work in the rabbit (Borg, 1973) is shown in Figure 4-2A, B. Monoaural acoustic stimulation of high intensity is followed by bilateral reflex contraction of the stapedius muscle. The pathways for the ipsi- and contralateral stapedius reflex are not identical and they are therefore illustrated separately in Figure 4-2.

PATHWAYS OF THE IPSILATERAL STAPEDIUS REFLEX (FIGURE 4-2A).

During acoustic stimulation, electric impulses from the sensory cells in the cochlea are transmitted through the primary acoustic neuron to the ventral cochlear nucleus. The primary acoustic neurons constitute the acoustic nerve. The trophic center for the second acoustic neuron is in the ventral cochlear nucleus. The majority of axons from the ventral cochlear nucleus pass through the trapezoid body to the medial part of the facial motor nucleus, and from this nucleus the electric impulses are transmitted through the facial nerve to the ipsilateral stapedius muscle. In addition, some nerve fibers pass from the ventral cochlear nucleus through the trapezoid body to the ipsilateral medial superior olive. From this nucleus the electrical impulses are transmitted via a third neuron to the medial part of the ipsilateral facial motor nucleus. The ipsilateral stapedius reflex arc thus consists of mainly three but to some extent four neurons.

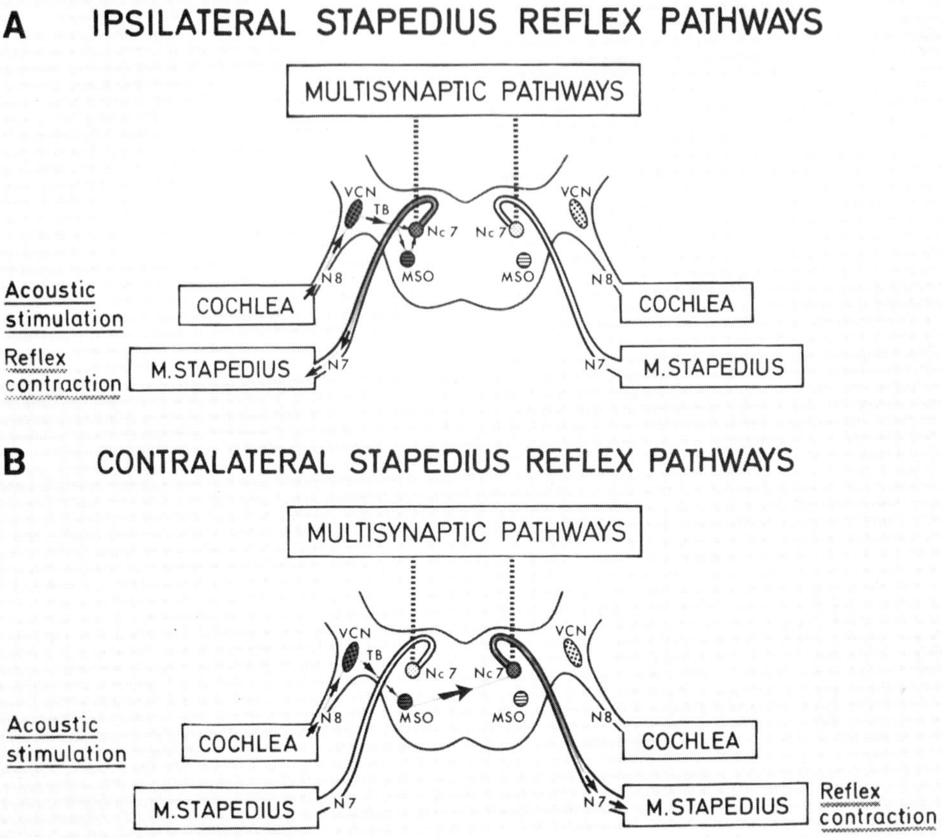

Figure 4-2. Schematic diagram over ipsi- and contralateral stapedius reflex pathways, based on experimental work in rabbits (Borg, 1973). N8, acoustic nerve; VCN, ventral cochlear nucleus; TB, trapezoid body; MSO, medial superior olive; N7, facial nerve.

PATHWAYS OF THE CONTRALATERAL STAPEDIUS REFLEX (FIGURE 4-2B).

The electrical impulses from the sensory cells in the cochlea pass via the primary acoustic neuron to the ventral cochlear nucleus as in the ipsilateral stapedius reflex. From the ventral cochlear nucleus the electric impulses are transmitted through a second neuron to the region of the medial superior olive. A third neuron connects the medial superior olive to the medial part of the contralateral facial motor nucleus. A fourth neuron transmits the electric impulses from the facial motor nucleus to the contralateral stapedius muscle. Thus, the ipsilateral stapedius reflex arc contains three and partly four neurons; the contralateral reflex arc contains four neurons.

Parallel to this three-four neuron direct pathway there are multisynaptic chains of interneurons. Section of the trapezoid body in the midline results in interruption of the direct crossed pathway. However, a slow response remains which is very sensitive to anesthetics. The ipsilateral reflex is unaffected by this lesion (Borg, 1977). As shown in Figure 4-3, there is no significant difference in threshold values for the ipsi- and contralateral reflex arcs before and after section of the trapezoid body in the midline. Above the threshold, however, the impedance changes elicited are smaller and have a slower onset in the crossed arc. The after-discharge is, however, unchanged or

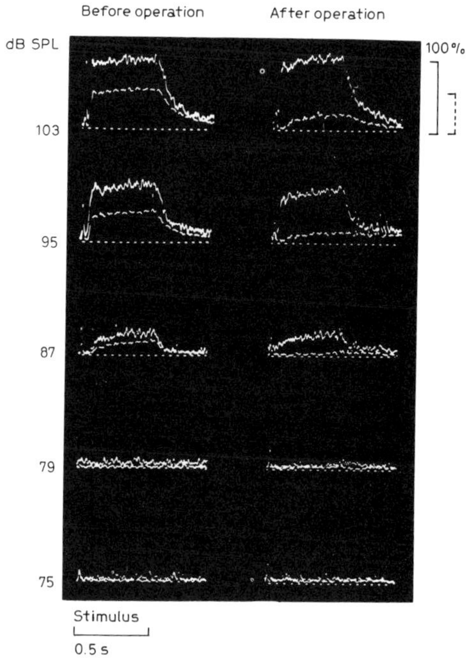

Figure 4-3. Impedance change as function of time recorded in unanesthetized rabbit before and after induction of chronic lesion to trapezoid body in midline. In right ear (upper trace) both stapedius and tensor tympani were active, in left ear (lower trace) tensor tympani had previously been cut. Right ear and left ear reflex responses were both normalized to one maximum value (scales upper right). Stimulus in right ear: 2000 Hz pure tone, 0.5 s duration. (Borg, 1977.)

relatively increased. This persisting after-discharge indicates that interneural chains are involved and these are not influenced by the lesion.

THRESHOLD OF THE ACOUSTIC STAPEDIUS REFLEX

The acoustic stapedius reflex threshold is defined as the intensity in dB hearing level at which the reflex response can first be detected. According to this definition, the reflex threshold value depends on the sensitivity of the apparatus used for detection of an elicited impedance change. In some subjects the impedance change has a well defined threshold. In other subjects, however, the impedance change has an unstable character over a stimulus intensity range of as much as 10 dB, during which the impedance change does not exceed 10 percent of the maximal obtainable impedance change. As illustrated in Figure 4-4, there are random variations in the reflex responses near the abscissa, and therefore, when determining the sensitivity of the acoustic stapedius reflex for scientific purposes, an intensity giving at least 10 percent of the maximum obtainable change should be used as "threshold value" (Møller, 1962, 1964; Borg, 1972).

The acoustic stapedius reflex thresholds are also influenced by the probe tone intensity and the frequency of the impedance equipment (Terkildsen et al., 1970; Peterson and Lidén, 1972). Using extratympanic manometry, Brask (1978) observed that a probe tone of subreflex threshold intensity used in impedance measurements

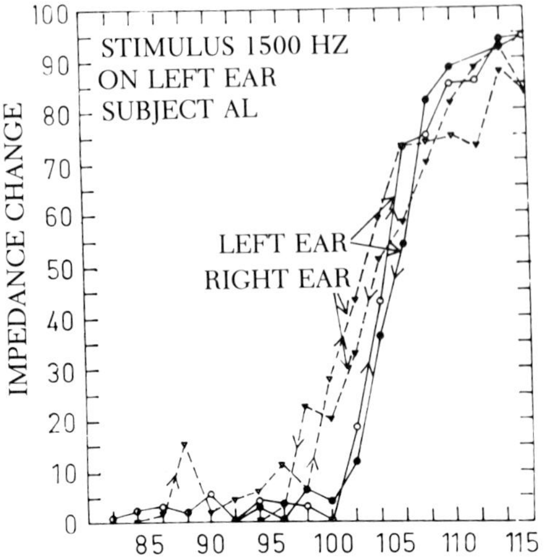

Figure 4-4. Impedance change vs stimulus intensity from experiment in which stimulus intensity is raised from below threshold to a level that gives maximum impedance change and then lowered again to below threshold. (In part from Mϕller, Aa: *Ann. Otol. Rhinol. Laryngol.* 70: 735, 1961.)

strengthens the effect on the acoustic stapedius reflex response. The size of this effect depends on: (1) the intensity of the probe tone; (2) the intensity of the stimulus; (3) the difference in frequency between the stimulus and the probe tone; and (4) the use of ipsi- or contralateral stimulation.

Reflex threshold measurements by means of the impedance methods currently in use are therefore not the result of "pure" ipsi- or contralateral stimulation. The thresholds tend to be "too low" (Brask, 1978). On the other hand, the reflex threshold values are 5 to 6 dB higher when measured by the impedance method than those obtained by measuring integrated electromyographic activity in the stapedius muscle (Zakrisson et al., 1974). It therefore seems safe to conclude that measurement of impedance change gives an adequate measure of the stapedius muscle activity.

The acoustic stapedius reflex threshold for pure tones varies somewhat with frequency and also with the age of the subject (Jepsen, 1955; Jerger et al., 1978). Figure 4-5 and Table 4-1 show hearing thresholds and stapedius reflex thresholds in a group aged fifteen to thirtyfour years with normal hearing (Jepsen, 1955). In this age group

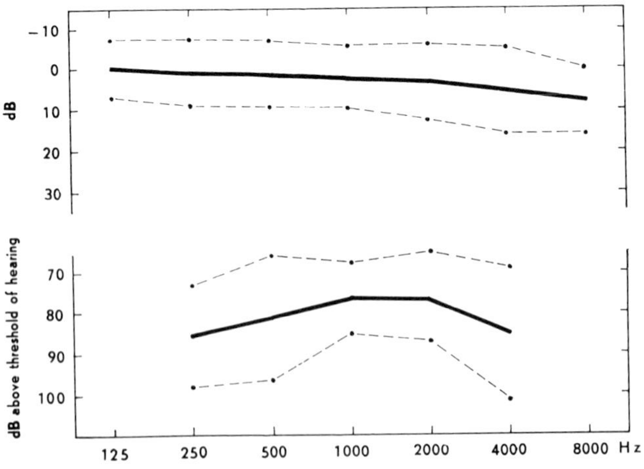

Figure 4-5. Thresholds of hearing and stapedius reflex, age groups 15-34 years (88 ears). (Jepsen, 1955.)

Table 4-1. Threshold of hearing and of stapedius reflex in age groups 15-34 years (88 ears.)

Hz	Threshold of hearing		Threshold of stapedius reflex	
	Mean	S.D.	Mean	S.D.
125	−0.4	3.5		
250	0.4	4.2	85.1	6.3
500	0.7	4.4	81.3	7.6
1000	1.6	3.6	76.5	3.9
2000	2.7	4.5	76.6	5.6
4000	5.1	5.1	84.7	8.4
8000	7.7	4.1		

the mean stapedius reflex thresholds for frequencies 250 to 4000 Hz varied between 76.5 and 85.1 dB HL, high and low frequency tones having somewhat higher thresholds than those of middle frequency.

Figure 4-6 shows the average reflex threshold (HL for pure tones, SPL for broadband noise) for various signals in relationship to age decades (Jerger et al., 1978). A systematic age effect is present with pure tones. At 1000 Hz the average reflex threshold level decreases from 90.5 dB in the zero to nine year group to 84 dB in the fifty to fifty nine year group. With the exception of 4000 Hz, all pure tones show the same decline with age. At 4000 Hz the expected trend occurs in the younger groups but seems to end abruptly in the decade from age thirty to thirty nine.

However, the age effect almost disappears when the reflex-eliciting signal is broadband noise. The stapedius reflex threshold for broad-band noise declines slightly between the age groups zero to nine and forty to forty nine years, but the total average change is only 2 dB, and the trend reverses abruptly in the age group fifty to fifty nine years.

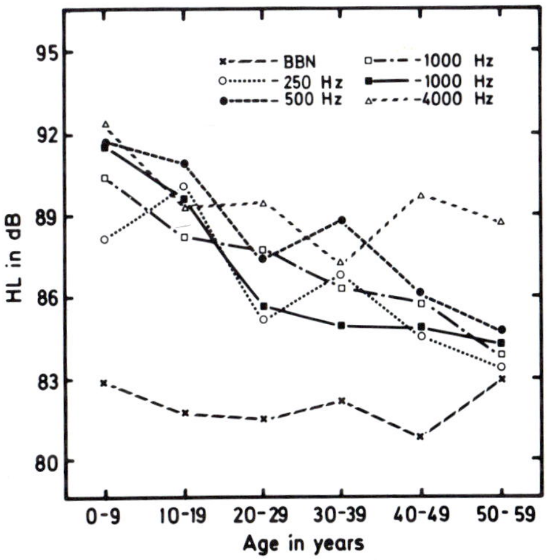

Figure 4-6. Effect of age on reflex thresholds of various test signals (HL pure tones, SPL for BBN) (Jerger et al., 1977.)

The data in Figures 4-5, and 4-6 and Table 4-1 were obtained by acoustic stimulation of the contralateral ear (Jepsen, 1955; Jerger et al., 1978). Measurements have shown that ipsilateral stimulation is more effective than contralateral stimulation, and further, that binaural stimulation is even more effective (summation) (Mϕller, 1962, 1964; Zakrisson et al., 1974; and Brask, 1978). The relation between stimulus strength and reflex activity, measured in terms of impedance change is shown in Figure 4-7. The diagram also illustrates the relative effectiveness of ipsilateral, contralateral, and bilateral stimulation.

In people with normal hearing, the acoustic stapedius reflex threshold is 1 to 10 dB lower for broad-band noise than for pure tones (the intensity of both signals is expressed in dB re hearing threshold level) (Mϕller, 1962; Djupesland et al., 1966; Flottorp et al., 1971; Niemeyer and Sesterhenn, 1974; Jerger et al., 1977; and Sesterhenn and Breuninger, 1976, 1977).

In patients with sensorineural hearing loss the difference between the stapedius reflex thresholds for noise (broad-band or filtered) and pure tones is smaller than in people of the same age with normal hearing. This reflex threshold difference depends on the degree of hearing loss. Stapedius reflex measurements can therefore be used for objective evaluation of hearing losses (see Chapter 8).

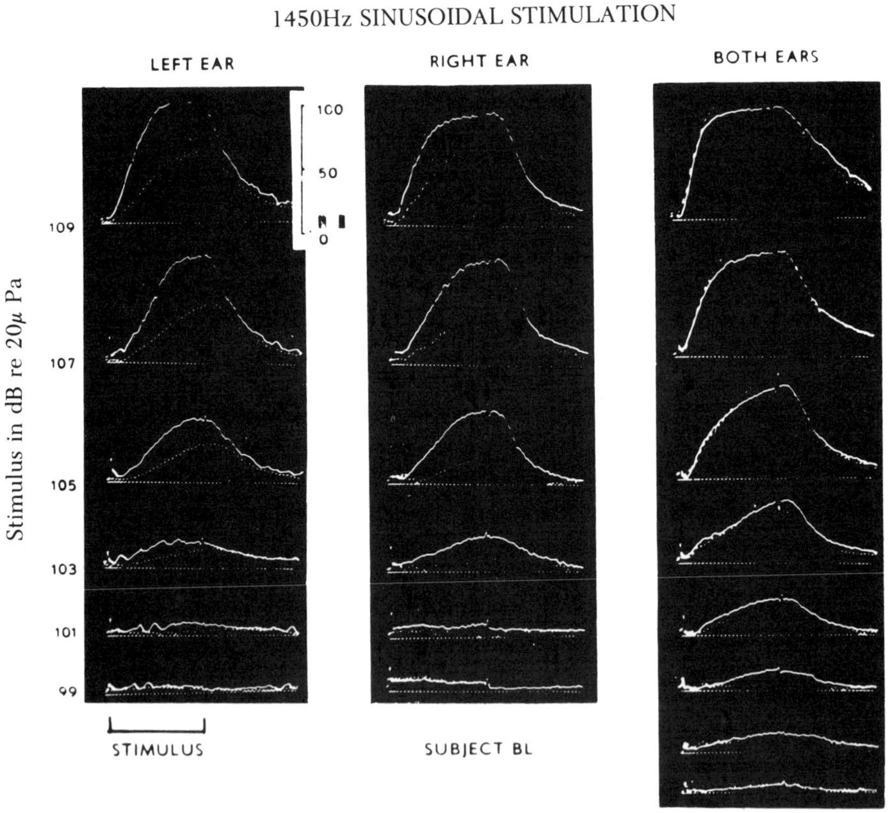

Figure 4-7. Acoustic impedance change vs time for monaural and binaural stimulation by 1450 Hz sinusoids. Impedance change was recorded simultaneously in both ears. Monaural stimulation: interrupted lines are recordings of impedance change in contralateral ear, solid lines are impedance change in ipsilateral ear. Binaural stimulation: interrupted lines indicate impedance change in left ear. Stimulus duration was 500 ms. (Mϕller, 1962a.)

Ethyl alcohol and sodium pentobarbital both have a pronounced effect on the acoustic stapedius reflex (Borg and Møller, 1967, 1975). Both the reflex threshold and the stimulus response curves are changed. Other common drugs may have a similar effect, and therefore a possible drug effect should be considered when evaluating acoustic stapedius reflex data.

DECAY AND RECOVERY OF THE ACOUSTIC STAPEDIUS REFLEX

Adaptation, defined as decrease of response to a persisting sensory stimulus, is a fundamental property of all sensory systems. The acoustic stapedius reflex is especially advantageous for studying this property, as the course of its adaptation (decay) can be studied objectively. In man this decay can provide useful information for (1) the evaluation of the possible role of the stapedius reflex as a protective mechanism (Borg et al., 1978), and (2) the establishment of diagnostic procedures with the stapedius reflex tool (Anderson et al., 1969).

Borg and Ødman (1978) have recently studied the time course of decay and recovery of ipsi- and contralateral stapedius reflex responses to a 2000 Hz pure tone in subjects with normal hearing. In simultaneous bilateral recordings the reflex responses were found to follow an almost identical time course with respect to both decay and recovery. This similarity is compatible with the assumption that decay and recovery originate in the afferent auditory system and not in the muscles. Recovery was 50 percent complete 250 ms after the end of the stimulus, and in most subjects the reflex responses had reached their initial amplitude after 1 to 3 s. The individual correlation between decay and recovery was negative but weak. This may indicate that decay and recovery have a tendency to balance each other, and that they are based to some extent on different mechanisms which are probably located peripherally in the auditory system.

THE ACOUSTIC STAPEDIUS REFLEX IN RELATION TO CRITICAL BANDWIDTH

The critical band is the bandwidth at which certain subjective responses, for instance, loudness, rather abruptly begin to change as the bandwidth of noise or the spacing of complex tones increases, while the overall sound intensity remains constant (Feldtkeller, 1955; Feldtkeller and Zwicker, 1956; Bauch, 1956; Zwicker et al., 1957; Zwicker, 1960; and Scharf, 1961a, 1966). The critical bandwidth may be regarded as a measure of the frequency selectivity of the ear (Zwicker, 1975; Evans, 1975). Several psychophysical methods have been used to study the critical bandwidth. In one type of experiment the loudness of a band of noise or of a complex of four pure tones at a constant sound pressure level was found to remain constant as the bandwidth increased up to the critical point, whereas with a broader bandwidth the loudness increased (Zwicker et al., 1957, 1975). The critical bandwidth varies with frequency (Scharf, 1966) and is largely independent of the sound pressure level (Feldtkeller and Zwicker, 1956; Scharf, 1959, 1961b, 1966).

It has not yet been fully clarified where in the auditory system or how the discrimination between sound energy within and outside the critical band takes place.

The results of several experiments indicate, however, that the location of the critical band mechanism is peripheral, possibly in the cochlea (Niese, 1960; von Bekesy, 1960, 1962; van den Brink, 1964; and Flottorp et al., 1971).

As mentioned earlier the reflex center for the acoustic stapedius reflex is commonly assumed to be located in the pons, most probably in the superior olivary complex (Lorente de Nó, 1933b, 1935; Rasmussen, 1946; and Borg, 1973). It is suggested that reflex contraction of the stapedius muscle due to acoustic stimulation is elicited when the neural activity in the reflex center exceeds a certain level. Animal experiments have shown that the integrated neural response in the superior olivary complex is parallelled by the loudness function (Boudreau, 1965). A correlation between the threshold of the acoustic stapedius reflex and the loudness of the eliciting stimulus may therefore be expected. Thus, measurement of the acoustic stapedius reflex threshold by observation of impedance changes should demonstrate indirectly the existence of a critical band in loudness summation. In normal ears such experiments have been carried out by McRobert and colleagues (1968), Flottorp and colleagues (1971), Djupesland and Zwislocki (1973), and Popelka and colleagues (1974, 1976). In the experiments described by Flottorp and colleagues (1971), the contralateral ear was stimulated by bands of noise and complex tones of various bandwidths. It was found that the reflex threshold, expressed in dB re 20μPa remained almost constant for bandwidths of less than a specific value, designated as the "critical bandwidth." When the bandwidth was incréased further, a decrease in the reflex threshold of approximately 3 to 6 dB/octave was observed (Fig 4-8). The breaking point shown in Figure 4-8 was interpreted as the critical bandwidth for a band-limited integrating mechanism in the acoustic stapedius reflex arc. Compared with the results obtained by psychophysical experiments, the reflex threshold examinations showed a larger critical bandwidth at middle and high center frequencies. In the low-frequency range better agreement was found (Fig. 4-9).

Djupesland and Zwislocki (1973) investigated the critical band in the stapedius

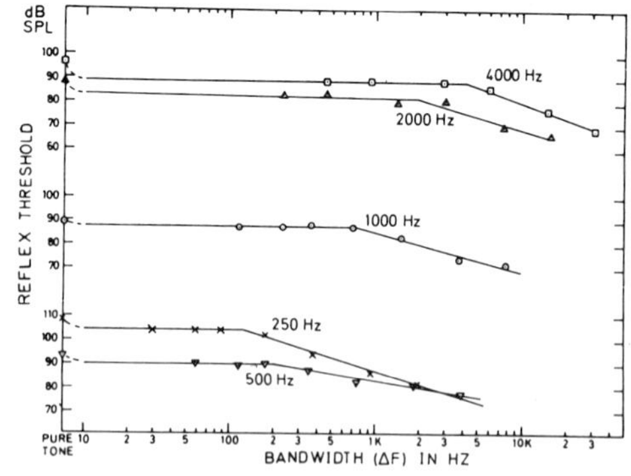

Figure 4-8. Threshold of acoustic stapedius reflex as a function of stimulus bandwidth (△ F). (Flottorp et al., 1971.)

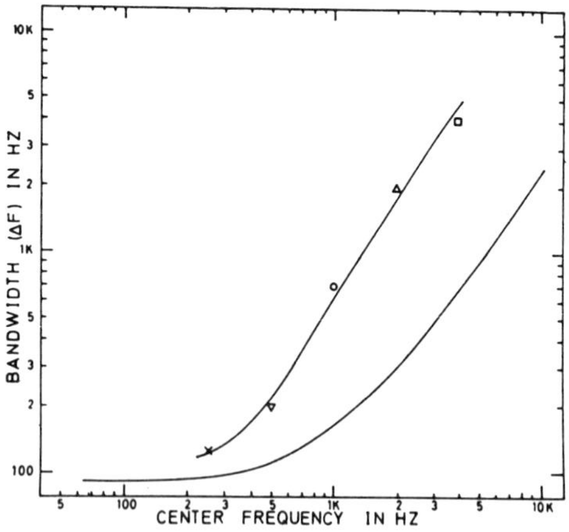

Figure 4-9. Critical bandwidth as function of frequency. Lower curve is derived from four kinds of experiments as referred to by Zwicker, Flottorp, and Stevens (1957). Upper curve is based on results obtained by measuring threshold of acoustic stapedius reflex. (Flottorp et al., 1971.)

muscle reflex by means of two tone complexes of variable frequency separation. It was found that the reflex thresholds at wide bandwidth conditions were higher for tonal complexes compared with those obtained with filtered Gaussian noise. For example, the difference between reflex thresholds for a tonal signal and for a signal with a very wide bandwidth centered around the tone was found to be approximately 10 dB when using two component tonal complexes (Djupesland and Zwislocki, 1973) and up to 28 dB when using filtered Gaussian noise (Flottorp et al., 1971). All the critical bandwidth data obtained using the stapedius reflex measurements agree very well (Flottorp et al., 1971; Djupesland and Zwislocki, 1973; and Popelka et al., 1976).

The discrepancy between the results obtained by reflex studies and those obtained by psychophysical methods may be due to the different neural levels involved. The acoustic stapedius reflex is a subcortically controlled neuromuscular mechanism, whereas the psychophysical methods involve cerebral function at the highest cortical level. There may be a modifying mechanism in the higher auditory pathways influencing loudness sensation and reducing the size of the critical bandwidth found in the reflex arc examinations. Improvement of the signal-to-noise ratio is known to occur in the higher auditory pathways (Katsuki, 1961; Goldstein et al., 1968; and Zwislocki, 1969). A similar or even identical neural mechanism may be responsible for the fact that the critical bandwidth found using psychophysical methods is narrower than that found with the reflex arc procedure.

Assuming that the stapedius reflex mechanism in people with normal hearing is governed by loudness, the results obtained by Flottorp and colleagues (1971) confirm the existence of a critical bandwidth in loudness summation. Moreover, these observations indicate that the basis for the critical band mechanism is located in the peripheral part of the auditory system, probably in the cochlea.

Measurement of the critical bandwidth by means of the acoustic stapedius reflex has also been carried out, in ears with hearing loss of the cochlea type. Djupesland and colleagues (1975) examined nine patients with typical Menière's syndrome, and Popelka and colleagues (1976) saw seven patients with noise induced hearing loss. In both studies the critical bandwidth data differed from those obtained in normal ears. Djupesland and colleagues (1975) found no critical band mechanism in seven ears and an abnormal one in two ears. Popelka and colleagues (1976) reported that data from those with impaired hearing differed from the normal data in two ways. First, acoustic reflex thresholds for wide bandwidth activating signals were elevated, resulting in a flat function relating acoustic reflex threshold to signal bandwidth. Second, acoustic reflex threshold for narrow bandwidth activating signals tended to be elevated as center frequency approached the region of greatest hearing loss (4000 Hz).

The fact that the critical bandwidth is different in normal and pathologic ears makes it possible to use measurement of critical bandwidths using the acoustic stapedius reflex as a topodiagnostic test.

TEMPORAL SUMMATION IN THE ACOUSTIC STAPEDIUS REFLEX MECHANISM

Numerous psychophysical experiments have established that the loudness of short sounds grows with increasing stimulus duration. This can be explained in terms of temporal summation. The loudness level increases by roughly 10 dB when the duration of the stimulus is increased by a factor of 10 (Zwislocki, 1960, 1969). This relationship is established for sounds with narrow frequency spectra at all practical intensity levels, including the threshold level. Broad-band noise at threshold level constitutes an exception (Zwislocki, 1969).

The exact location of the auditory temporal summation is unknown. Nevertheless, several experiments have indicated that it is in the central nervous system (Zwislocki, 1960, 1969).

As mentioned earlier, reflex contraction of the stapedius muscle is produced by neural activity in the superior olivary complex, considered to be the center of the reflex arc. Accordingly, activity in the stapedius muscle should reflect the temporal auditory summation if the summation occurs at or below the level of the superior olivary complex.

The effect of temporal summation on the human stapedius reflex has been studied by varying the duration of a sound eliciting a predetermined impedance change in the contralateral ear (Djupesland and Zwislocki, 1971; Djupesland et al., 1973b). The results show that the duration of short acoustic stimuli (2000 Hz tone, "white noise," and 1/1 octave bands of noise) has a pronounced effect on the stapedius reflex response. The sound intensity necessary to produce impedance changes of a predetermined size ("criterion response") was found to be a function of stimulus duration. The relationship between sound intensity and stimulus duration eliciting this "criterion response" (50 percent of maximal obtainable impedance change) is presented in Figure 4-10. With a tenfold increase in stimulus duration the intensity level could be lowered about 22 to 25 dB. This is about 2.5 times as much as would be required for maintaining constant loudness.

Using "white noise" and 1/1 octave bands of noise as stimuli, the relationship between sound intensity and stimulus duration was unchanged up to a certain stimulus duration (Fig. 4-10). With longer durations the relationship changed. In most cases the change occurred abruptly, appearing as a "knee" in the diagram (Fig. 4-10). The time corresponding to the "knee point" and the relationship between sound intensity and stimulus duration longer than the "knee point" time varied with the type of stimulus. As shown in Figure 4-10, the "knee point" time was shorter with low than with high-frequency sounds.

With stimulus durations shorter than 50 to 80 ms, the relationship between sound intensity and stimulus duration was about the same with all types of stimuli. This indicates that with such short stimuli, temporal summation in the acoustic stapedius reflex is independent of type of stimulus.

Temporal summation in the acoustic reflex has been measured by Gknewikow

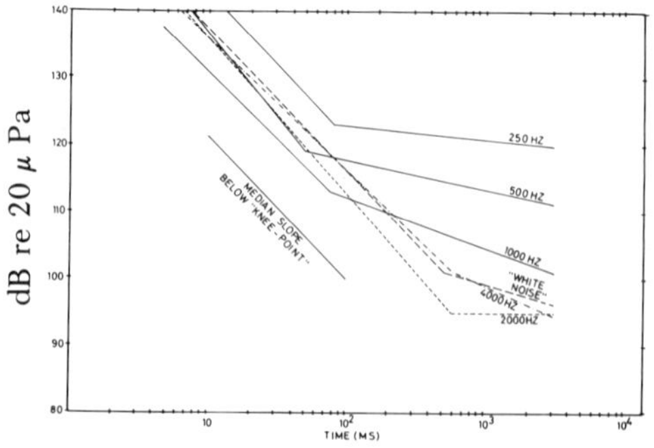

Figure 4-10. Relationship between sound pressure level and stimulus duration required to elicit criterion response (50 percent of maximal obtainable impedance change) for different types of stimuli. Median of mean values (three measurements on each subject) for five normal-hearing subjects. (Djupesland et al., 1973b.)

(1974), Bazarov and Moroz (1975), Woodford and colleagues (1975), Richards (1976), Morgan and colleagues (1975), and Jerger and colleagues (1977) with divergent results. The acoustic monitoring systems commonly employed for reflex detection are characterized by poor signal-to-noise ratios, and efforts to improve the noise problem by selective filtering inevitably introduces a time constant into the measurement system which may obscure observation of short-duration events (Sundby et al., 1971; Morgan et al., 1977; and Jerger et al., 1977). It is therefore likely that the discrepancies between both different investigators and reflex and theshold slope functions are due to artifacts of instrumentation and measurement technique. Jerger and colleagues (1977) have overcome the measurement problem by means of a signal-averaging technique. A measurement system was designed, characterized by a small time constant and high background-level noise level, and the signals were analyzed by an averaging technique in order to improve the signal-to-noise ratio. Temporal summation in the acoustic reflex mechanism was studied in ten subjects with normal hearing by Jerger and colleagues (1977), who concluded:

1. The rate at which the amplitude of the acoustic reflex grows as a function of signal intensity varies with the signal duration.
2. This slope variation calls into question the validity of temporal summation data based on either visual detection threshold or constant proportion of maximum observable amplitude models.
3. Differences in degree of temporal summation at the visual detection threshold reported by various investigators, and differences due to bandwidth can be explained as interaction between variation of slopes and noise in the measurement system.
4. The family of functions relating reflex amplitude to signal duration at various signal levels is an alternative, possibly more fruitful method for analyzing the interaction of signal intensity and signal duration.
5. Analysis of the amplitude duration function indicates that the initial reflex contraction is governed by the signal intensity, independently of the duration. The subsequent amplitude of the reflex response is governed by interaction between the signal duration and the time constant of the reflex mechanism.
6. The reflex time constant probably decreases with increasing signal intensity to a limiting value of 100 ms.

Temporal summation of acoustic energy can also be measured by means of hearing threshold determination. Pure tones (500, 1000, 2000, 4000, 8000 Hz) with durations varying from 1 to 1000 ms have been used [Brahe Pedersen and Elberling, 1972; Brahe Pedersen, 1975]. This method ("brief tone audiometry") can be used to differentiate between some types of hearing loss (Brahe Pedersen, 1975). It is therefore possible that with an adequate technique, studies of temporal summation in the acoustic reflex mechanism could be used as an objective diagnostic test. Research is in progress, but no conclusive results have yet been obtained.

THE ACOUSTIC STAPEDIUS REFLEX ELICITED BY BONE-CONDUCTED PURE TONES

Using air-conducted pure tones as stimuli, the theshold of the acoustic stapedius reflex in man is found to be 60 to 105 sensation level (Jepsen, 1955; Jerger et al., 1972). The corresponding reflex threshold for bone-conducted pure tones has been measured by Djupesland and colleagues (1973a). In this study, the sensitivity of the acoustic stapedius reflex was measured by monitoring changes in the acoustic impedance of the ear. The reflex threshold was defined as the stimulus intensity giving approximately 10 percent of the maximal obtainable impedance change.

A Mini Shaker (Brüel and Kjaer, Type 4810) was placed on the contralateral mastoid process. The hearing thresholds for the frequencies 250, 500, 1000, 2000, 3000, 4000, and 6000 Hz were measured by the method of limit. In addition, the reflex thresholds for the same frequencies were measured. Later on, identical hearing and reflex threshold measurements were carried out in the same subjects using an ear phone (Telephonics TDH 39) connected to the contralateral ear. A loudness balance test between air- and bone-conducted sounds using Fowler's (1936) method was also performed.

The results of the loudness balance tests are presented in Figure 4-11. The rate of loudness increase as a function of sensation level was approximately the same for air- and bone-conducted pure tones.

As shown in Figure 4-11, a considerable difference between reflex thresholds for air- and bone-conducted pure tones was found, especially in the low-frequency range where the difference amounted to 5 to 25 dB. In the high-frequency range, reflex contraction of the stapedius muscle could not be elicited in all the subjects tested, even when the maximum intensity was used (circled symbols 2000 to 6000 Hz). Control experiments excluded artifacts, for instance the possibility that the bone vibrator elicited a tactile stapedius reflex.

At high-intensity levels with frequencies 250, 500, and 1000 Hz the Mini Shaker always produced a tingling sensation in the area below the bone vibrator. The threshold of the tingling sensation coincided with the reflex threshold. It is possible that unusual overload of the inner ear starts at the tingling sensation threshold. A possible difference in the inner ear distortion for air- and bone-conducted pure tones may therefore be responsible for the difference in reflex thresholds. The results of a preliminary investigation seem to support this hypothesis (Sundby et al., 1978). If this observation is correct, the acoustic stapedius reflex elicited by bone-conducted pure tones could be used as a diagnostic test by comparing the degree of inner ear distortion in normal and abnormal ears. Preliminary experiments carried out in patients with Menière's syndrome have shown that the reflex threshold for low-frequency, bone-conducted pure tones is lower than in normal ears (Djupesland, 1964a), thus indicating abnormal inner ear distortion as a result of inner ear pathologic factors. Abnormal inner ear distortion in patients suffering from Menière's syndrome has also been demonstrated by other methods (Opheim and Flottorp, 1955).

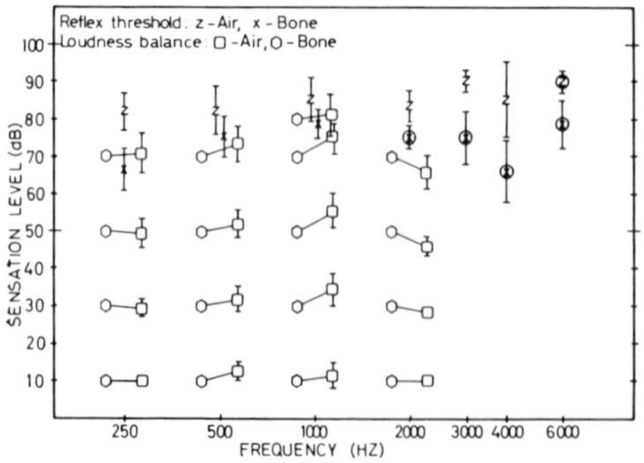

Figure 4-11. "Reflex threshold" an equal loudness for air- and bone-conducted tones in normal-hearing persons. Circled symbols indicate that for bone-conducted stimuli in high frequency range impedance changes could not be elicited in all subjects. (Djupesland et al., 1973a.)

Another possibility is nonlinear distortion of skull structures involved in normal bone conduction. Arlinger and colleagues (1977) seem to have confirmed such a hypothesis in their measurements on human cadavers.

REFERENCES

Anderson, H., Barr, B. and Wedenberg, E.: Intra-aural reflexes in retrocochlear lesions. In Hamberger, C.A. and Wersall, J. (Eds.): *Nobel Symposium 10, Disorders of the Skull Base Region*. Stockholm, Almqvist & Wiksell, p. 490.

Arlinger, S.D., Kylén, P. and Hellqvist, H.: Skull distortion of bone conducted signals. *Acta. Otolaryng. (Stockh.)* 85: 318, 1978.

Bauch, H.: Die Bedeutung der Frequenzgruppe für die Lautheit von Klangen. *Acustica* 6: 40, 1956.

Bazarov, V. and Moroz, B.: Dependence of the acoustic reflex threshold on the duration of the noise stimulus. *Vestn. Oto-rino-laring.* 3: 13, 1975.

von Bekesy, G.: Neural inhibitory units of the eye and skin. Quantitative description of contrast phenomenon. *J. Opt. Soc. Amer.* 50: 1060, 1960.

von Bekesy, G.: Lateral inhibition of heat sensations on the skin. *J. Appl. Physiol.* 17: 1003, 1962.

Borg, E. and Møller, Aa.R.: Effect of ethylalcohol and pentobarbital sodium on the acoustic middle ear reflex in man. *Acta. Otolaryng. (Stockh.)* 64: 415, 1967.

Borg, E.: A quantitative study of the effect of the acoustic stapedius reflex on sound transmission through the middle ear of man. *Acta Otolaryng. (Stockh.)* 66: 461, 1968.

Borg, E.: Acoustic middle ear reflexes. A sensory control system. Thesis. *Acta Otolaryng. (Stockh.)* Suppl. 304, 1972.

Borg, E.: On the neuronal organization of the acoustic middle ear reflex. A physiological and anatomical study. *Brain Res.* 49: 101, 1973.

Borg, E. and Zakrisson, J.E.: Stapedius reflex and speech features. *J. Acoust. Soc. Amer.* 54: 525, 1973.

Borg, E. and Zakrisson, J.E.: Stapedius reflex and monaural masking. *Acta Otolaryng.* 78: 155, 1974.

Borg, E. and Møller, Aa.R.: Effect of central depressants on the acoustic middle ear reflex in rabbit. *Acta Physiol.* Scand. 94: 327, 1975.

Borg, E.: The intra-aural muscle reflex in retrocochlear pathology: a model study in the rabbit. *Audiol.* 16: 316, 1977.

Borg, E. and Ødman, B.: Decay and recovery of the acoustic stapedius reflex in humans. *Acta Otolaryng.(Stockh.)* 8F: 421, 1979.

Borg, E., Nilsson, R. and Lidén, G.: Fatique and recovery of the human acoustic stapedius reflex in industrial noise. *J. Acoust. Soc. Amer.* 65: 846,1979.

Boūdreaū, F. C.: Stimulus correlates of nerve activity in the superior-olivary complex of the cat. *Acoust. Soc. Amer.* 37: 779, 1965.

Brahe Pedersen, C. and Elberling C.: Temporal integration of acoustic energy in normal hearing persons. *Acta Otolaryng. (Stockh.)* 74: 398, 1972.

Brahe Pedersen, C.: Korttone audiometri. Thesis. University of Copenhagen, FADL's Forlag, Copenhagen. Århus, Odense., 1975.

Brask, T.: Extratympanic manometry in man. Clinical and experimental investigations of the acoustic stapedius and tensor tympani contractions in normal subjects and in patients. Thesis. *Scand. Audiol.* (Suppl. 7), 1978.

van der Brink, G.: Experiments on cochlear stimulation. *J. Acoust. Soc. Amer.* 36: 1213, 1964.

Cajal, S.R.: Histologie du système nerveux de l'homme et des vertébrés. Vol. I. Paris, Maloine, 1909.

Cemach, A.J.: Beitrage zur Kenntnis der kochlearen Reflexe. *Beitr. Anat. Ohr.* 14: 1, 1920.

Dallos, P.J.: Dynamics of the acoustic reflex: phenomenological aspects. *J. Acoust. Soc. Amer.* 36: 2175, 1964.

Davis, R.C.: Motor effects of strong auditory stimuli. *J. Exp. Psychol.* 38: 257, 1948.

Djupesland, G.: Intra-aural muscular reflexes elicited by air current stimulation of the external ear. *Acta Otolaryng. (Stockh.)* 54: 143, 1962.

Djupesland, G.: Mechanical component to deafness in Menière's disease. *Acta Otolaryng. (Stockh.)* Suppl. 188: 206, 1964a.

Djupesland, G.: Middle ear muscle reflexes elicited by acoustic and non-acoustic stimulation. *Acta Otolaryng. (Stockh.)* Suppl. 188: 287, 1964b.

Djupesland, G.: Electromyography of the tympanic muscles in man. *Int. Audiol.* 4: 33, 1965.

Djupesland, G.: Contractions of the tympanic muscles in man. Thesis. Oslo, Universitetsforlaget, 1967.

Djupesland, G., Flottorp, G. and Winther, F.Ø.: Size and duration of acoustically elicited impedance changes in man. *Acta Otolaryng. (Stockh.)* Suppl. 224: 220, 1966.

Djupesland, G. and Zwislocki, J.J.: Effect of temporal summàtion on the human stapedius reflex. *Acta Otolaryng. (Stockh.)* 71: 262, 1971.

Djupesland, G. and Zwislocki, J.J.: On the critical band in the acoustic stapedius reflex. *J. Acoust. Soc. Amer.*, 54: 1157, 1973.

Djupesland, G., Flottorp, G., Sundby, A. and Szalay, M.: A comparison between middle-ear muscle reflex thresholds for bone- and air-conducted pure tones. *Acta Otolaryng. (Stockh.)* 75: 178, 1973a.

Djupesland, G., Sundby, A. and Flottorp, G.: Temporal summation in the acoustic stapedius reflex mechanism. *Acta Otolaryng. (Stockh.)* 76: 305, 1973b.

Djupesland, G. and Kvernvold, H.: Acoustic impedance measured on ears with normal and diphasic impedance changes. *Scand. Audiol.* 4: 39, 1975.

Djupesland, G., Sundby, A. and Hogstad, K.E.: A study of critical bandwidth in Menière's syndrome using the acoustic stapedius reflex. *Scand. Audiol.* 4: 127, 1975.

Evans, E.F.: Cochlear nerve and cochlear nucleus. In Keidel, W.D. and Neff W.D. (Eds.): *Handbook of Sensory Physiology* Vol. V: 2. Berlin, Springer Verlag, 1975.

Ewertsen, H., Filling, S., Terkildsen, K. and Thomsen, K.A.: Comparative recruitment testing. *Acta Otolaryng. (Stockh.)* Suppl. 140: 116, 1958.

Feldtkeller, R.: Über die Zerlegung des Schallspektrums in Frequenzgruppen durch das Gehör. *Elektron. Rundschau* 9: 387, 1955.

Feldtkeller, R. and Zwicker, E.: *Das Ohr als Nachrichten-empfanger* Stuttgart, Hirzel, 1956.

Fick, A.: Cited by Lucae, A., 1874, p. 164.

Flottorp, G., Djupesland, G. and Winther, F.Ø. The acoustic stapedius reflex in relation to critical bandwidth. *J. Acoust. Soc. Amer.* 49: 457, 1971.

Fowler, E.P.: A method for the early detection of otosclerosis; a study of sound well above the threshold. *Arch. Otolaryng.* 24: 731, 1936.

Fria, T., Le Blanc, J., Kristensen, R. and Alberti, P.W.: Ipsilateral acoustic reflex stimulation in normal and sensorineural impaired ears: A preliminary report. *Can. J. Otolaryng.* 4: 695, 1975.

Gknewikow, D.: Temporal auditory summation in the acoustic stapedial reflex. Ph. D. dissertation, Vanderbilt University, Unpublished.

Goldstein, M.H., Jr., Hall, J.L. and Butterfeld, B.O.: Single-unit activity in the primary auditory cortex of unanesthetized cats. *J. Acoust. Soc. Amer.* 43: 444, 1968.

Hammerschlag, V.: Ueber die Reflexbewegung des Musculus tensor tympani and ihre centralen Bahnen. *Arch Ohrenheilk.* 47: 251, 1899.

Hammerschlag, V.: Die Lage des Reflexcentrums für den Musculus tensor tympani. *Arch. Ohrenheilk.* 56: 157, 1902.

Holst, H., Ingelstedt, S. and Örtegren, U.: Ear drum movements following stimulation of the middle ear muscles. *Acta Otolaryng. (Stockh.)* 182: 73, 1963.

Hung, I.J. and Dallos, P.: Study of the acoustic reflex in human beings. I. Dynamic characteristics. *J. Acoust. Soc. Amer.*, 52: 1168, 1972.

Jepsen, O.: The threshold of the reflexes of the tympanic muscles in a normal material examined by means of the impedance method. *Acta Otolaryng. (Stockh.)* 39: 406, 1951.

Jepsen, O.: Studies on the acoustic stapedius reflex in man. Measurements of the acoustic impedance of the tympanic membrane in normal individuals and in patients with peripheral facial palsy. Thesis. Universitetsforlaget, Aarhus, Denmark, 1955.

Jerger, J., Jerger, S. and Mauldin, L.: Studies in impedance audiometry. I. Normal and sensorineural ears. *Arch. Otolaryng. (Chicago)* 96: 513, 1972.

Jerger, J., Burney, P., Mauldin, L. and Crump, B.: Predicting hearing loss from the acoustic reflex. *J. Speech and Hearing Dis.* 39: 11, 1974.

Jerger, J., Mauldin, L. and Lewis, N.: Temporal summation of the acoustic reflex. *Audiol.* 16: 177, 1977.

Jerger, J., Hayes, D., Anthony, L. and Mauldin, L.: Factors influencing prediction of hearing level from the acoustic reflex. *Monographs in Contemporary Audiology.* Vol. 1, Sept. 1978.

Katsuki, Y.: Neural mechanism of auditory sensation in cats. In Rosenblith, W. A., (Ed.): *Sensory Communication.* New York, John Wiley Co., 1961.

Kawata, S.: Judgement of recruitment by means of measuring the retraction grade of the tympanic membrane. *Acta Otolaryng. (Stockh.)* 49: 517, 1958.

Klockhoff, I.: Middle ear muscle reflexes in man. A clinical and experimental study with special reference to diagnostic problems in hearing impairment. Thesis. *Acta Otolaryng. (Stockh.)* Suppl. 164, 1961.

Kobrak, H.G.: Experimental observations and sound conduction in the middle and inner ear. *Ann. Otol. (St. Louis)* 62: 748, 1953.

Koehler, W.: Die Funktion des Trommelfells und des M. tensor tympani. *Dtsch. Med. Wschr.* 36: 1153, 1910.

Lidén, G: The stapedius muscle reflex used as an objective recruitment test: a clinical and experimental study. In Wolstenholme, G.E.W. and Knight, J., (Eds.): *Ciba Foundation Symposium on Sensorineural Hearing Loss.* London, J. & A. Churchill, 1970.

Lidén, G., Peterson, J.L. and Harford, E.R.: Simultaneous recording of changes in relative impedance and air pressure during acoustic and non-acoustic elicitation of the middle-ear reflexes. *Acta Otolaryng. (Stockh.)* 263: 208, 1970.

Lorente De Nó, R.: Anatomy of the eighth nerve. III. General plan of structure of the primary cochlear

nuclei. *Laryngoscope (St. Louis)* 43: 327, 1933a.
Lorente De Nó, R.: The reflex contractions of the muscles of the middle ear as a hearing test in experimental animals. *Trans. Amer. Laryng. Rhinal. Otol. Soc.* 39: 26, 1933b.
Lorente De Nó, R.: The function of the central acoustic nuclei examined by means of the acoustic reflexes. *Laryngoscope (St. Louis)* 45: 573, 1935.
Lüscher, E: Über reflektorische Trommelfellbewegungen und über die Funktion des Musculus tensor tympani beim Menschen. *Z. Hals, Nas Ohrenheilk.* 28: 40, 1931.
Mach, E. and Kessel, J.: Versuch über die Accomodation des Ohres. *S. -B. Akad. Wiss. Wien* 66: 337, 1872.
Mangold, E.: *Wilkürliche* Kontraktionen des Tensor tympani und die graphische Registrierung von Druckschwankungen im ausseren *Gehörgang. Pflügers Arch. ges. Physiol.* 149: 539, 1913.
Mangold, E. and Eckstein, A.: Reflektorische Kontraktionen des Tensor tympani beim Menschen. *Pflügers Arch. ges. Physiol.* 152; 528, 1913.
McRobert, H., Bryan, M.E. and Tempest, W.: The acoustic stimulation of the middle ear muscles. *J. Sound Vib.* 7; 129, 1968.
Mendelson, E.S.: A sensitive method for registration of human intratympanic muscle reflexes. *J. Appl. Physiol.* 11; 499, 1957.
Mendelson, E.S.: Improved method for studying tympanic reflexes in man. *J. Acoust. Soc. Amer.* 33: 147, 1961.
Metz, O.: The acoustic impedance measured on normal and pathological ears. Thesis. *Acta Otolaryng. (Stockh.)* Suppl. 63, 1946.
Metz, O.: Studies on the contraction of the tympanic muscles as indicated by changes in the impedance of the ear. *Acta Otolaryng. (Stockh.)* 39: 397, 1951.
Metz, O.: Threshold of reflex contractions of muscles of middle ear and recruitment of loudness. *Arch. Otolaryng. (Chicago)* 55: 536, 1952.
Mϕller, Aa.: Bilateral contraction of the tympanic muscles in man. Speech Transmission Laboratory Royal, Institute of Technology Report No. 18, Stockholm.
Mϕller, Aa.: Acoustic reflex in man. *J. Acoust. Soc. Amer.*, 34: 1524, 1962a.
Mϕller, Aa.: The sensitivity of contraction of the tympanic muscle in man. *Ann. Otol. (St. Louis)* 77: 86, 1962b.
Mϕller, Aa.: The acoustic impedance in experimental studies on the middle ear. *Int. Audiol.* 3: 123, 1964.
Morgan, D.E., Gilman, S. and Dirks, D.D.: Temporal integration at the "threshold" of the acoustic reflex. *J. Acoust. Soc. Amer.* 62: 168, 1977.
Niemeyer, W. and Sesterhenn, G.: Calculating the hearing threshold from the stapedius reflex threshold for different sound stimuli. *Audiol.* 13: 421, 1974.
Niese, H.: Subjektive Messung der Lautstärke von Bandpassrauschen. *Hochfrequenztech. Elektroakust.* 68: 202, 1960.
Opheim, O. and Flottorp, G.: The aural harmonics in normal and pathological hearing. *Acta Otolaryng. (Stockh.)* 45: 513, 1955.
Ostmann: Über die Reflexerregbarkeit des Musculus tensor tympani durch Schallwellen und ihre Bedeutung für den Höract. *Arch. Anat. Physiol. (Physiol. Abteilung)* 22: 75, 1898.
Peterson, J.L. and Lidén, G: Some static characteristics of the stapedial muscle reflex. *Audiol.* 11: 97, 1972.
Popelka, G., Karlovich, R. and Wiley, T.: Acoustic reflex and critical bandwidth. *J. Acoust. Soc. Amer.* 55: 883, 1974.
Popelka, G., Margolis, R. and Wiley, T.: Effect of activating signal bandwidth on acoustic-reflex thresholds. *J. Acoust. Soc. Amer.* 59: 153, 1976.
Rasmussen, G.L.: The olivary peduncle and other fiber projections of the superior olivary complex. *J. Comp. Neurol.* 84: 141, 1946.
Richards, A: Threshold of the acoustic stapedius reflex for short-duration tone bursts. *J. Aud. Res.* 15: 87, 1976.
Salomon, G. and Starr, A.: Electromyography of middle ear muscles in man during motor activities. *Acta Neurol. Scand.* 39: 161, 1963.
Scharf, B.: Critical bands and the loudness of complex sounds near threshold. *J. Acoust. Soc. Amer.* 31: 365, 1959.
Scharf, B.: Complex sounds and critical bands. *Psychol. Bull.* 58: 205, 1961a.
Scharf, B.: Loudness summation under masking. *J. Acoust. Soc. Amer.* 33: 503, 1961b.
Scharf, B.: Critical bands. Special Report from the Laboratory of Sensory Communication, Syracuse University, New York, 1966.
Sesterhenn, G. and Breuninger, H.: The acoustic reflex at low sensation levels. *Audiol.* 15: 523, 1976.
Sesterhenn, G. and Breuninger, H.: Determination of hearing threshold for single frequencies from the acoustic reflex. *Audiol.* 16: 210, 1977.
Sundby, A., Flottorp, G. and Djupesland, G: Time constants of registrating equipment in middle ear impedance investigation. In *Proceedings of the Second Nordic Meeting on Medical and Biological Engineering*, 1971.
Sundby, A., Flottorp, G. and Djupesland, G.: A comparison of aural harmonic thresholds for air- and bone-conducted pure tones. 1978. In preparation.

Terkildsen, K.: Movements of the ear drum following intraaural muscle reflexes. *Arch. Otolaryng. (Chicago)* 66: 484, 1957.
Terkildsen, K.: Acoustic reflexes of the human musculus tensor tympani. *Acta Otolaryng. (Stockh.)* Suppl. 158: 230, 1960a.
Terkildsen, K.: The intra-aural muscle reflexes in normal persons and in workers exposed to intense industrial noise. *Acta Otolaryng. (Stockh.)* 52: 384, 1960b.
Terkildsen, K.: Akustiske impedansmålinger og mellomørets funktion. Thesis. The University of Copenhagen, Denmark, 1962.
Terkildsen, K.: Osterhammel, P. and Scott Nielsen, S: Impedance measurements. Probe-tone intensity and middle-ear reflexes. *Acta Otolaryng. (Stockh.)* 263: 205, 1970.
Thomsen, K.A.: Case of psychogenic deafness demonstrated by measuring of impedance. *Acta Otolaryng. (Stockh.)* 45: 82, 1955a.
Thomsen, K.A.: The Metz recruitment test. *Acta Otolaryng. (Stockh.)* 45: 544, 1955b.
Tsukamoto, H.: Zur Physiologie der Binnenohrmuskeln. *Z. Biol.* 95: 146, 1934.
Waar, A.C.H.: Mikroskopische Wahrnehmungen der Funktion der Mittelohrmuskeln beim Menschen. *Acta Otolaryng. (Stockh.)* 5: 335, 1923.
Weiss, H.S., Mundie, J.R., Cashin, J.L. and Shinabarger, E.W.: The normal human intra-aural muscle reflex in response to sound. *Acta Otolaryng. (Stockh.)* 55: 505, 1962
Woodford, C., Henderson, D., Hamernik, R. and Feldman, A.: Threshold-duration function of the acoustic reflex in man. *Audiol.* 14: 53, 1975.
Yonovitz, A. and Harris, J.D.: Eardrum displacement following stapedius muscle contraction. Naval submarine medical research laboratory. Report No. 723, 1972.
Yonovitz, A. and Harris, J.D.: Eardrum displacement following stapedius muscle contraction. *Acta Otolaryng. (Stockh.)* 81: 1, 1976.
Zakrisson, J.E., Borg, E. and Blom, S.: The acoustic impedance change as a measure of stapedius muscle activity in man. A methodological study with electromyography. *Acta Otolaryng. (Stockh.)* 78: 357, 1974.
Zakrisson, J.E.: The role of the stapedius reflex poststimulatory auditory fatigue. *Acta Otolaryng. (Stockh.)* 79: 1, 1975.
Zakrisson, J.E., Borg, E., Diamant, H. and Møller, Aa.R.: Auditory fatigue in patients with stapedius muscle paralysis. *Acta Otolaryng. (Stockh.)* 79: 228, 1975.
Zwicker, E., Flottorp, G. and Stevens, S.S.: Critical bandwidth in loudness summation. *J. Acoust. Soc. Amer.* 29: 548, 1957.
Zwicker, E.: Über die Rolle der Frequenzgruppe beim Hören. *Ergeb. Biol.* 23: 187, 1960.
Zwicker, E.: Scaling. In Keidel, W.D. and Neff, W. D. (Eds.): *Handbook of Sensory Physiology*, Vol. V: 2. Berlin, Springer Verlag, 1975.
Zwislocki, J.J.: Temporal summation of loudness: an analysis. *J. Acoust. Soc. Amer.*, 46: 431, 1969.

Chapter Five

ASSESSMENT OF EUSTACHIAN TUBE FUNCTION

CHARLES D. BLUESTONE, M.D.

INTRODUCTION

Eustachian tube dysfunction appears to be one of the most important factors in the pathogenesis of middle ear disease. Primary mucosal disease of the middle ear is a distinct possibility in some patients but is not the major etiologic factor in most. Mucosal disease may be due to allergy (controversial and unproven) or rarely to an abnormality of the mucociliary transport, e.g., Kartagener's syndrome (Fisher et al., 1978). In any event, abnormal function of the Eustachian tube appears to be the problem in the majority of patients with otitis media and certain related conditions. The Eustachian tube has at least three physiologic functions with respect to the middle ear (Fig. 5-1): *ventilation* of the middle ear to equilibrate air pressure in the middle ear with atmospheric pressure and to replenish oxygen which has been absorbed, *protection* from nasopharyngeal sound pressure and secretions, and *clearance* into the nasopharynx of secretions produced within the middle ear. Assessment of these functions can be helpful in the diagnosis and prevention of middle ear disease, as well as in management of patients. Protective and drainage functions can be evaluated by roentgenographic techniques utilizing radiopaque media (Aschan, 1954; Compere, 1958; Bluestone, 1971; and Bluestone et al., 1972a, 1972d). However, the methods are not physiologic and are technically difficult. Of all the tests of ventilation function which are available clinically, tympanometry offers the most physiologic approach and is technically simple (Holmquist, 1969; Brooks, 1969). When the tympanic membrane is not intact, the manometer portion of the electroacoustic impedance bridge can be employed (Bluestone et al., 1972a, 1972b). Methods of assessment of Eustachian tube function will be discussed in this chapter, but before attempting to understand the significance of the results obtained, some basic background knowledge of Eustachian tube anatomy and physiology is necessary. Also, some newer concepts of pathophysiology of Eustachian tube function and pathogenesis of middle ear disease will be discussed.

ANATOMY OF THE EUSTACHIAN TUBE

The Eustachian tube connects the middle ear cavity to the nasopharynx. In the

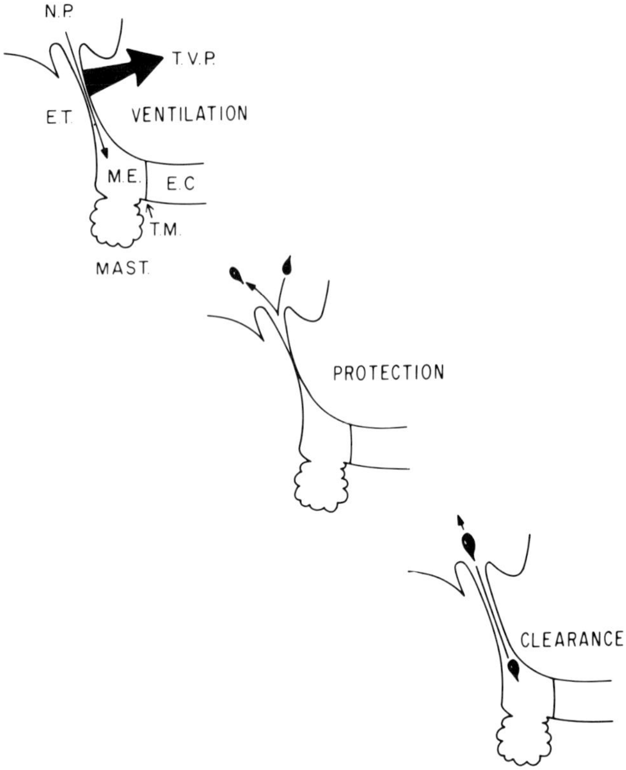

Figure 5-1 Three physiologic functions of Eustachian tube in relation to middle ear. N.P., nasopharynx; E.T., Eustachian tube; T.V.P., tensor veli palatini muscle; M.E., middle ear; Mast., mastoid; T.M., tympanic membrane; E.C., external canal.

adult, the anterior two thirds is cartilaginous and the posterior third bony, but in the infant, the bony portion is relatively longer. The direction of the tube in the adult inclines superiorly with the horizontal plane at an angle of 30 to 40°. In the infant, this inclination is only 10° (Proctor, 1967). The lumen of the Eustachian tube is shaped like two cones with the apex of each directed toward the middle. The aural orifice of the tube is oval in shape, measuring 5 mm high and 2 mm wide in the adult. The nasopharyngeal orifice in the adult is a vertical slit at right angles to the base of the skull, but in the infant this opening is oblique, owing to the more horizontal position of the cartilage. The diameter of the orifice is 8 to 9 mm in the adult and 4 to 5 mm in the infant. In the newborn, the nasopharyngeal orifice lies in the plane of the hard palate, but in the adult it is situated 10 mm above this plane. The middle portion of the Eustachian tube, or isthmus, is not sharply constricted but is relatively long, with gradual widening at each end, forming the aural and nasopharyngeal orifices. The diameter of the isthmus in the adult is 1 to 2 mm; in the infant it is somewhat larger. The mucosal lining of the cartilaginous portion is similar to that of the nasopharynx and contains mucous glands. The mucosa in the protympanic portion of the Eustachian tube is similar to that of the middle ear and contains both mucous-producing elements and cilia.

Usually the Eustachian tube is closed, but it opens during swallowing, yawning, and sneezing, permitting the air pressure in the middle ear to equalize with atmospheric pressure. This opening mechanism is muscular and involves the cartilaginous portion. As elucidated by Rich (1920), the levator palatini, palatopharyngeus, internal pterygoid, and superior constrictor muscles have no influence upon the patency of the orifice or the lumen of the tube. The tensor veli palatini is the only muscle related to active tubal opening (Cantekin et al., 1978). No constrictor muscle of the tube has ever been demonstrated, and closure is the result of relaxation of the tensor muscle with passive return of the tubal walls to a condition of approximation.

The tensor veli palatini muscle is composed of two fairly distinct bundles of muscle fibers divided by a layer of fibroelastic tissue. The bundles lie lateral to the Eustachian tube, in a superficial-deep relationship to one another. The fibers of the superficial bundle run in an inferosuperior direction from their attachment in the inferior margin of the sphenoid bone, around the hamulus, to an attachment along the posterior border of the hard palate. The fibers of the deep bundle run from an inferolateral attachment in the fibroelastic layer to a superomedial attachment on the lateral membranous tubal wall, forming an acute angle with the wall. The tendinous portion of the deep bundle passes around the hamulus and inserts along the posterior margin of the hard palate (Rood and Doyle, 1978).

PHYSIOLOGY AND PATHOPHYSIOLOGY OF THE EUSTACHIAN TUBE

Radiographic Studies

The protective and clearance functions of the Eustachian tube have been assessed by a radiographic technique (Bluestone et al., 1972a, 1972d). Radiopaque material was instilled through the nose of patients to observe the retrograde flow of the medium from the nasopharynx into the Eustachian tube. Patients were considered to have normal protective function when radiopaque material entered only the nasopharyngeal or isthmic portion of the tube but did not enter the bony portion of the tube or middle ear cavity. The normal Eustachian tube protected the middle ear from the contrast material even when the liquid was under increased nasopharyngeal pressure during closed-nose swallowing (Fig. 5-2). If, during the retrograde study, contrast medium traversed the entire Eustachian tube and refluxed into the middle ear during swallowing, the tube was considered to have increased distensibility and poor protective function (Fig. 5-3). The effectiveness of the Eustachian tube in clearing the radiopaque medium instilled into the middle ear was taken as an indication of the effectiveness of the Eustachian tube in the clearance of secretions. Rapid and complete clearance of the medium into the nasopharynx was considered to indicate normal drainage function, while failure of the contrast material to drain from the middle ear into the nasopharynx indicated mechanical obstruction of the Eustachian tube (Fig. 5-4), especially when contrast material also failed to enter the nasopharyngeal portion of the tube during the retrograde study (Fig. 5-5). These abnormal functions of the tube were found in patients with otitis media when compared with a small group of normal subjects. Infants and children with both repaired and unrepaired cleft palate were found to have abnormal Eustachian tube function when assessed by this radiographic technique, which suggested a poor opening mechanism in the infants with an unrepaired cleft palate (Fig. 5-6) (Bluestone, 1971; Bluestone et al., 1972c), and either a persistent failure of the Eustachian tube to open actively or increased distensibility of

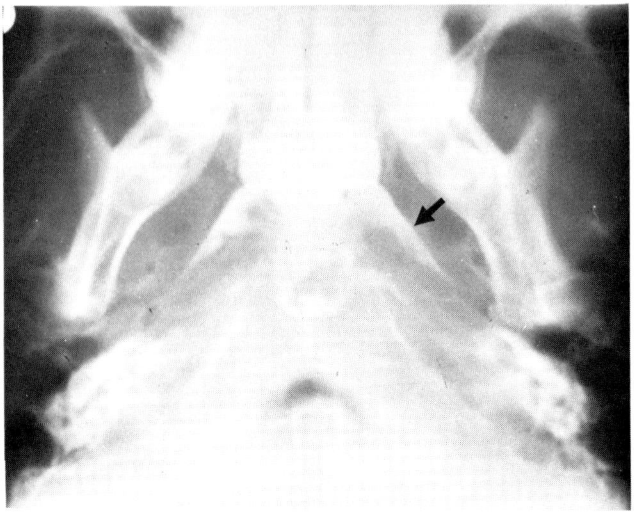

Figure 5-2 Normal retrograde function. During both open-nose and closed-nose swallowing, radiopaque contrast material filled nasopharyngeal portion of Eustachian tube (arrow) of child with normal tympanic membranes and negative otologic history.

the Eustachian tube, or both, after the repair of the soft palate (Bluestone et al., 1972b).

Model of Protective and Clearance Functions

The understanding of these radiographic studies can be enhanced if a model of the system is constructed (Bluestone and Beery, 1976). The Eustachian tube, middle ear, and mastoid can be likened to a flask with a long, narrow neck (Fig. 5-7), the mouth of the flask representing the nasopharyngeal end, the narrow neck the isthmus of the Eustachian tube, and the bulbous portion the middle ear and mastoid air chamber. Figure 5-7a shows that when a small amount of liquid is instilled into the mouth of the

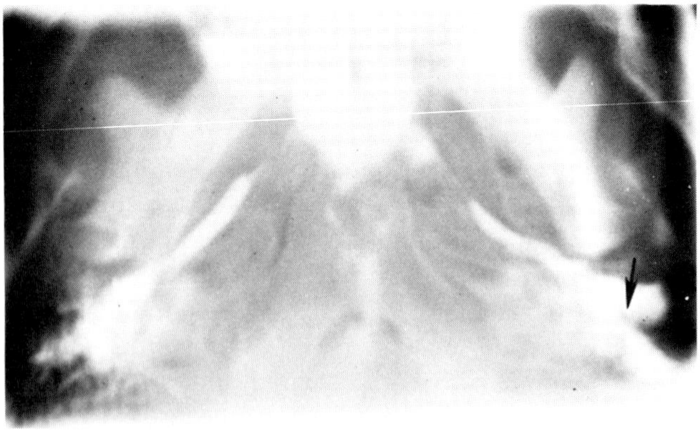

Figure 5-3 Retrograde reflux. Radiograph of six-year-old boy with otitis media. On open-nose swallowing, contrast material traversed entire Eustachian tube and entered middle ear and mastoid (arrow).

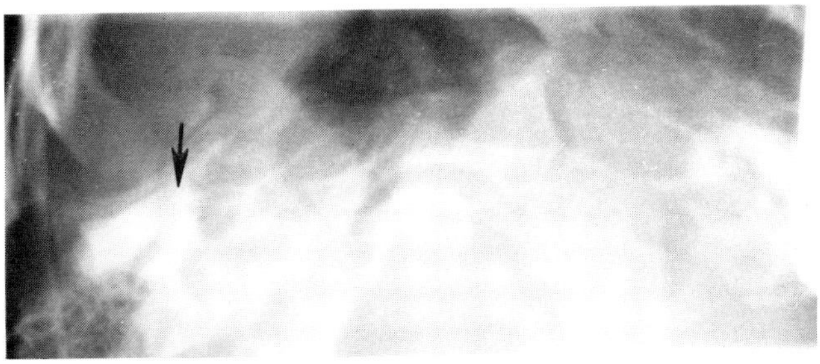

Figure 5-4 Roentgenogram showing prograde obstruction (arrow). Radiopaque contrast material failed to flow from middle ear into nasopharynx.

flask, liquid flow will stop somewhere in the narrow neck, owing to capillarity within the neck and the relative positive air pressure that develops in the chamber of the flask. This basic geometric design is considered to be critical for the protective function of the Eustachian tube-middle ear system. Reflux of the liquid into the vessel occurs if a hole is made in the bulbous portion of the flask (Fig. 5-7b), since the pressure in the bottom of the flask remains unchanged. This is analogous to the condition in which a perforation of the tympanic membrane or the presence of a tympanostomy tube could allow reflux of nasopharyngeal secretions as a result of loss of the middle ear-mastoid air cushion. Similarly, following a radical mastoidectomy the presence of the patent Eustachian tube could cause troublesome otorrhea (Bluestone et al., 1978). Figure 5-7c shows the effect of the application of a negative pressure to the bottom of the flask: The liquid is aspirated into the vessel. In the clinical situation represented by the model, high negative middle ear air pressure could lead to the aspiration of nasopharyngeal secretions into the middle ear. Figure 5-7d shows the effect of applied positive pressure to the mouth of the flask: The liquid is insufflated into the vessel. Nose-blowing, crying, or closed-nose swallowing could create a high positive nasopharyngeal pressure and result in a similar condition in the human system.

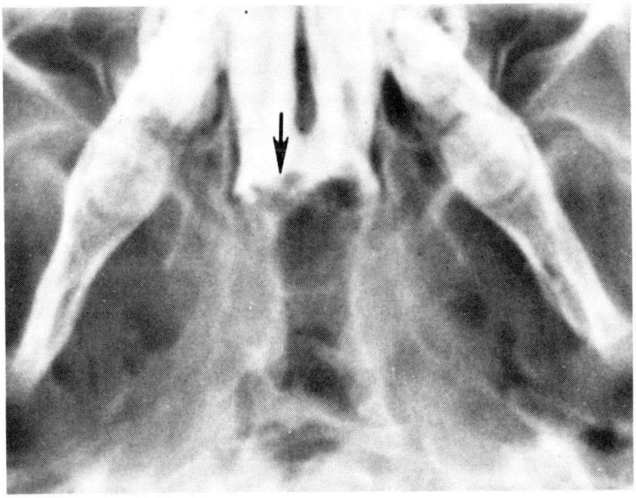

Figure 5-5 Retrograde obstruction. Radiograph of five-year-old boy with otitis media. Radiopaque media failed to enter nasopharyngeal portion of Eustachian tube during both open- and closed-nose swallowing. Note enlarged adenoids (arrow).

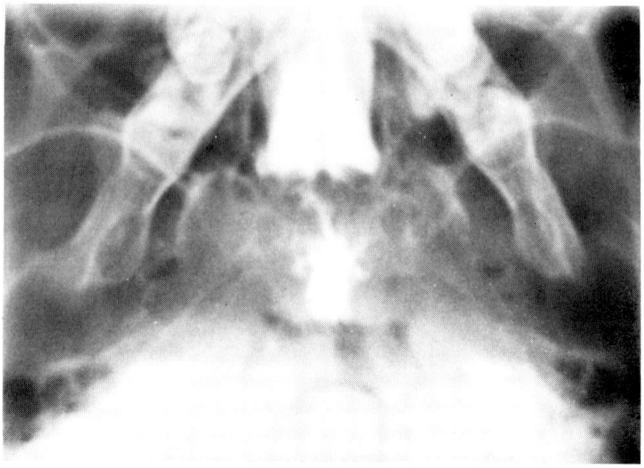

Figure 5-6 Roentgenogram of infant with unrepaired cleft palate. During both open-nose and closed-nose swallowing, radiopaque contrast material failed to enter Eustachian tube, demonstrating retrograde obstruction.

However, one of the major differences between a flask with a rigid neck and a biologic tube such as the Eustachian tube is that the isthmus (neck) of the human tube is compliant. Application of positive pressure at the mouth of the flask with a compliant neck would distend the neck, enhancing fluid flow into the vessel. The effect of applied negative pressure in a flask with a compliant neck is shown in Figure 5-8; liquid flow through the neck would not occur (Fig. 5-8a) until a negative pressure was slowly applied to the bottom of the flask (Fig. 5-8b). In this case fluid flow would occur even if the neck was collapsed, but if the negative pressure were applied suddenly, temporary locking of the compliant neck would prevent flow of the liquid (Fig. 5-8c). Therefore, the speed of the application of the negative pressure as well as the compliance in such a system would appear to be critical factors in the results obtained. Clinically, aspiration of gas into the middle ear would be possible, since negative middle ear pressure would develop slowly as the gas was absorbed by the middle ear mucous membrane. However, sudden application of negative middle ear pressure, such as would occur with rapid alterations in atmospheric pressure (as in an airplane

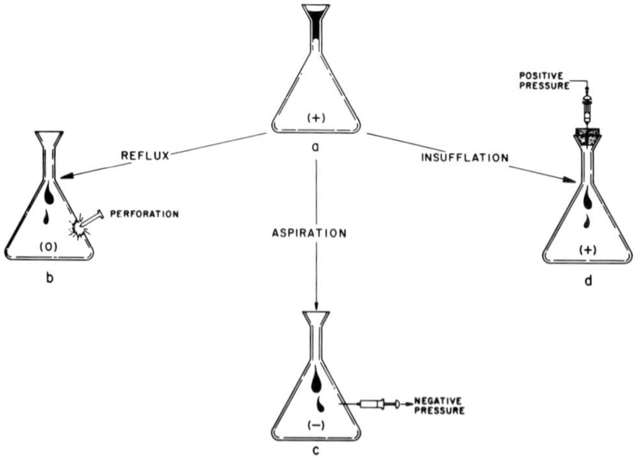

Figure 5-7 Fluid flow into flask.

changing altitude, when diving, or when attempting to test the ventilatory function of the Eustachian tube) could lock the tube, thus preventing the flow of air.

Certain aspects of fluid flow from the middle ear into the nasopharynx can be demonstrated by inverting the flask of the model. Figure 5-9a shows that a liquid trapped in the bulbous portion of the flask does not flow out of the vessel as a result of the relative negative pressure that develops inside the chamber. However, if a hole is "made" in the vessel the liquid drains out of the flask the suction is broken (Fig. 5-9b). Clinically these conditions occur in cases of middle ear effusion in which pressure is relieved by myringotomy. Insufflation of air into the flask releases pressure, which may explain the frequent success of politzerization or the Valsalva maneuver in clearing a middle ear effusion.

The foregoing description of fluid flow through a flask presents only some of the mechanical aspects of the physiology of the human middle ear system. Other factors that probably affect the flow of liquid and air through the middle ear in the physiologic state include (1) the mucociliary transport system of the Eustachian tube and middle ear, (2) contraction of the tensor tympani muscle and tympanic membrane movement, (3) active tubal opening mechanisms, and (4) surface tension factors.

Ventilatory Function of the Eustachian Tube

The ventilatory function of the Eustachian tube can be assessed employing manometry, sonometry, and tympanometry. Early in the 1960s, Ingelstedt and coworkers described the inflation-deflation test (a measure of the subject's ability to equilibrate applied over or under middle ear pressure by swallowing) to assess the function of the Eustachian tube in adults with perforation of the tympanic membrane and a history of chronic otitis media (Flisberg, Ingelstedt, and Ortegren, 1963). These direct measurements suggested that the Eustachian tube in these subjects could not equilibrate applied negative pressure, which was considered abnormal and suggested Eustachian tube dysfunction. Following the original description of the inflation-deflation test by Ingelstedt, Miller (1965) tested children with tympanostomy tubes and found they also could not equilibrate applied negative middle ear pressure.

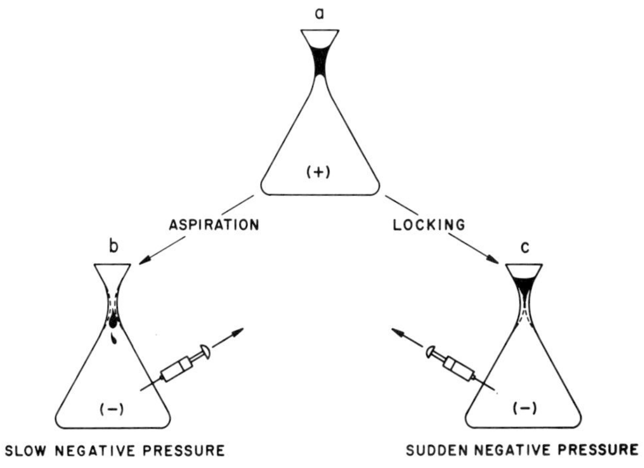

Figure 5-8 Fluid flow through flask with compliant neck.

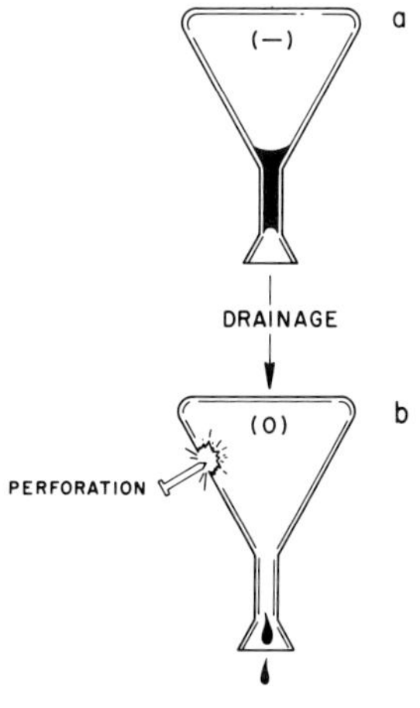

Figure 5-9 Fluid flow from inverted flask.

The inflation-deflation test, which was modified after the Ingelstedt method (which can be performed employing the currently available electroacoustic impedance bridges and will be described in detail later in this chapter) was employed in children who had had tympanostomy tubes inserted for recurrent or chronic otitis media with effusion by Bluestone and coworkers (Bluestone et al., 1974). When compared with the findings of subjects with a traumatic perforation of the tympanic membrane and a negative otologic history, the Eustachian tube function of those children with recurrent or chronic otitis media with effusion was abnormal. These ventilation function studies were also found to be abnormal in children with cleft palate (Bluestone et al., 1972b; Bluestone et al., 1975b). The radiographic Eustachian tube function test (Bluestone et al., 1972d) and the modified inflation-deflation test (Bluestone et al., 1975a) were also employed in an attempt to determine the efficacy of adenoidectomy in children. Cantekin and colleagues (1976) employed a specially designed manometric system and performed the modified inflation-deflation function test in a large number of children with tympanostomy tubes in place who had had recurrent or chronic otitis media with effusion. They compared their findings with a small number of subjects who had traumatic perforations and a negative otologic history and described abnormal function of the Eustachian tube when compared with the "normal" subjects.

In 1978, Cantekin and coworkers described a technique called the forced-response test to evaluate tubal function in subjects with nonintact tympanic membranes. This method is unique in that it eliminates the "mucous forces" in the Eustachian tube lumen which may interfere with the results of the inflation-deflation test when attempts are made to assess the active opening mechanisms and the compliance of the tube. In this test the passive resistance is assessed and the active resistance can also be determined during swallowing. With this method, patients with nonintact tympanic membranes secondary to a chronic perforation or tympanostomy tube can be distinguished from apparently normal subjects with a traumatic perforation of the tympanic membrane and a negative otologic history. The ratio of the passive and active resistance correctly separates a normal from an abnormally functioning Eustachian tube. Subsequent studies in a large number of patients with tympanostomy tubes in place or a perforation secondary to otitis media have revealed that all of the abnormal ears had either a poor active function (as demonstrated by weak or absent dilation of the Eustachian tube during swallowing activity) or in many instances, a constricted tube upon swallowing. Constriction of the Eustachian tube upon swallowing was frequently found in patients with cleft palate and has been attributed to the opposing force of the internal pterygoid muscle (Cantekin et al., 1978). At the present time, the forced-response test can be performed only when the tympanic membrane is not intact and not with the currently available electroacoustic impedance bridge manometric systems.

The microflow technique of Ingelstedt and colleagues (1967) is the only method that has been used to obtain quantitative Eustachian tube function assessment of tubal function in adults with intact tympanic membranes; however, a pressure chamber is required. This technique permits continuous recording of the volume deviation of the tympanic membrane with respect to its neutral position with changes of ambient pressure and changes of pressure within the middle ear. The tympanic membrane is in permanent and free contact with ambient air inside. Within the elastic limits of the tympanic membrane ($\pm$ 150 mm H_20 pressure differential between the middle ear and ear canal), very accurate assessment of the inflation-deflation test can be conducted.

However, this technique cannot be used for the forced-response test because the middle ear pressures to be determined are beyond the elastic limits of the tympanic membrane.

In an effort to determine normal function employing the microflow technique inside a pressure chamber, Elner and colleagues (1971) studied 102 adults with intact tympanic membranes and an apparently negative otologic history. The patients were divided into four groups according to their ability to equilibrate a static relative positive and negative pressure of 100 mm H_20 in the middle ear (Table 5-1). Group I equilibrated pressure differences across the tympanic membrane completely. Group II equilibrated positive pressure, but a small residual negative pressure remained in the middle ear. Group III was capable only of equilibrating relative positive pressure with a small residual remaining, but not negative pressure; and group IV was incapable of equilibrating any pressure. Toynbee's test was negative and Valsalva's test positive in all patients in groups III and IV. These data probably indicate decreased stiffness of the Eustachian tube in groups II-IV when compared with group I. This study also showed that 95 percent of normal adults could equilibrate an applied positive pressure, and 93 percent could equilibrate applied negative pressure by active swallowing, to some extent. However, 28 percent of the subjects could not completely equilibrate applied positive or negative pressure or both.

Sound conduction through the Eustachian tube has been employed as a test of tubal function for over a hundred years (Politzer, 1869), but only recently have reliable data been reported. Virtanen (1977) employed sound at six, seven, and eight kHz into the nose and recorded the sound conduction through the Eustachian tube during swallowing, employing a receiver in the external ear. This method, called sonometry, appears to be promising but cannot be performed with the electroacoustic impedance bridge.

Determination of middle ear pressure and acoustic impedance by electroacoustic impedance equipment was introduced three decades ago (Metz, 1946). This technique has been widely used since then, especially tympanometry, which is the measurement of the acoustic driving point-admittance, looking into the ear canal as a function of the static pressure in the canal. If low-frequency tones are used for the measurement, the value of static pressure producing the maximum acoustic admittance is approximately the pressure in the middle ear. Some tests of Eustachian tube ventilation can be performed using the electroacoustic impedance bridge, and these tests will be described in detail later.

Parameters of middle ear pressure have been studied. Brooks (1969) determined

Table 5-1. EUSTACHIAN TUBE FUNCTION TESTS IN 102 NORMAL SUBJECTS WITH INTACT TYMPANIC MEMBRANES*

Tubal Function Group	No. of Cases (%)	Equilibration when the Middle Ear Pressure is: 100 mm H_20	-100 mm H_20	Toynbee Pos./No.	(%)	Valsalva Pos./No.	(%)
I	74/72	Yes	Yes	67/69	97	63/73	86
II	21/21	Yes	Residual	7/18	39	16/21	76
III	2/2	Residual	No	0/2	0	2/2	100
IV	5/5	No	No	0/5	0	5/5	100
Total	102/100			74/94	79	86/100	86

*From Elner et al., 1971.

the resting middle ear pressure by tympanometry in a large group of apparently normal children as being from 0 to -175 mm H_2O. However, pressures outside this parameter have been reported following screening of large populations of apparently asymptomatic children (Jerger, 1970). High negative middle ear pressure does not necessarily indicate disease but may indicate only temporary tubal obstruction. Ventilation occurs, but only after the nasopharynx-middle ear pressure gradient reaches an opening pressure. It has been suggested that these children probably should be considered "at risk" for middle ear problems until our body of knowledge increases (Bluestone et al., 1973). In normal adults, Alberti and Kristensen (1970) obtained resting middle ear pressures between +50 and -50 mm H_2O. Again, a pressure outside this range does not necessarily mean the patient has ear disease.

From these studies of fluid flow through a vessel and studies in children and adults, the following physiology of the Eustachian tube has been postulated (Bluestone, 1976). Figure 5-10 shows that the normal Eustachian tube is functionally obstructed or collapsed at rest with probably a slight negative pressure existing in the middle ear (Fig. 5-10a). In ideal tubal function, intermittent active opening of the Eustachian tube maintains near-ambient pressures in the middle ear (Fig. 5-10b). It is suspected that in cases in which active function is inefficient in opening the Eustachian tube, functional collapse of the tube persists (Fig. 5-10c). The interval between openings would then depend on the establishment of a pressure gradient between the middle ear cavity and the nasopharynx which passively assists tubal function (Fig. 5-10d). Physiologically, this gradient is achieved by the absorption of middle ear gas, which results in progressive negative middle ear pressure. This type of ventilation appears to be quite common in children, as moderate-to-high negative middle ear pressures have been identified by tympanometry in many who are apparently normal (Beery et al., 1975).

PATHOGENESIS OF OTITIS MEDIA AND CERTAIN RELATED CONDITIONS

There appear to be two major types of abnormal function of the Eustachian tube which can cause a middle ear effusion: obstruction or abnormal patency—or both. Eustachian tube obstruction can be either functional or mechanical. Functional

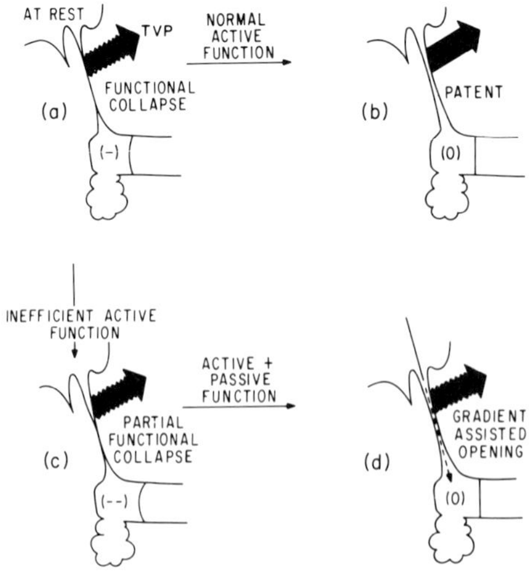

Figure 5-10 Diagrammatic representation of physiologic ventilation of middle ear by active opening of Eustachian tube by tensor veli palatini muscle. An alternative mechanism is by gradient assisted opening of Eustachian tube (see text).

obstruction results from persistent collapse of the Eustachian tube owing to increased tubal compliance, or an inadequate active opening mechanism, or both. Functional Eustachian tube obstruction is common in infants and younger children, since the amount and stiffness of the cartilage support of the Eustachian tube is less than in older children and adults, and since there appear to be marked age differences in the craniofacial base which render the tensor veli palatini muscle less efficient prior to puberty. Figure 5-11 depicts the chain of events in the pathogenesis of otitis media with effusion when the Eustachian tube is functionally obstructed. This type of obstruction may result in persistent high negative middle ear pressure, and when associated with marked collapse or retraction of the tympanic membrane has been termed *atelectasis* (Fig. 5-11a). If ventilation occurs when there is high negative middle ear pressure, nasopharyngeal secretions could be aspirated into the middle ear and result in an acute bacterial otitis media with effusion (Fig. 5-11b). To test this hypothesis in the experimental animal, an investigation in the Rhesus monkey was instituted (Cantekin et al., 1977). Unilateral transection of the tensor veli palatini muscle posterior to the hamulus of the pterygoid bone resulted in persistent high negative middle ear pressure with effusion, while in the opposite, unoperated side, middle ear pressure remained normal. Forty-eight hours after instillation of pneumococcus into the nasopharynx of the monkey, acute otitis media with effusion developed in the ear with the high negative middle ear pressure but not in the unoperated side.

Figure 5-11c shows that if ventilation does not occur, persistent functional Eustachian tube obstruction could result in a sterile otitis media with effusion. The occurrence of an otitis media with effusion at this stage might depend upon the degree and duration of the negative pressure as well as on middle ear hypoxia or hypercarbia. Since tubal opening could be possible in a middle ear with an effusion, aspiration of nasopharyngeal secretions might occur, thus creating the clinical condition in which persistent otitis media with effusion and recurrent acute bacterial otitis media with effusion occur together. All infants with unrepaired palatal clefts and many children with repaired palates have otitis media with effusion, as a result of functional obstruction of the Eustachian tube (Bluestone, 1971).

Intrinsic mechanical obstruction of the Eustachian tube is the result of inflammation. Figure 5-12 illustrates the sequence of events in which intrinsic inflammation of the Eustachian tube may result in an abnormal middle ear condition.

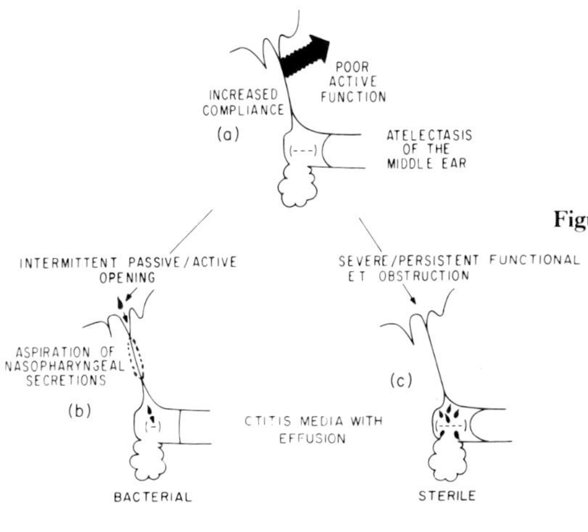

Figure 5-11 Diagrammatic representation of mechanism by which functional obstruction of Eustachian tube can result in atelectasis of middle ear or bacterial or sterile otitis media with effusion (see text).

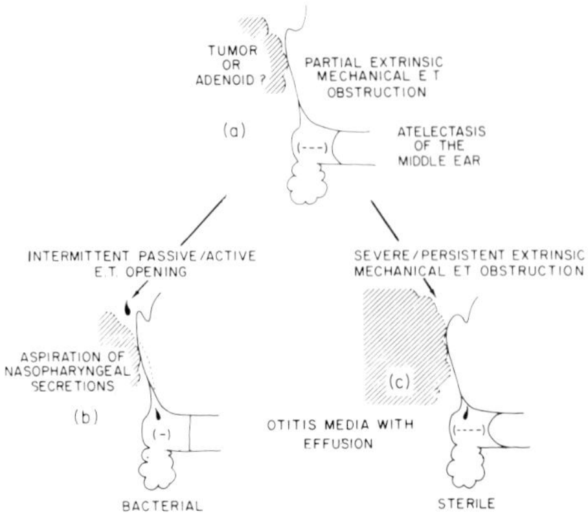

Figure 5-12 Diagrammatic representation of mechanism by which intrinsic mechanical obstruction of Eustachian tube can result in atelectasis of tympanic membrane-middle ear or bacterial or sterile otitis media with effusion (see text).

Most ears at risk for developing atelectasis or otitis media with effusion when inflammation is present probably have a significant degree of functional obstruction (Fig. 5-12a). An upper respiratory tract infection in such children has been shown to significantly decrease Eustachian tube function (Bluestone et al., 1977). Periods of upper respiratory tract infection may then result in either atelectasis of the middle ear (Fig. 5-12b), bacterial otitis media with effusion (Fig. 5-12c), or a sterile otitis media with effusion (Fig. 5-12d) due to swelling of the Eustachian tube lumen. The mechanisms are similar to those described for functional Eustachian tube obstruction. Allergy as a cause of intrinsic mechanical Eustachian tube obstruction has not been demonstrated.

Extrinsic mechanical obstruction of the Eustachian tube may be the result of extrinsic compression by nasopharyngeal tumors or adenoids (Bluestone et al., 1972d, Bluestone et al., 1975). Figure 5-13 shows the possible mechanisms by which extrinsic obstruction may result in ear disease. Partial Eustachian tube obstruction may result only in atelectasis of the tympanic membrane-middle ear (Fig. 5-13a) or a bacterial otitis media with effusion (Fig. 5-13b), but more severe obstruction could result in a sterile otitis media with effusion (Fig. 5-13c). Otitis media with effusion has been produced in animal models when the Eustachian tube was mechanically obstructed (Paparella et al., 1970). However, verification that adenoids actually obstruct the Eustachian tube remains unproven.

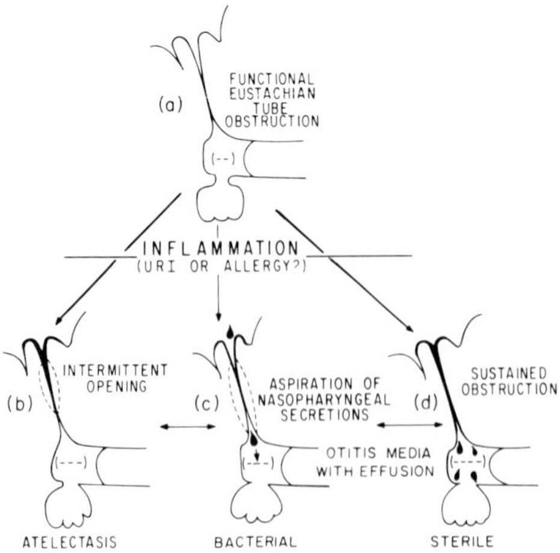

Figure 5-13 Diagrammatic representation of mechanism by which extrinsic mechanical obstruction of Eustachian tube can result in atelectasis of tympanic membrane-middle ear or bacterial or sterile otitis media with effusion (see text).

Nasal obstruction may also be involved in the pathogenesis of otitis media with effusion. Swallowing when the nose is obstructed (due to inflammation or obstructed adenoids) results in an initial positive nasopharyngeal air pressure, followed by a negative pressure phase. When the tube is pliant, positive nasopharyngeal pressure might insufflate infected secretions into the middle ear, especially when the middle ear has a high negative middle ear pressure; or with negative nasopharyngeal pressure, such a tube could be prevented from opening and be further obstructed functionally ("Toynbee phenomenon") (Bluestone et al., 1974; Bluestone et al., 1975a).

The other major type of dysfunction of the Eustachian tube is abnormal patency. In its extreme form, the tube is open even at rest, i.e., patulous. Lesser degrees of abnormal patency of the tube occur when the tube actively opens owing to the pull of the tensor veli palatini muscle or conceivably even in the absence of active dilation of the tube. The Eustachian tube in this instance has very low resistance in comparison with the normal Eustachian tube. Not only can air flow easily from the nasopharynx into the middle ear, but also, unwanted nasopharyngeal secretions can readily traverse the tube and cause "reflux otitis media." This type of tube—having an increased susceptibility to nasopharyngeal secretion—appears to be quite common in the native American population (American Indians), in that they have been shown to have tubal resistance that is lower than the normal Caucasian population (Beery et al., 1978) and to have ear disease that is characterized by recurrent acute otitis media, frequently associated with perforation and drainage.

Some individuals may have functional obstruction at times and at other times have increased patency of the Eustachian tube . As an example, functional obstruction may be present and result in high negative pressure, or otitis media with effusion, or both, but the tube is abnormally patent (distensible) when copious nasopharyngeal secretions are present. This is especially true in association with increased nasopharyngeal pressure, e.g., nose-blowing, sneezing, crying, or closed-nose swallowing. This then can result in reflux, aspiration, or insufflation of secretions into the middle ear and cause an acute bacterial otitis media with effusion.

TESTS OF EUSTACHIAN TUBE VENTILATORY FUNCTION EMPLOYING THE ELECTROACOUSTIC IMPEDANCE BRIDGE

The tests of Eustachian tube ventilatory function which can be performed with the electroacoustic impedance bridge are (1) resting middle ear pressure, (2) inflation-deflation, (3) Toynbee's, and (4) Valsalva's. During all tests of Eustachian tube function, the patient should remain in the sitting position unless the effect of positional change is desired. Ingelstedt and colleagues (1969) evaluated Eustachian tube function in healthy adult volunteers in both the sitting and supine position and found dysfunction in the latter. Jonson and Rundcrantz (1969) related this to their findings of increased capillary venous engorgement in the tubal mucosa when the head and neck were elevated less than 20° from the horizontal plane. The presence of a middle ear effusion or mucosal edema may interfere with an accurate assessment of the functional portion of the Eustachian tube owing to possible mechanical obstruction at the aural end. If possible, the middle ear should be free of effusion, otorrhea, or mucous membrane swelling prior to testing.

Inflation-Deflation Test

The normal Eustachian tube should be able to equilibrate the negative pressure that develops in the middle ear as gas is absorbed. This is probably the most important physiologic function of the tube. To test this function, the pressure within the middle ear is reduced—deflation—by a direct method when the tympanic membrane has a perforation or a tympanostomy tube is present. The applied negative pressure should be equilibrated by swallowing activity. Since the application of a sudden negative middle ear pressure is not physiologic, the tube may lock, making equilibration impossible. This frequently occurs in the "floppy" Eustachian tube. Therefore, tubal function must also be assessed by increasing — inflation — the middle ear pressure. Swallowing should equilibrate the middle ear pressure. Locking will not occur when the middle ear has a relative positive pressure.

When the tympanic membrane is intact, inflation-deflation tests of Eustachian tube function must be assessed by indirect methods. This can be accomplished by increasing the external canal pressure, pushing the tympanic membrane inward, creating a slight positive middle ear pressure. Reducing the external canal pressure will distend the tympanic membrane, decreasing the middle ear pressure. Swallowing activity should equilibrate both positive and negative middle ear pressures.

Toynbee's Test

The effect of nasal obstruction on Eustachian tube ventilatory function can be simulated by having the patient swallow when the nose is manually compressed. This is Toynbee's test. The maneuver usually results in a positive pressure within the nasopharynx, followed by a negative pressure phase (Perlman, 1951). If the Eustachian tube opens during the test, the middle ear pressure will change depending upon the timing of the tubal opening and the pressure gradient. The test is usually considered positive when an alteration in middle ear pressure results. The finding of negative middle ear pressure after Toynbee's test usually indicates excellent tubal function, since the Eustachian tube actively opens and is sufficiently stiff to withstand nasopharyngeal negative pressure. However, some Eustachian tubes that are patulous or have very low resistance will also transfer gas from the middle ear into the nasopharynx during Toynbee's test (as well as with "sniffing").

Valsalva's Test

The effect of high positive nasopharyngeal pressures on the Eustachian tube can be evaluated qualitatively by Valsalva's test. The test is considered positive when the Eustachian tube and middle ear can be inflated by a forced expiration, the mouth being closed and the nose held by thumb and forefinger. A positive Valsalva test indicates a distensible tube and by itself is not a reliable test of Eustachian tube function.

TECHNIQUE

Nonintact Tympanic Membrane

INFLATION-DEFLATION TESTS

When a perforation of the tympanic membrane or a tympanostomy tube is present, inflation-deflation tests of the ventilatory function of the Eustachian tube can be studied by employing the pump-manometer portion of the impedance bridge (Bluestone et al., 1972a). Figure 5-14 is a simplified explanation of the combined passive and active function test when positive pressure is applied to the middle ear—inflation. This test is similar to ascending in an airplane until the Eustachian tube passively opens (Fig. 5-14a). The test consists of the application of enough positive pressure into the middle ear to force open the Eustachian tube (Fig. 5-14b). The pressure remaining in the middle ear after passive opening and closing is termed the closing pressure (Fig. 5-14c). Further equilibration of pressure is achieved by swallowing—active function—which is the result of contraction of the tensor veli palatini muscle (Rich, 1920; Cantekin et al., 1978). When the muscle contracts, the lumen of the Eustachian tube is opened and air flows down the tube (Fig. 5-14d). The pressures can be monitored on a strip chart recorder (Fig. 5-14e); the pressure remaining in the middle ear after passive and active function is termed the residual positive pressure. Figure 5-15 shows the deflation phase of the study, which is similar to descent in an airplane (Fig. 5-15a). Low negative pressure is applied to the middle ear (Fig. 5-15b), which is then equilibrated by active function (Fig. 5-15c). The pressure remaining in the middle ear after swallowing is termed the residual negative pressure (Fig. 5-15d). In certain instances active function to applied low positive pressure is also assessed (Fig. 5-16). This is similar to ascent in an airplane but to an altitude lower than a pressure that would force open the Eustachian tube (Fig. 5-16a).

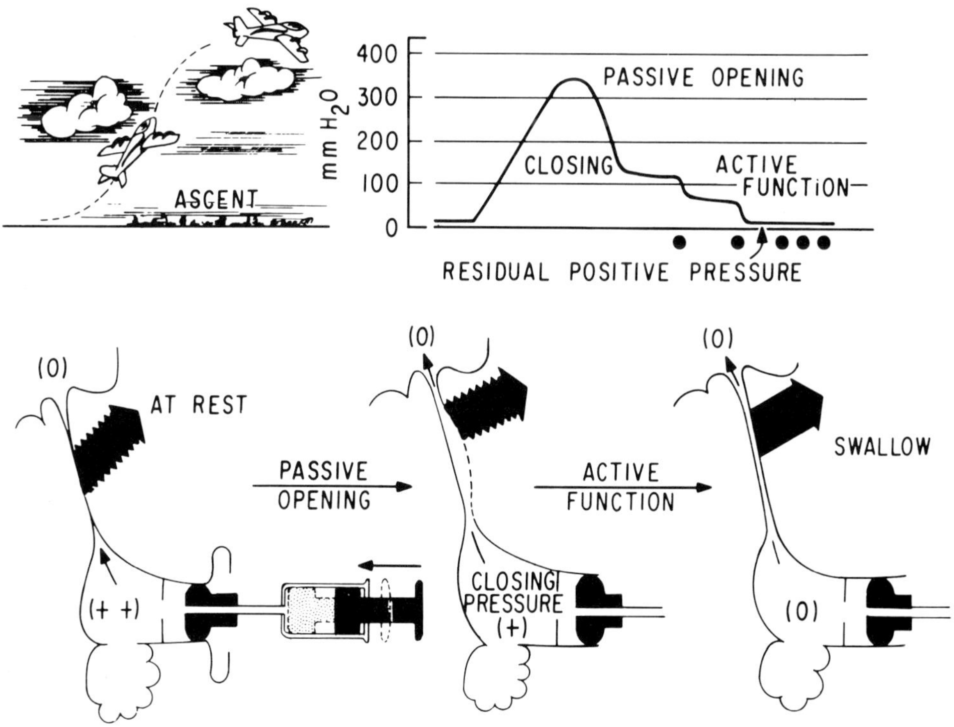

Figure 5-14 Passive and active function test of Eustachian tube is similar to ascending in an airplane. Passive function is assessed by application of sufficient middle ear positive pressure to force open Eustachian tube. Remaining positive pressure after passive closing of Eustachian tube is equilibrated by swallowing—active function. Marks under strip chart recorder represent swallows (see text).

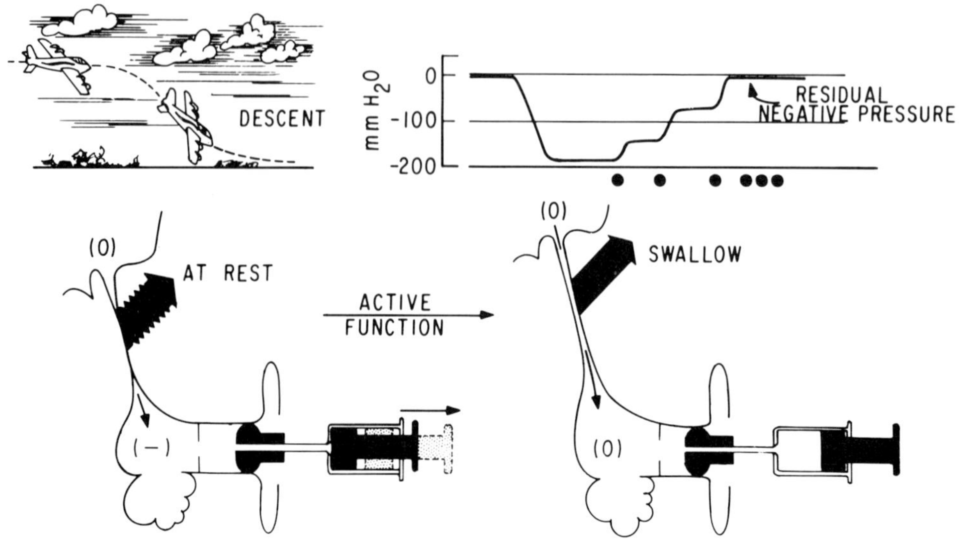

Figure 5-15 Active function of Eustachian tube to applied negative pressure—deflation—is similar to descending in an airplane (see text).

The patient is asked to swallow in an attempt to equilibrate the pressure by active function (Fig. 5-16b,c).

Figure 5-17 shows the symbols employed and examples of results obtained in ventilation studies. Example A describes a typical study of a patient with normal function. Following passive opening and closing of the Eustachian tube during the inflation phase of the study, the patient is able to equilibrate completely the remaining positive

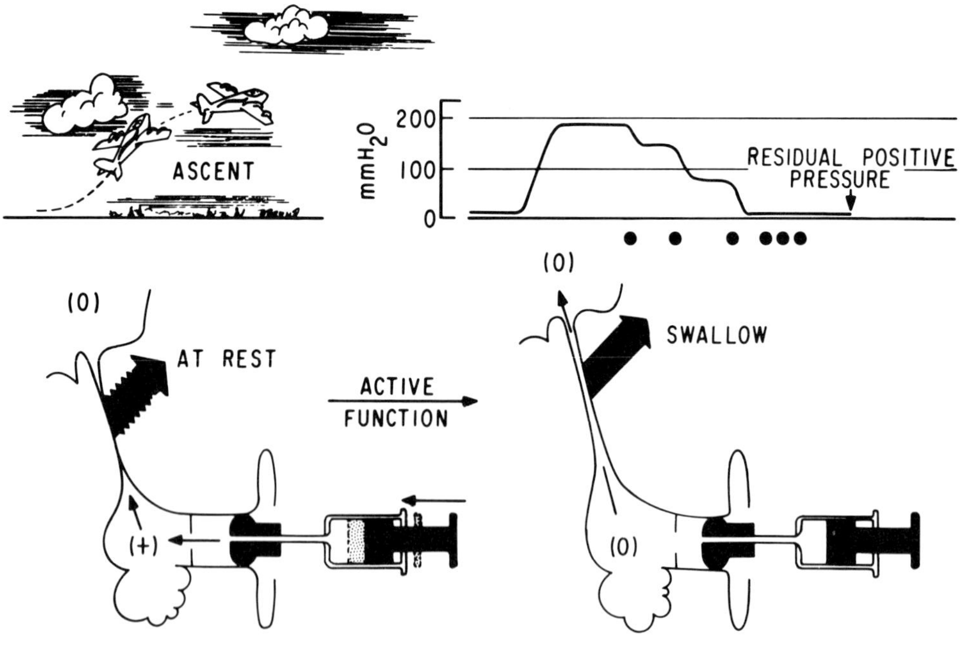

Figure 5-16 Active function of Eustachian tube to applied positive pressure is also tested by inflation to pressure below opening pressure but above closing pressure (see text).

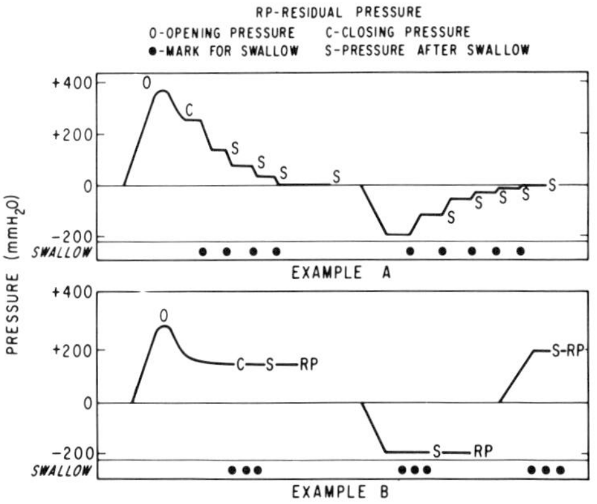

Figure 5-17 Symbols and examples of results of inflation-deflation ventilation studies employing strip chart recorder. (A) Normal adult with traumatic perforation; (B) four-year-old male with functioning tympanostomy tube who had persistent otitis media with effusion.

pressure. Active swallowing also completely equilibrates applied negative pressure—deflation. Example B describes a typical study of a child who had had otitis media with effusion. The Eustachian tube passively opens and closes following inflation, but subsequent swallowing fails to equilibrate the residual positive pressure. In the deflation phase of the study, the child is unable to equilibrate negative pressure. Inflation to a pressure below the opening pressure but above the closing pressure cannot be equilibrated by the active swallowing function.

Failure to equilibrate the applied negative pressure during the test indicates *locking* of the Eustachian tube during the test. This type of tube is considered to have *increased compliance* or is "floppy" in comparison to the tube with perfect function. A stiff tube will neither distend in response to high positive pressures nor collapse in response to negative pressures; however, a tube that lacks stiffness is collapsed, and this in turn results in functional tubal obstruction. The tube would collapse even further, and might lock entirely, in response to negative pressures; it might not open in response to low positive pressure, but as pressure progressively increases, it would open and might ultimately distend.

The speed of the application of the positive and negative pressure is an important variable in testing the Eustachian tube function employing this test. The faster the application of the positive pressure, the higher the opening pressure. During the deflation phase of the study, the faster the application of the negative pressure, the more likelihood of the "locking phenomenon."

Figure 5-18 describes elements of the procedure and the symbols used in recording the results of these ventilatory studies when a strip chart is not available, in which case the pressures are noted on the manometer. Example A is similar to example A in Figure 5-17. However, as shown in the figure, the tube did not passively open. Depending upon the type of electroacoustic impedance bridge, the pump-manometer may not produce pressures greater than 400 mm H_20. The mean opening pressures for apparently normal subjects with a traumatic perforation and negative otologic history reported by Cantekin and coworkers (1977)was 330 mm H_20 ($\pm$ 70 mm H_20). Many subjects open above 400 mm H_20, which is above the limit of the manometers used in the most commonly available bridges. Again, the opening pressure is dependent on the speed of the pump. Example B is another example of functional obstruction of the Eustachian tube function. The diagnosis of total mechanical obstruction of the Eustachian tube (air cannot flow out or into the middle ear) cannot be made if the pressures cannot be elevated greater than 400 mm H_20. If the tube does not open to 1000 mm H_20 one can assume that total obstruction is present. This pressure is not

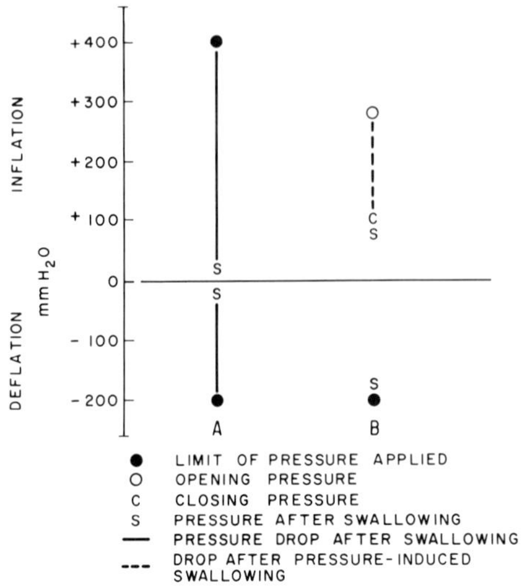

Figure 5-18 Procedure and symbols used in describing ventilatory (inflation-deflation) studies when strip chart recorder is not employed. Two illustrative examples are shown (see text).

hazardous to the middle ear or inner ear windows if the pressure is slowly applied.

During each equilibration, the time interval between each swallow should be approximately 20 seconds to avoid strain on the pharyngeal muscles. The subject should swallow "dry," but in patients with reduced function of the Eustachian tube swallowing water may be tried.

The diagnosis of a nonintact tympanic membrane can frequently be made with the electroacoustic impedance bridge in the absence of a otoscopic examination. When tympanometry is attempted, either the bridge cannot be balanced or a larger than expected volume is noted. Another indication would be the finding of a sudden loss of pressure (opening pressure) during the attempt to pump 200 mm H_20 pressure in the external canal. If the diagnosis of a nonintact tympanic membrane is suspected but not confirmed by these findings, the external canal pressure should be raised to 400 mm H_20 in an attempt to reach an opening pressure. Most Eustachian tubes will open before this limit is reached. If not, the subject should be asked to swallow, and if reduction in presure results the diagnosis is confirmed. These findings can be helpful to the clinician in detecting microscopic perforations of the drum and determining the patency of tympanostomy tubes.

PATULOUS EUSTACHIAN TUBE

The Eustachian tube is considered patulous when, after the probe tip is adequately fitted in the external canal, applied positive and negative pressure cannot be held in the middle ear. Low opening pressures, when both positive and negative pressures are applied, would indicate the same condition. The tube is abnormally open at rest.

Intact Tympanic Membrane

RESTING MIDDLE EAR PRESSURE

When the tympanic membrane is intact, tympanometric determination of the

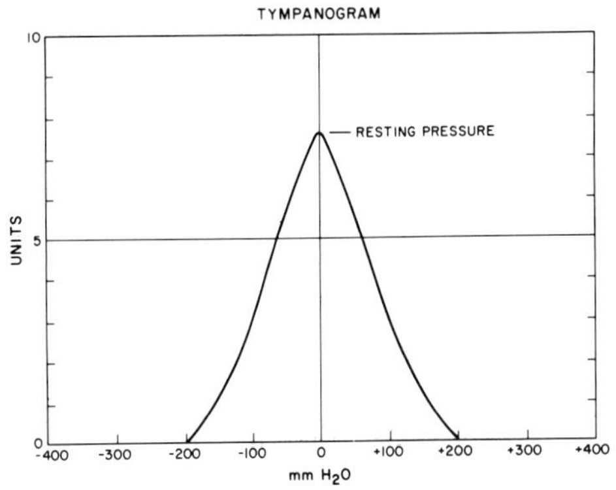

Figure 5-19 Tympanogram in which resting middle ear pressure is normal.

middle ear pressure is an excellent assessment of Eustachian tube ventilatory function and is the most physiologic function test clinically available. Figure 5-19 is an example of a tympanogram of a patient with normal middle ear resting pressure. Figure 5-20 is an example of what happens in a patient with high negative middle ear resting pressure that is indicative of obstruction of the Eustachian tube, which may be functional or mechanical or both. However, these determinations only represent the middle ear pressure at one moment. The finding of normal resting middle ear pressure does not necessarily indicate normal Eustachian tube function, but the finding of negative middle ear pressure is presumptive evidence of Eustachian tube dysfunction. Serial determinations would be more indicative of the dynamics of tubal function in any one patient. Since the tympanic membrane is intact, the response of the Eustachian tube to positive and negative middle ear pressures must be induced by indirect methods. Because the alteration in the middle ear pressure may be slight, an xy plotter or strip chart recorder is necessary.

INFLATION-DEFLATION TEST

Figure 5-21 is an example of the inflation-deflation technique when the tympanic membrane is intact. Following the tympanometric determination of the resting middle ear pressure, with the probe tip still in place, the pressure in the external ear canal is increased to 200 mm H_20. The subject is asked to swallow several times. In this way,

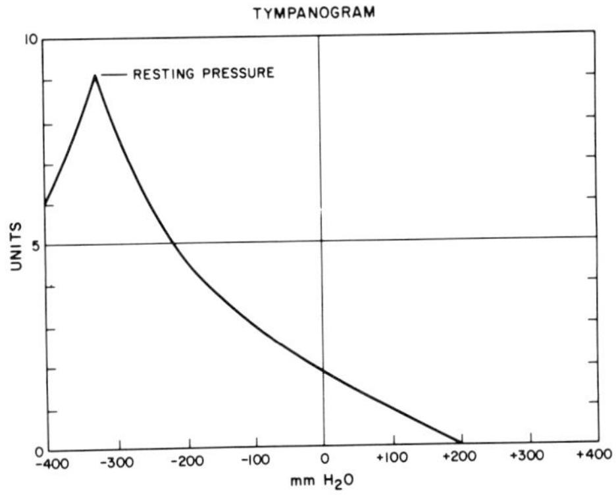

Figure 5-20 Tympanogram of patient with high negative resting middle ear pressure.

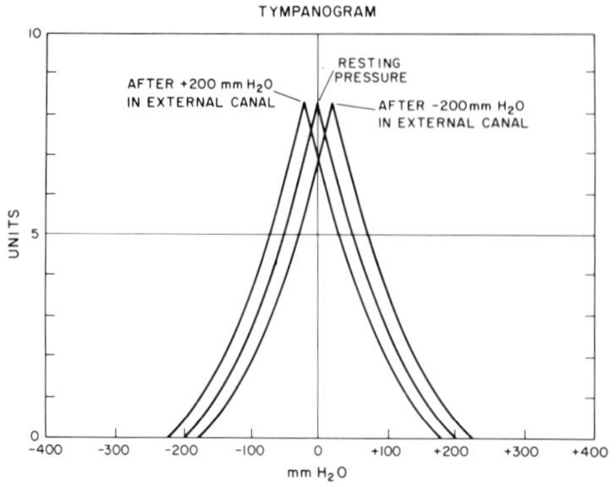

Figure 5-21 Normal inflation-deflation Eustachian tube function test when tympanic membrane is intact, employing tympanometry.

the middle ear pressure is increased—inflation—by the pressure applied against the tympanic membrane, and if the Eustachian tube function is normal, gas will go down the tube into the nasopharynx during swallowing. Equilibration of gas pressure between the middle ear and nasopharynx should result. The middle ear pressure following this maneuver can then be determined by asking the patient to refrain from swallowing while the tympanogram is repeated. If the test is successful, a slight negative middle ear pressure as compared with the resting pressure will result. Following this procedure, the pressure in the middle ear is then decreased—deflation—by lowering the external canal pressure to -200 mm H_20. The tympanic membrane will be pulled toward the probe, creating a greater volume in the middle ear cavity. A relative negative middle ear pressure compared with that in the nasopharynx is produced. The subject is asked to swallow several times. Following this, another typanometric peak is obtained while the patient refrains from swallowing. A slight positive pressure will be found, since gas is transferred from the nasopharynx into the middle ear, equilibrating the pressures. This test may be successful in subjects with excellent Eustachian tube function but is not useful in differentiating between normal and abnormal function when it is not successful. Unfortunately, since most subjects, both normal and those with varying degrees of middle ear disease, have no change in middle ear pressure during this test, its clinical value is severely limited.

TOYNBEE'S AND VALSALVA'S TESTS

When the tympanic membrane is intact, the effect of the Toynbee maneuver on the Eustachian tube and middle ear can be assessed by tympanometry. The resting middle ear pressure is initially determined. With the probe tip still in place, the pump-manometer portion of the instrument should be open to the atmosphere to eliminate pressure against the tympanic membrane. This can be accomplished by either temporarily disengaging the plastic tubing from the back of the instrument or holding the purge button on the pump, depending upon the instrument model. The patient is then asked to compress the nose manually and swallow several times. The pressure remaining in the middle ear following this maneuver can be determined by repeating the tympanogram while the patient refrains from swallowing. Figure 5-22 is an example of the procedure. The subject was able to develop negative middle ear pressure following the Toynbee maneuver. Since a negative pressure is present in the middle ear, the patient's ability to equalize is assessed (deflation test). Following one

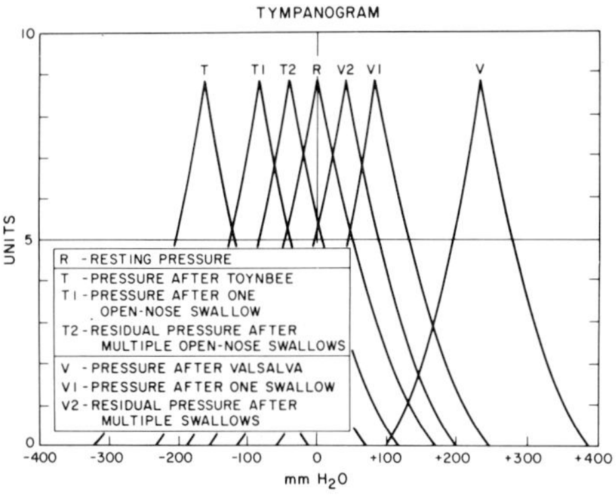

Figure 5-22 Toynbee's and Valsalva's tests of Eustachian tube function when tympanic membrane is intact employing tympanometry.

swallow, another tympanometric peak is obtained which reveals partial equilibration of the negative pressure. The pressure remaining in the middle ear following multiple swallows is the residual negative pressure.

Following the Toynbee maneuver, the patient's ability to inflate the middle ear is then tested by the Valsalva maneuver. Again, the pump-manometer portion of the instrument should be open to the atmosphere. The patient is asked to blow against the manually compressed nose and closed lips, creating a high nasopharyngeal positive pressure. Pressure remaining in the middle ear can then be evaluated by obtaining a tympanometric peak. If the test is successful, positive middle ear pressure results. Subsequent swallows reduce the positive pressure (inflation test). The pressure remaining in the middle ear following multiple swallows is the residual positive pressure. Figure 5-23 illustrates Toynbee's and Valsalva's test results shown on a strip chart recorder. This test is helpful if the subject is able to develop negative pressure within the middle ear during Toynbee's test and then is able to equilibrate the negative pressure to the initial resting pressure. This would indicate excellent function of the Eustachian tube. However, inability to develop negative middle ear pressure following Toynbee's test or positive intratympanic pressure after Valsalva's test does not differentiate between normal and abnormal tubal function.

PATULOUS EUSTACHIAN TUBE

If a patulous Eustachian tube is suspected, the diagnosis can be confirmed by tympanometry when the tympanic membrane is intact. A tympanogram is first obtained while the patient is breathing normally and is repeated during breath-holding. The fluctuation in the tympanometric line should coincide with breathing

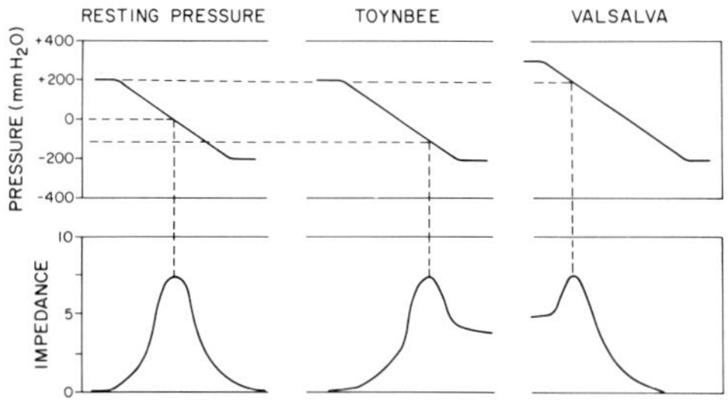

Figure 5-23 Strip chart tympanometric recording of Toynbee's and Valsalva's tests of Eustachian tube function when tympanic membrane is intact.

(Fig 5-24). The fluctuation can be exaggerated by asking the patient to occlude one nostril with the mouth closed during forced inspiration and expiration or by Toynbee's test (Fig. 5-25).

INDICATIONS FOR TESTING EUSTACHIAN TUBE FUNCTION

Since the determination of resting middle ear pressure may be an indication of how well the Eustachian tube is functioning, serial testing of certain patients by tympanometry may be helpful. One of the most important indications to assess Eustachian tube function is in the differential diagnosis of a patient who does not have otitis media but has symptoms that might be related to Eustachian tube dysfunction. Symptoms such as fullness, snapping or popping in the ear, fluctuating hearing loss, tinnitus, or vertigo may be indicative of abnormal Eustachian tube function. When the tympanic membrane is intact, a tympanogram that reveals high negative pressure would be presumptive evidence of abnormal tubal function, whereas normal resting middle ear pressure would not be a diagnostic aid. However, when the resting intratympanic pressure is within normal limits but the patient can develop negative middle ear pressure during the deflation test (Fig. 5-21) or following Toynbee's test (Fig. 5-22) the Eustachian tube is probably functioning normally. Unfortunately, failure to develop negative middle ear pressure during either or both of these tests does not indicate poor Eustachian tube function.

Screening for the presence of high negative pressure in certain high-risk populations, i.e., children with known sensorineural hearing loss, developmentally delayed and mentally impaired children, children with cleft palate or other craniofacial anomalies, native American children (Indian and Eskimo), and children with Down's syndrome, appears to be helpful in identifying those patients who may need to be closely monitored for the occurence of otitis media (Harford et al., 1978).

The value of otoscopy as a method for screening children for middle ear disease is limited, since it depends on the availability of clinicians and their expertise. Air-conduction audiometry has generally been employed for such screening, but its accuracy has been challenged (Eagles et al., 1967). Tympanometry, however, appears to be a reliable method for detecting the presence of high negative pressure as well as otitis media with effusion in children (Brooks, 1968, 1971; Beery et al., 1975). The

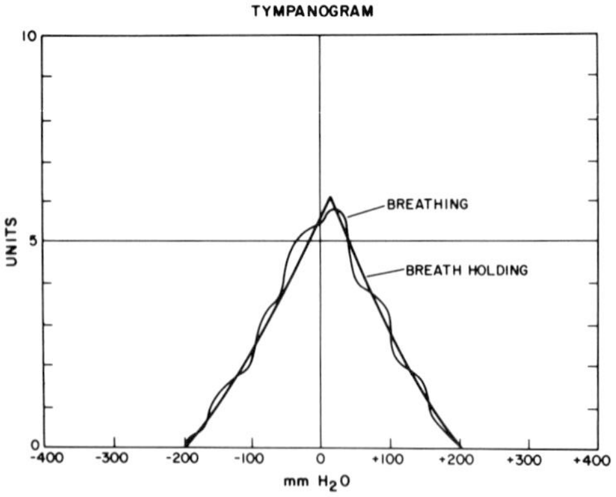

Figure 5-24 Tympanogram of patient with patulous Eustachian tube. Wavy line was obtained while subject was breathing. Steady line taken while breath-holding.

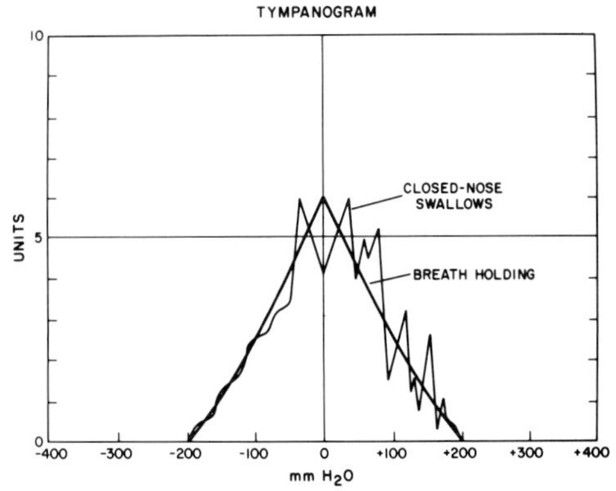

Figure 5-25 Tympanogram of same patient as in Figure 5-24. Wide fluctuations obtained while patient swallowed several times with mouth and nose closed (Toynbee's test). Steady line taken while breath-holding.

identification of high negative pressure without effusion in children is indicative of some degree of Eustachian tube obstruction. These children, as well as children with middle ear effusion, should have follow-up serial tympanograms.

Any patient with recurrent acute or chronic otitis media with effusion should have, as part of their otolaryngological and audiological workup, Eustachian tube function studies. The management of such patients may depend on the findings. Mechanical obstruction of the Eustachian tube may indicate treatment different from that of functional obstruction. Adenoidectomy may not be indicated in a child with a small adenoid mass and a tubal function test indicating functional obstruction. However, the operation *may* benefit the child with marked mechanical obstruction (Bluestone et al., 1975).

Patients in whom tympanostomy tubes have been inserted may benefit from serial Eustachian tube function studies. Improvement in function as indicated by inflation-deflation tests might aid the clinician in determining the proper time to remove the tubes. Cleft palate repair (Bluestone et al., 1972b), adenoidectomy (Bluestone et al., 1975), elimination of nasal and nasopharyngeal inflammation (Bluestone et al., 1977), or growth and development of a child (Holborow, 1970), may be associated with improvement in Eustachian tube function.

Eustachian tube function of the patient with a chronic perforation of the tympanic membrane may be helpful in preoperatively determining the success or failure of tympanoplasty surgery. Holmquist (1970) studied adults prior to tympanoplasty and

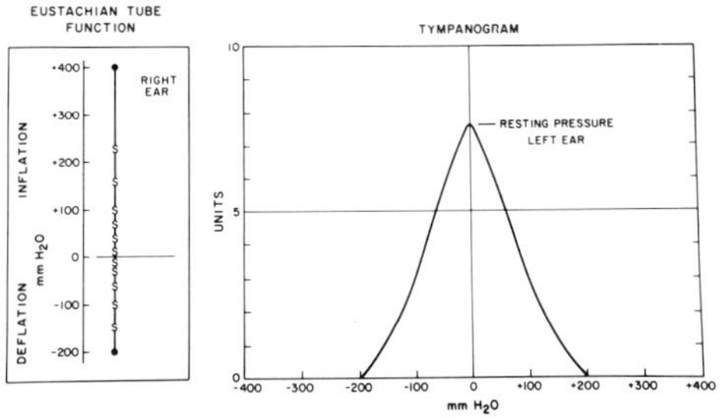

Figure 5-26 Pretympanoplasty evaluation of patient who demonstrated normal inflation-deflation Eustachian tube function test in perforated ear and normal resting pressure in contralateral ear with intact typanic membrane.

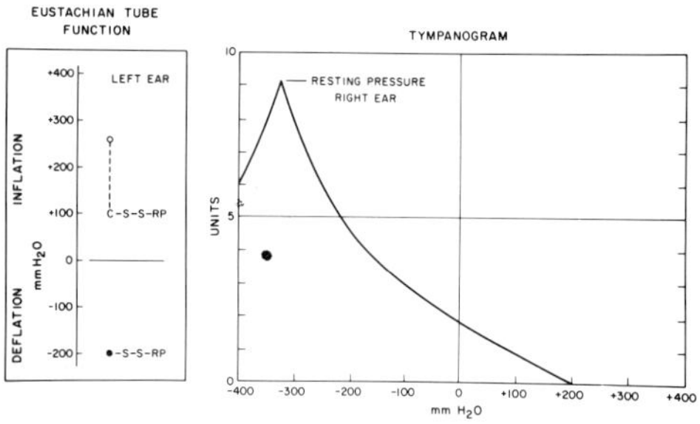

Figure 5-27 Pretympanoplasty evaluation of patient who couldn't equilibrate applied positive or negative pressure during inflation-deflation Eustachian tube test in ear with perforation. Tympanogram of contralateral ear with intact tympanic membrane revealed high negative pressure.

reported a high percentage of success in patients with good Eustachian tube function—i.e., equilibration of applied negative pressure—while in those without this function, surgery frequently failed to close the perforation. Bluestone and colleagues (1978) assessed children prior to tympanoplasty and found that in addition to inflation-deflation studies in the ear with a perforation, tympanometric assessment of a contralateral ear with an intact tympanic membrane may be helpful. Figure 5-26 is an example of such an evaluation. The ear with the perforated tympanic membrane had perfect Eustachian tube inflation-deflation studies. The contralateral ear with an intact tympanic membrane had normal middle ear pressure that was noted on several occasions. Tympanoplasty surgery in such a case was frequently successful. Figure 5-27 is an example of a child with a perforation of the left tympanic membrane whose Eustachian tube function studies revealed no active function. Serial tympanograms in the contralateral ear consistently revealed high negative pressure. Tympanoplasty was usually unsuccessful, i.e., there was graft failure, development of high negative middle ear pressure, or otitis media with effusion when these findings were present. Aside from these extremes, however, neither inflation-deflation Eustachian tube function tests nor tympanometry could be used as a reliable predictor of the results of tympanoplasty in children.

SUMMARY

Even though the present state of our knowledge of Eustachian tube physiology is limited and our testing far from an exact science, the evaluation of patients with middle ear disease, using these techniques, should be performed. A more rational and effective clinical management of patients with middle ear disease should become possible as we gain further understanding of the Eustachian tube and develop improved ways to assess its function.

REFERENCES

Alberti, R. and Kristensen, R.: The clinical application of impedance audiometry. *Laryngoscope* 80:635, 1970.

Aschan, A.: The Eustachian tube. *Acta Otolaryngol. (Stockh.)* 44:295, 1954.

Beery, Q., Bluestone, C.D. and Cantekin, E.I.: Otologic history, audiometry and tympanometry as a case finding procedure for school screening. *Laryngoscope* 85:1976, 1975.

Beery Q., Doyle, W., Wiet, R., Cantekin, E. and Bluestone, C.: Eustachian function in an American Indian population. *Ann. Otol., Rhinol. Laryngol.* 1979. In press.

Bluestone, C.: Eustachian tube obstruction in the infant with cleft palate. *Ann. Otol. Rhinol. Laryngol.* 80 (Suppl. 2): 1, 1971.
Bluestone, C., Paradise, J. and Beery, Q.: Physiology of the Eustachian tube in the pathogenesis and management of middle ear effusions. *Laryngoscope* 82:1654, 1972a.
Bluestone, C., Paradise, J., Beery, Q. and Wittel, R.: Certain effects of cleft palate repair on Eustachian tube function. *Cleft Palate Journ.* 9:183, 1972b.
Bluestone, C., Wittel, R. and Paradise, J.: Roentgenographic evaluation of Eustachian tube function in infants with cleft and normal palates. *Cleft Palate Journ.* 9:93, 1972c.
Bluestone, C., Wittel, R., Paradise, J. and Felder, H.: Eustachian tube function as related to the adenoidectomy for otitis media. *Trans.*AAOO 76:1325, 1972d.
Bluestone, C., Beery, Q. and Paradise, J.: Audiometry and tympanometry in relation to middle ear effusions in children. *Laryngoscope* 83:594, 1973.
Bluestone, C., Beery, Q. and Andrus W.: Mechanics of the Eustachian tube as it influences susceptibility to and persistence of middle ear effusions in children. *Ann. Otol. Rhinol, Laryngol.* 83 (Suppl. 11):27, 1974.
Bluestone, C., Cantekin, E. and Beery, Q.: Certain effects of adenoidectomy on Eustachian tube ventilatory function. *Laryngoscope* 85:113, 1975a.
Bluestone, C., Cantekin, E., Beery, Q. and Paradise, J.: Eustachian tube ventilatory function in relation to cleft palate. *Ann. Otol. Rhinol. Laryngol.* 84:333, 1975b.
Bluestone, C. and Beery, Q.: Concepts on the pathogenesis of middle ear effusions. *Ann. Otol. Rhinol.* Laryngol. 85 (Suppl. 25): 182, 1976.
Bluestone, C., Cantekin, E. and Beery, Q.: Effect of inflammation on the ventilatory function of the Eustachian tube. *Laryngoscope* 87:493, 1977.
Bluestone, C., Cantekin, E., Beery, Q. and Stool, S.: Function of the Eustachian tube related to surgical management of acquired aural cholesteatoma in children. *Laryngoscope* 87:1155, 1978.
Brooks, D.: An objective method of detecting fluid in the middle ear. *J. Internat. Audiol.* 7:280, 1968.
Brooks, D.: The use of the electro-acoustic impedance bridge in the assessment of middle ear positions. *J. Internat. Audiol.* 8:563, 1969.
Brooks, D.: Electro-acoustic impedance bridge studies on normal ears of children. *J. Speech Hearing Res.* 14:247, 1971.
Cantekin, E., Bluestone, C. and Parklin, L.: Eustachian tube ventilatory function in children. *Ann. Otol. Rhinol. Laryngol.* 85 (Suppl. 25):171, 1976.
Cantekin, E., Bluestone, C., Saez, C., Doyle, W. and Phillips, D.: Normal and abnormal middle ear ventilation. *Ann. Otol. Rhinol. Laryngol.* 86 (Suppl. 41):1, 1977.
Cantekin, E., Doyle, W., Reichert, T., Phillips, D. and Bluestone, C.: Dilation of the Eustachian tube by electrical stimulation of the mandibular nerve. *Ann. Otol. Rhinol. Laryngol.* 88:40, 1979.
Compere, W., Jr.: Tympanic cavity clearance studies. *Trans. AAOO* 62:444, 1958.
Doyle, W., Phillips, D., Cantekin, E., Bluestone, C. and Siegel, M.: A non-human primate model of cleft palate and its implications to middle ear pathology. *Ann. Otol. Rhinol. Laryngol.* In press.
Eagles, E., Wishik, S. and Doerfler, L.: Hearing sensitivity and ear disease in children: a prospective study. *Laryngoscope* (Suppl.), 1967.
Elner, A., Ingelstedt, S. and Ivarsson, A.: The normal function of the Eustachian tube. *Acta Otolaryngol. (Stockh.)* 72:320, 1971.
Fisher, R., McAdams, J., Entis, G., Cotton, R., Ghory, J. and Avsden-Moore, R.: Middle ear ciliary defect in Kartagener's syndrome. *Pediatrics* 62:443, 1978.
Flisberg, K., Ingelstedt, S. and Ortegren, U. Controlled "ear aspiration" of air: a "physiological" test of the tubal function. *Acta Otolaryngol. (Stockh.)* 82 (Suppl.):35, 1963.
Harford, E., Bess, R., Bluestone, C. and Klein, J., (Eds.): *Impedance Screening for Middle Ear Disease in Children.* New York, Grune & Stratton, 1978.
Holborow, C.: Eustachian tube function. *Arch. Otolaryngol.* 92:624, 1970.
Holmquist, J.: Eustachian tube function assessed with tympanometry: a new testing procedure in ears with intact tympanic membrane. *Acta Otolaryngol. (Stockh.)* 68:501, 1969.
Holmquist, J.: Middle ear ventilation in chronic otitis media. *Arch. Otolaryngol.* 92:617, 1970.
Ingelstedt, S., Ivarsson, A. and Jonson, B.: Mechanics of the human middle ear; pressure regulation in aviation and diving, a non-traumatic method. *Acta Otolaryngol. (Stockh.)* Suppl. 228, 1967.
Ingelstedt, S., Ivarsson, A. and Jonson, B.: Mechanics of the human middle ear. *Acta Otolaryng. (Stockh.)* Suppl. 228, 1969.
Jerger, J.: Clinical experience with impedance audiometry. *Arch. Otolaryngol.* 92:311, 1970.
Jonson, B. and Rundcrantz, H.: Posture and pressure within the internal jugular vein. *Acta Otolaryngol. (Stockh.)* 68:271, 1969.
Metz, O.: The acoustic impedance measured normal and pathological ears. *Acta Otolaryngol. (Stockh.)* Suppl. 63, 1946.
Miller, G.: Eustachian tube function in normal and diseased ears. *Arch. Otolaryngol.* 81:41, 1965.
Paparella, M., Hiraida, F., Juhn, S. et al.: Cellular events involved in middle ear fluid production. *Ann. Otol. Rhinol. Laryngol.* 79:766, 1970.

Perlman, H.: Observations on the Eustachian tube. *Arch. Otolaryngol.* 55:370, 1951.
Politzer, A.: Ueber die Willkurlichen Bewegungen des Trommelfells. *Weiner Med. Halle. Nr.* 18:103, 1862.
Proctor, B.: Embryology and anatomy of the Eustachian tube. *Arch. Otolaryng.* 86:503, 1967.
Renvall, U., Lidén, G., Jungert, S., Nilsson, E.: Impedance audiometry as screening method in school children. *Scand. Audiol.* 2:133, 1973.
Rich, A.: Physiological study of Eustachian tube and its related muscles. *Bulletin, Johns Hopkins Hospital* 31:206, 1920.
Rood, S. and Doyle, W.: Morphology of M. tensor veli palatini, tensor tympani and dilator tubae muscles. *Ann. Otol. Rhinol. Laryngol.* 87:202, 1978.
Virtanen, H.: Eustachian tube sound conduction—sonotubometry, an acoustical method for objective measurement of auditory tubal opening. Thesis, Department of Otolaryngology, University of Helsinki, Helsinki, Finland, 1977.

Chapter Six

DIAGNOSTIC APPLICATIONS OF IMPEDANCE AUDIOMETRY: MIDDLE EAR DISORDER; SENSORINEURAL DISORDER

JAMES JERGER, Ph.D.
DEBORAH HAYES, Ph.D.

INTRODUCTION

In the diagnostic application of impedance audiometry there are no absolutes. The results of any single measurement—the static compliance, the tympanogram, or the acoustic reflex threshold hearing level—are usually ambiguous and have little individual diagnostic value. We can define ranges of expected normal and abnormal results for each of these measures individually, but the overlap among different clinical groups is usually so large that the absolute values determined for an individual patient are almost uniformly ambiguous.

In spite of this ambiguity in each of the absolute measures, the patterns formed by combinations of different measures are usually unique to specific clinical entities. Within this paradox lies the diagnostic value of impedance audiometry. Individually, each measure lacks specificity, but the combination formed by a suitable test battery often defines a distinct clinical entity.

Learning to use impedance measures diagnostically is an exercise in pattern recognition. The clinician must learn all possible patterns of test results and the clinical entities with which they are associated. Throughout this chapter, the emphasis will be on patterns, their recognition and interpretation. Absolute scores, values, and outcomes will be introduced only insofar as they contribute to the recognition of significant patterns. Specifically, we will discuss the identification of middle ear disorder, the nature of middle ear disorder, and the nature of sensorineural disorder.

IDENTIFICATION OF MIDDLE EAR DISORDER

Middle ear disorder refers to any pathologic alteration in the physical characteristics of the middle ear system. This alteration may or may not result in a conductive hearing loss. A conductive hearing loss refers to a loss in threshold sensitivity resulting from a middle ear disorder. A middle ear disorder does not necessarily produce a conductive hearing loss, but a conductive hearing loss implies middle ear disorder.

The expected pattern (Klockhoff, 1961; Lidén, 1969a; Djupesland, 1969; Jerger, 1970; Lidén et al., 1970; and Jerger et al., 1974a) of results in middle ear disorder is (1) abnormal static compliance; (2) abnormal tympanogram; and (3) elevated or absent acoustic reflexes. Whenever this pattern occurs in its entirety, one can be confident that a middle ear disorder is present. The expected pattern does not, however, always appear in its entirety.

Of the three individual measures, the static compliance is least sensitive to middle ear disorder, the tympanogram is intermediate, and the acoustic reflex is most sensitive (Sheehy, cited in Jerger, 1974; Orchik et al., 1978a).

In general, the absolute value of the static compliance is diagnostically useful only if it is very large or very small. For example, otitis media is a clinical entity in which the static compliance almost always falls below the normal range (Paradise et al., 1976; Haughton, 1977). Values below 0.30 cc are the rule. Whenever the static compliance falls into this low range, the presence of a middle ear disorder and consequent conductive hearing loss may be reasonably inferred.

Similarly, discontinuity of the ossicular chain usually produces static compliance values well above the normal limit of 1.60 cc. Values in the range from 1.80 to 2.55 cc are not uncommon and usually indicate the presence of a substantial middle ear disorder.

Unfortunately, with the exception of these two extreme categories, the static compliance values of middle ear disorders tend to overlap the normal range to a disconcerting degree (Terkildsen and Nielsen, 1960; Bicknell and Morgan, 1968; Jerger, 1970; and Jerger et al., 1974a). In otosclerosis, for example, values in the normal range are not uncommon (Segers, 1974). Thus, the observation of abnormal static compliance indicates a possible middle ear disorder, but the observation of static compliance within the normal range does not necessarily rule out a middle ear disorder.

The shape of the tympanogram is a somewhat more sensitive indicator of middle ear disorder than the static compliance, but major ambiguities exist. Negative pressure in the middle ear space usually produces a type C tympanogram, and a variety of disorders produce the type B, but two important categories of middle ear disorder, otosclerosis and ossicular discontinuity, produce type A configurations. Again, we must conclude that the presence of an abnormal tympanogram argues for a middle ear disorder, but the presence of a normally shaped tympanogram does not rule one out.

The acoustic reflex is much more sensitive to the presence of a middle ear disorder than either the static compliance or the tympanogram. When the reflex-eliciting signal is delivered to an ear with a middle ear disorder and the probe is coupled to the opposite, normal, ear, the reflex threshold hearing level (HTL) typically will be elevated by the amount of the conductive hearing loss (Jerger et al., 1974a). A conductive hearing loss of 30 dB, for example, will raise the reflex HTL from a normal level of 85 dB to an elevated level of 115 dB (85 plus 30). When the probe is coupled to an ear with a middle ear disorder of even the slightest degree, the acoustic reflex typically is absent altogether. The acoustic reflex is thus sensitive to middle ear disorder in both the signal-eliciting (sound) and recording (probe) conditions. Because of this sensitivity, it is usually safe to conclude that there is no middle ear disorder in either ear if reflex HTLs are normal in both ears.

Although normal reflex levels usually argue against a middle ear disorder, abnormal reflex findings do not necessarily argue for middle ear disorder. The reflex abnormalities may very well be symptoms of either cochlear or retrocochlear disorder.

Each of the three measures is individually ambiguous. Normal static compliance does not rule out a middle ear disorder; normal tympanogram does not rule out a middle ear disorder; abnormal reflex thresholds do not necessarily confirm a middle ear disorder. It is not surprising, therefore, that previous attempts to use any of these measures individually, even in screening applications, have led to certain frustrations (Bicknell and Morgan, 1968; Lidén, 1969a; Alberti and Jerger, 1974; Beery et al., 1975; Paradise et al., 1976; Orchik et al., 1978a; and Orchik et al., 1978b).

In combination, however, these measures define patterns uniquely sensitive to middle ear disorder and conductive hearing loss. In practice, it is almost impossible to miss a middle ear disorder if the overall pattern of impedance results is carefully scrutinized. If any one impedance measure is abnormal, the presence of a middle ear disorder must be strongly suspected. Within this framework, we can consider the patterns of impedance test results and how they relate to specific types and configurations of hearing disorder.

THE NATURE OF MIDDLE EAR DISORDER

Impedance audiometry can yield valuable information on the nature of middle ear disorder, but it is important to emphasize two related principles in the interpretation of any impedance pattern.

First, impedance alterations do not result from a disease process per se, but from its effect on the physics of the middle ear vibratory mechanism. Thus, the impedance pattern associated with otosclerosis, for example, is not caused by the otosclerotic disease process but by the effect of ossicular chain fixation on the impedance characteristics of the middle ear system. This important distinction is easily lost as our discussion turns toward the impedance results associated with specific types of middle ear disorder.

The second related principle is that impedance patterns do not diagnose a particular disease process. We can predict, with a reasonable degree of accuracy, that a particular pattern of impedance results is consistent with a particular ear disease. However, the practice of diagnosing a middle ear disorder (i.e., serous otitis, cholesteatoma) from the impedance results alone should be scrupulously avoided. Usually you will be right, but you will also be embarrassingly wrong on those rare occasions when an obscure anatomic variant mimics a more common affliction.

With these two important principles in mind, we can now consider the constellation of impedance findings associated with different types of middle ear disorder.

Otosclerosis

In patients with otosclerosis and related ossicular chain fixation, the tympanogram is usually a shallow type A, the static compliance is usually in the range from 0.20 to 0.40 cc, and the acoustic reflex is usually not observed in either ear (Bicknell and Morgan, 1968; Lidén, 1969a; Jerger, 1970; Lidén et al., 1970; Alberti and Kristensen, 1970; Jerger et al., 1974a; Bel et al., 1975; Dancer et al., 1977; and Dieroff, 1978).

The type A tympanogram is the "impedance signature" of ossicular fixation. There is virtually no other type of middle disorder that does not show some abnormality in the tympanogram. The very fact of a type A tympanogram in an ear with a conductive hearing loss, then, is pathognomonic of ossicular fixation. There may be, however, considerable variation in the depth of the tympanogram. Many patients with otosclerosis will show tympanograms with no obvious abnormality (Dancer et al., 1977; Dieroff, 1978).

Similarly, although the static compliance is usually below the range of normal, in some patients with otosclerosis the static compliance will be well within the normal range (Segers, 1974). Thus, a normal tympanogram and normal static compliance values, associated with a conductive hearing loss, are particularly characteristic of ossicular fixation.

Also characteristic of ossicular fixation is the absence of acoustic reflexes. Rarely, in the very early stages of stapes fixation, the acoustic reflex may be elicited at relatively normal hearing levels. Usually, however, these reflexes will show a uniquely abnormal time course characterized by a negative deflection (decrease in impedance) at both the onset and conclusion of the eliciting signal (Djupesland, 1963, 1969; Terkildsen et al., 1973; Causse et al., 1974; and Bel et al., 1974). Negative deflections at the onset of the eliciting signal are not abnormal; they occur in most normal ears. Negative deflections at the end of the eliciting signal, however, are definitely abnormal. Figure 6-1 compares the time course of a typical normal and a typical "otosclerotic" reflex. This double negative deflection pattern seems to result from early ossicular chain fixation (Bel et al., 1974, 1975). The clinician should remember, however, that it is not otosclerosis per se, but ossicular fixation that produces the abnormal temporal pattern. Its presence, therefore, does not necessarily mean otosclerosis. Other disorders producing ossicular chain fixation may produce the same result.

In summary, otosclerosis is characterized by a type A tympanogram that may or may not be exceedingly shallow; static compliance that may or may not be somewhat below the normal range; and reflexes that may or may not be present. If present, however, reflexes tend to show a "double negative" time course with well-defined negative deflections at both the onset and termination of the reflex-eliciting signal.

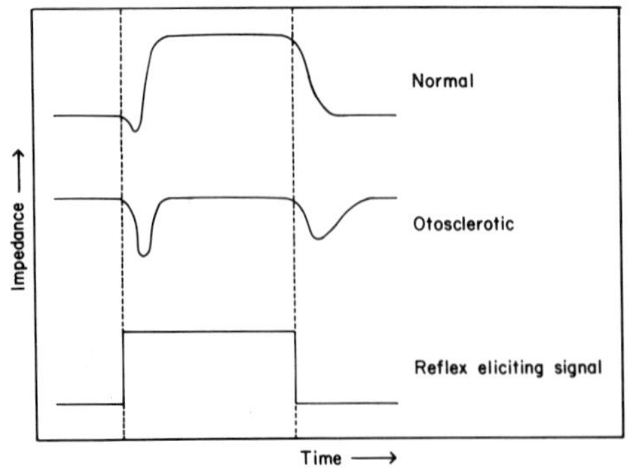

Figure 6-1 Time course of acoustic reflex in normal ear and in otosclerotic ear. Note that both show negative deflection at onset, but only "otosclerotic" reflex shows negative deflection at conclusion.

Ossicular Discontinuity

The expected outcome in discontinuity is an abnormally deep type A tympanogram, static compliance well above the normal range, and absent acoustic reflexes (Lidén, 1969b; Jerger et al., 1974a; Lidén et al., 1974, 1977; Lidén, 1975; and Chesnutt et al., 1975). There are, however, several qualifications and exceptions.

Although abnormally deep tympanograms characterize ossicular discontinuity, they are not unique to this disorder (Feldman, 1974; Alberti and Jerger, 1974; and Keller, 1976). Any condition that increases the flaccidity of the tympanic membrane (TM) will produce the same effect on the tympanogram. A good example is the monomeric membrane. This will almost always produce an abnormally deep tympanogram indistinguishable from ossicular discontinuity.

Several investigators have described "W-shaped" tympanograms, believed to be unique to ossicular discontinuity, when the frequency of the probe tone is raised from 220 Hz to 660 to 900 Hz (see Chapter 3). We now know (Alberti and Jerger, 1974), however, that the "W" configuration at higher probe-tone frequencies can be produced by so many varieties of TM disease that its diagnostic value, especially with respect to ossicular discontinuity, is extremely limited.

Although static compliance values well above the range of normal characterize ossicular discontinuity, they, too, are not unique to this disorder. Similar to the case of the abnormally deep tympanogram, any condition that increases the flaccidity of the TM will produce aberrant static compliance values. Furthermore, static compliance values within the high range of normal (i.e., 1.00 to 1.60 cc) have frequently been observed in ossicular discontinuity.

While the acoustic reflex is typically absent in an ear with an ossicular discontinuity, it may infrequently be observed when sound is presented to the opposite, normal ear (Hayes, 1977). In other words, the reflex is observed even though the probe tip is coupled to an ear with a significant middle ear disorder. This unusual situation arises when there is a functional connection between the stapedius tendon and that portion of the ossicular chain still attached to the tympanic membrane. This case may occur, for example, when only the anterior crus of the stapes is fractured. In this case, the partial discontinuity may produce a substantial conductive hearing loss, but the contraction of the stapedius muscle can alter the impedance of the remainder of the chain still attached to the TM.

Thus, although the tympanogram, static compliance, and acoustic reflex may not produce the classic pattern of ossicular discontinuity, the degree of conductive hearing loss is a helpful consideration in identifying this disorder. The combination of an abnormally deep type A tympanogram, static compliance above the range of normal, and a substantial air-bone gap (30 to 50 dB) even in the presence of relatively normal acoustic reflex threshold hearing levels with the probe in the conductive ear, points decisively to ossicular discontinuity, since other conditions likely to produce abnormally deep tympanograms and aberrant static compliance seldom produce concomitant conductive hearing loss.

In summary, the overall pattern of results in ossicular discontinuity is an abnormally deep type A tympanogram, static compliance well above the normal range, and a substantial conductive hearing loss. The acoustic reflex is usually absent to sound in the opposite ear but may be present if a functional connection exists between the stapedius tendon and the TM.

Here, again, we have a good example of the importance of pattern. The abnormally deep tympanogram, per se, is ambiguous; the acoustic reflex is ambiguous; the sizable conductive hearing loss is ambiguous. The combination of all three, however, is virtually unique to ossicular discontinuity.

Otitis Media

In general, impedance measures reflect the various stages in the development of middle ear infection. As the air in the middle ear space is exhausted, owing to blockage or faulty function of the Eustachian tube, negative air pressure causes retraction of the tympanic membrane. The effect on the tympanogram is immediate. The peak of the tympanogram is shifted in the region of negative air pressure by an amount equivalent to the static negative pressure in the middle ear space. This is, of course, the familiar type C tympanogram. It is a fundamental type A shape, but with the peak occurring at a significant negative air pressure. As the air in the middle ear space becomes more and more exhausted and the drum becomes more and more retracted, the peak of the type C tympanogram moves systematically downward into the region of negative pressure. The peak may occur at a negative pressure as low as -600 mm/$H_2$0.

Eventually, however, the lack of sufficient air causes effusion from the tissue lining the middle ear space. As fluid fills the middle ear space, the first effect on the tympanogram is a rounding of the peak, a blunting of its usually sharp definition. As the fluid level increases, the mobility of the ossicular chain decreases, and the middle ear impedance increases, usually to a fairly substantial extent. This increase in impedance, with consequent decrease in compliance, causes the rounded peak of the tympanogram to drop lower and lower. In a completely fluid-filled ear the tympanogram may be almost a flat line, with little or no evidence of compliance maximum. We refer to all such tympanograms as type B. They represent a later or more serious stage of otitis media than the type C, eardrum-retracted stage. Figure 6–2 shows a series of tympanograms illustrating the various stages through which the tympanogram progresses during the development of acute serous otitis media.

In the early, type C stage of otitis media, the static compliance, measured at the peak of the tympanogram, will of course be well within normal limits. As the tympanogram goes into the type B configuration, however, the static compliance drops, usually to an extremely low value. Results in the range of 0.10 to 0.21 cc are not uncommon. This is one of the few middle ear conditions in which the static compliance typically falls well below the normal range of 0.30 to 1.60 cc.

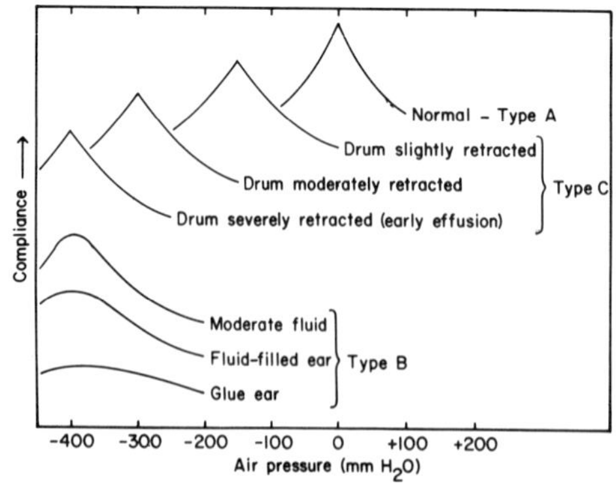

Figure 6–2 Series of tympanograms illustrating various stages through which tympanogram progresses during development of acute serous otitis media.

The acoustic reflex usually disappears at a very early stage of otitis media, owing to the gross increase in impedance. In the very early stages, however, when the tympanogram is still type C, one may observe the reflex if care is taken to hold air pressure at the exact peak of the tympanogram. In some patients this is easily done and reflexes can be demonstrated. In other patients, however, with similar tympanograms and audiograms, the peak pressure is less easily maintained and reflexes are difficult—sometimes impossible—to demonstrate. In later stages, when the tympanogram is type B, reflexes are virtually eliminated.

Tympanogram shape, static compliance, and the acoustic reflex are all useful in monitoring the patient's recovery from otitis media. If ventilating tubes are inserted in the TMs, the static compliance measures immediately tell whether the tube is patent. If the initial volume measurement is consistent with normal values for the volume of the external ear canal (0.50 to 1.50 cc), the tube is blocked. If, however, the initial volume measurement is grossly larger (2.00 to 3.00 cc), one may then infer that the tube is patent and the combined volume of external canal and middle ear space is being measured. This analysis is especially useful when, because of faulty Eustachian tube function, the air pressure introduced to the external canal does not leak out of the middle ear space. The only drawback to the above observation is that similarly large air volumes are also encountered in ears with mastoid cavities.

As the otitic ear heals, the tympanogram gradually changes from type B to type C to type A and progress can be usefully monitored. Finally, when the acoustic reflex returns, a near-normal middle ear mechanism may be assumed.

In summary, otitis media produces a characteristic sequence of changes in the tympanogram, a marked lowering of the static compliance, and early disappearance of the acoustic reflex. In the early stage, with the type C tympanogram, the reflex may be demonstrable if air pressure can be successfully maintained at the peak of the tympanogram. All three impedance measures are useful in monitoring the success of therapy for otitis media.

Cholesteatoma

Ears with cholesteatoma clearly illustrate the principle that impedance measures reflect the alteration in middle ear physics caused by a particular disease process rather than the disease process itself. Cholesteatoma may mimic ossicular fixation, otitis media, or even discontinuity, depending on the nature and extent of ossicular chain involvement. If the cholesteatoma produces only slight pressure against the ossicular chain, the impedance pattern of early fixation (type A tympanogram, relatively normal or slightly reduced static compliance, elevated reflex thresholds) will appear. If, however, the tumor occupies much of the middle ear space and virtually envelops the vibratory mechanism, adding substantial mass to the system, then the impedance characteristic of serous otitis (type B tympanogram, low static compliance, absent acoustic reflexes) will usually be seen. Finally, if the cholesteatoma erodes through the lenticular process of the incus, or the incudostapedial articulation, the impedance pattern characteristic of discontinuity may well appear. In the latter case it is not unusual to find that the cholesteatoma itself forms a functional link between incus and stapes, leading to a characteristically rounded tympanogram and surprisingly little conductive hearing loss.

Perforation of the Tympanic Membrane

Perforation of the tympanic membrane is the unique condition when static compliance measurement is diagnostically significant. In this case, measurement of the volume of air in the external ear canal ("Z_1") may reveal the presence of a perforation not readily visible otoscopically. The typical volume measurement of air in the external canal is between 0.50 and 1.50 cc. A volume in excess of 2.00 cc usually means that the tympanic membrane is perforated, although a mastoid cavity may result in a similar reading. In the case of a perforated TM, neither the tympanogram nor acoustic reflexes can be recorded.

In summary, in evaluating any pattern of impedance results, it is important to remember the principle that impedance reflects not the eitologic factors of disease, but their effect on middle ear physics. Thus, congenital stapes fixation, malleolar fixation, or any other process that increases the stiffness of the ossicular chain, will produce an impedance picture indistinguishable from otosclerosis. Similarly, tympanosclerosis, monomeric membrane, atrophic scar—in short, virtually any residual damage following disease of the tympanic membrane—will present an impedance pattern not easily differentiated from ossicular discontinuity.

In reporting the results of impedance audiometry, then, it is best to describe the alterations or modifications in middle ear function, and perhaps to note their consistency with one or more common types of middle ear disorder. In most cases, however, it is hazardous to attempt to diagnose the middle ear disease on the basis of impedance results alone.

THE NATURE OF SENSORINEURAL DISORDER

Although impedance testing was originally advocated primarily for the evaluation of middle ear disorders, clinical experience has shown that it makes an even more important contribution in the area of sensorineural hearing loss. The most exciting application is the differentiation of cochlear and eighth nerve disorders. More recent applications in facial nerve disorder and neuromuscular disease promise to increase the diagnostic value of impedance audiometry even further.

Patterns of Acoustic Reflexes

The acoustic reflex is the most important impedance measure in the diagnosis of sensorineural hearing loss. This does not imply in any way that the total test battery is not important. Rather, it is assumed that the clinician has first scrutinized the results of the static compliance, the tympanogram, the acoustic reflex tests, and all other audiometric data and has ruled out a middle ear disorder. It is now time to study even more carefully the pattern of acoustic reflex results to arrive at a diagnostic impression.

In sensorineural evaluation, the important diagnostic patterns are formed by (1) the relationship of the uncrossed acoustic reflex to the crossed acoustic reflex, (2) the relationship of the acoustic reflex hearing threshold level (HTL) to the degree of hearing loss, and (3) the time-course of the reflex to sustained signals.

The importance of the uncrossed acoustic reflex cannot be overemphasized.

Before its standard clinical usage, certain ambiguities existed in the interpretation of reflex abnormalities. For example, an absent acoustic reflex might be the result of:

a. insufficient loudness in the ear to which the reflex eliciting signal is delivered;
b. a seventh nerve disorder in the recording (probe) ear; or
c. a middle ear disorder of even the mildest degree in the probe ear.

The uncrossed acoustic reflex allows differentiation of these effects. If a reflex cannot be elicited whenever sound is presented to one ear, irrespective of whether the probe is coupled to the same ear (uncrossed condition) or opposite ear (crossed condition), and all other reflexes are normal, then the problem is a "sound effect"; sound cannot be sufficiently loud to elicit a reflex contraction. A seventh nerve disorder or middle ear disorder can be effectively ruled out. Conversely, if a reflex is abnormal whenever the probe is in a particular ear, regardless of how the reflex-eliciting signal is delivered (crossed or uncrossed condition), then a "probe effect" must be strongly suspected. In this case the reflex abnormality is probably the result of either a seventh nerve disorder or a middle ear disorder in the recording ear. As with any impedance result, these patterns do not represent absolutes. Nonetheless, in the hands of a skilled clinician, they are invaluable in analyzing potentially ambiguous acoustic reflex situations.

One useful method for visualizing the results of the crossed and uncrossed acoustic reflex tests is shown in Figure 6–3. The top half of the figure (upper "face") represents the results of the crossed acoustic reflex test. The bottom half of the figure (lower "face") represents the results of the uncrossed acoustic reflex test. In both cases the results are recorded for the 1000 Hz reflex-eliciting signal only. When all reflexes are present at normal HTLs, the four boxes are left open. When a reflex is abnormal, however, the appropriate box is either hatched, if the reflex is present but abnormal, or filled in, if the reflex is absent altogether.

Figure 6–4A–D shows four distinct reflex patterns that may emerge when the results of acoustic reflex testing are presented in this fashion.

Figure 6–4A shows the absence of acoustic reflex whenever the probe is coupled to a particular ear, in this case, the left ear. An acoustic reflex cannot be recorded from the left ear regardless of whether the eliciting signal is delivered to the opposite

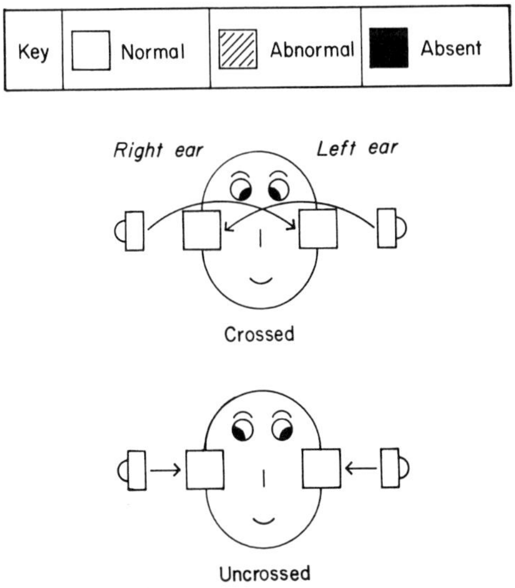

Figure 6–3 Form for recording crossed and uncrossed acoustic reflexes. Boxes are left open if reflex is normal, hatched if reflex is present but abnormal, filled-in if reflex is absent altogether.

ear (crossed acoustic reflex) or the same ear (uncrossed acoustic reflex). This vertical pattern is essentially a peripheral configuration. It suggests that the absence of the acoustic reflex is due to the efferent portion of the acoustic reflex arc (seventh nerve disorder or middle ear disorder). In the case presented in Figure 6–4A, this pattern

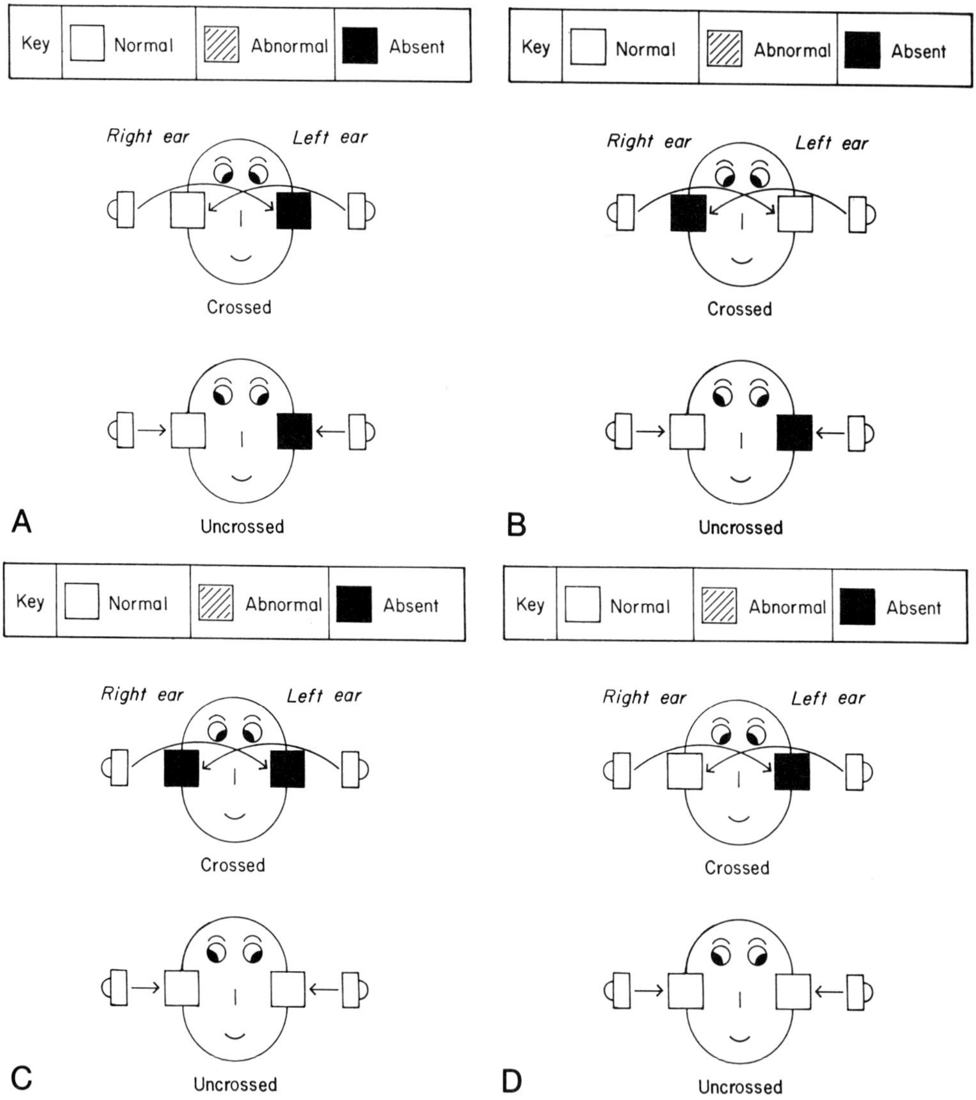

Figure 6–4 (A)Vertical acoustic reflex pattern representing absence of acoustic reflex whenever probe is coupled to left ear. This pattern is consistent with left seventh nerve or mild left middle ear disorder.
(B)Diagonal acoustic reflex pattern representing absence of acoustic reflex whenever sound is delivered to left ear. This pattern is consistent with left eighth nerve or severe left cochlear disorder.
(C)Horizontal acoustic reflex pattern representing absence of both crossed acoustic reflexes. Both uncrossed acoustic reflexes are normal. This pattern suggests brain stem pathway disorder.
(D)"Unibox" acoustic reflex pattern representing abnormality of one crossed acoustic reflex. The other crossed and both uncrossed reflexes are normal. This rare pattern is associated with brain stem disorder.

might represent the results from a subject with left facial paralysis or a mild middle ear disorder in the left ear.

Figure 6–4B shows the absence of the acoustic reflex whenever sound is delivered to the left ear. This diagonal pattern suggests abnormality in the afferent portion of the acoustic reflex arc (cochlear disorder or eighth nerve disorder). The pattern shown in Figure 6–4B might be expected in a patient with a severe cochlear disorder in the left ear or a left eighth nerve disorder. In either case, middle ear function is probably normal in both ears.

Figure 6–4C shows absence of the crossed acoustic reflex in both ears. Acoustic reflexes are present, however, to signals presented in the uncrossed condition. This relatively rare horizontal pattern is the result of an interruption of the crossed pathways of the acoustic reflex arc in the brain stem. It may be seen in patients with intra-axial brain stem disorders.

Finally, Figure 6–4D represents the rare "unibox" pattern (Jerger et al., 1979). It shows the absence of one crossed acoustic reflex. The other crossed reflex and both uncrossed acoustic reflexes, however, are present at normal levels. This pattern is typically seen in patients with specific brain stem disorders. Even in these patients the unibox pattern occurs only infrequently.

These four acoustic reflex patterns do not necessarily represent every possible case. Nevertheless, they are helpful in assessing and interpreting results of the acoustic reflex tests. By learning the various reflex configurations associated with different auditory disorders, the clinician can sharpen his or her diagnostic acumen.

DIFFERENTIATING COCHLEAR AND EIGHTH NERVE DISORDERS

The acoustic reflex is useful in differentiating cochlear from eighth nerve disorders in two ways. First, the acoustic reflex is characteristically present in ears with cochlear disorder (below a limiting degree of hearing loss) and characteristically absent in ears with an eighth nerve disorder. Second, when the acoustic reflex is unexpectedly present in an ear with an eighth nerve disorder, it typically exhibits an abnormal time course to sustained signals.

Cochlear

In the ear with a cochlear disorder, the reflex sensation level (SL) for pure tones in the 500 to 4000 Hz region declines in exact proportion to the degree of hearing loss (Jerger et al., 1974b, 1978). It is a decibel-for-decibel trade. This relationship is illustrated graphically in Figure 6–5. Data are based on reflex thresholds (SLs) of 515 patients with varying degrees of sensorineural (cochlear) hearing loss. Note that, at O dB hearing loss, the average reflex SL is 85 dB. At 40 dB hearing loss, however, the average reflex SL is only 45 dB. The function decelerates and levels off at an average limiting SL of 25 dB. This sets an upper limit on the degree of sensorineural hearing loss that will still show a reflex. If the upper limit of the audiometer producing the reflex-eliciting signal is 110 dB, then the maximum cochlear hearing loss still showing a reflex would be, on the average, 85 dB (110 minus 25). If the upper limit of the audiometer is 125 dB, then the maximum loss will be 100 dB (125 minus 25). This is usually a sufficient range to include most testable sensorineural losses.

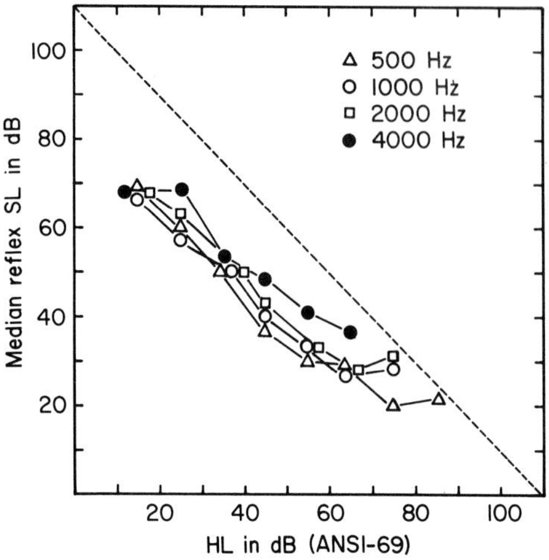

Figure 6–5 Reflex SL and degree of hearing loss (in dB HL) in 515 patients with sensorineural (cochlear) loss. (Reprinted by permission of A.M.A. *Arch. Otolaryngol.* 96:513, 1972.

The practical implication of this finding is that if a patient has a sensorineural loss that does not exceed 85 to 100 dB, and the loss is cochlear, he ought to show a reflex when a sufficiently intense sound is introduced into that ear.

Figures 6–6 through 6–8 show the expected acoustic reflex patterns in a variety of ears with a cochlear disorder on the left. Figure 6–6 represents the result of a mild-to-moderate (20 to 75 dB) hearing loss. All four boxes are left open because all crossed and uncrossed reflexes are present at normal levels (85 to 100 dB HTL). Figure 6–7 shows the expected result in a cochlear ear with a hearing loss ranging from 85 to 100 dB. The boxes representing sound to the normal (right) ear are left open, indicating normal acoustic reflexes when sound is presented to that ear. The boxes representing sound to the left ear, however, are hatched, indicating the elevation of the reflex HTL to 105 dB or more when sound is presented to that ear. Finally, Figure 6–8 represents the acoustic reflex result in an ear with a profound cochlear hearing loss. Reflexes with sound in the right ear are again normal, represented by open boxes. With sound in the left ear, however, all reflexes are absent, represented with blackened boxes. In profound sensorineural loss, this diagonal reflex pattern is the "signature" condition.

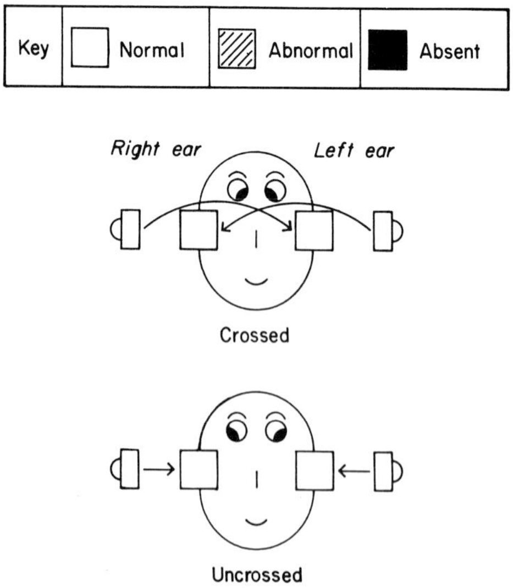

Figure 6–6 Crossed and uncrossed acoustic reflex results in patient with normal hearing in right ear and mild cochlear loss in left ear. All boxes are left open, indicating normal reflexes in both ears.

The observation of the second pattern (Fig. 6–7), elevated reflex HTLs associated with a mild hearing loss, or the third pattern (Fig. 6–8), absent acoustic reflexes, associated with a mild-to-moderate hearing loss, should always raise the strong suspicion of an eighth nerve disorder. Anderson and colleagues (1969) were the first investigators to describe essentially three abnormal acoustic reflex findings in patients with eighth nerve disorders. These are (1) elevated acoustic reflexes; (2) absent acoustic reflexes; and (3) acoustic reflex decay.

Eighth Nerve: Reflex Elevation and Absence

The phenomenon of "elevated" reflex thresholds in eighth nerve disorder refers to the elevation of the reflex HTL in relation to expectation based on normal and cochlear ears. In terms of reflex SL, however, the threshold is quite "normal." For example, in the normal ear, both reflex HTL and SL are 85 dB. In the ear with a 30 dB cochlear loss, reflex HTL will also be 85 dB, but reflex SL will be 55 dB (85 minus 30). In the ear with a 30 dB loss due to an eighth nerve disorder, however, reflex HTL will be 115 dB and reflex SL will be 85 dB (115 minus 30). These various relations are illustrated by a hypothetical example in Table 6–1.

Since the reflex SL tends to remain "normal" (i.e., 85 dB) in eighth nerve disorders, increasing hearing loss will eventually drive the reflex HTL beyond the upper limit of the audiometer. If the upper limit of the audiometer producing the reflex-eliciting signal is 100 dB, we would expect the reflex to disappear altogether when hearing loss exceeds 25 dB. It is not surprising, then, that reflexes are the exception rather than the rule in eighth nerve disorder. (Jerger et al., 1974b; Olsen et al., 1975; Sheehy and Inzer, 1976; and Johnson, 1977). Unless the audiometric loss is

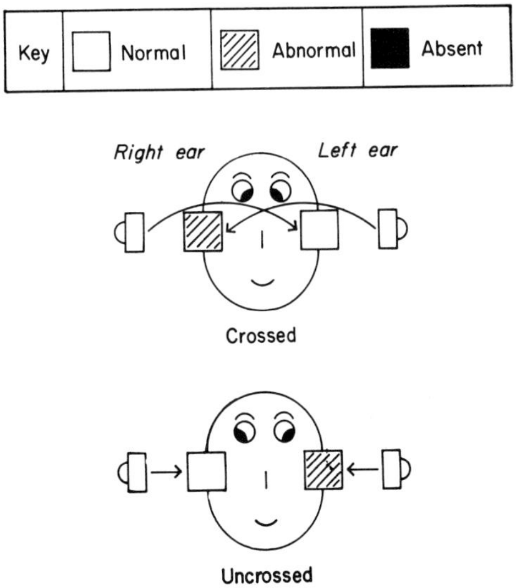

Figure 6–7 Crossed and uncrossed acoustic reflex results for patient with normal hearing in right ear and severe cochlear loss in left ear. Reflexes are normal with sound in right ear (open boxes) but elevated with sound in left ear (hatched boxes).

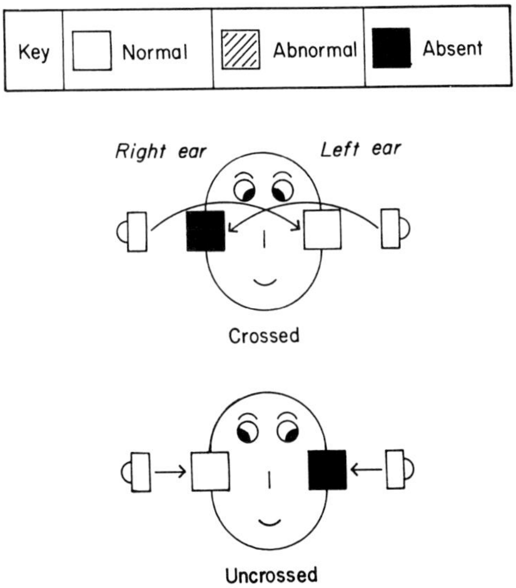

Figure 6–8 Crossed and uncrossed acoustic reflex results for patient with normal hearing in right ear and profound cochlear loss in left ear. Reflexes are normal with sound in right ear (open boxes) but absent with sound in left ear (filled-in boxes).

Table 6-1. Hypothetical reflex data*

Type of Ear	Threshold HL	Reflex HL	Reflex SL
Normal	0	85	85
Cochlear	30	85	55
Eighth Nerve	30	115	85

*These data illustrate threshold abnormality (abnormally small reflex SL) in cochlear disorder, and "elevated" reflex threshold (normal reflex SL) in eighth nerve disorder.

very slight, the acoustic reflex is usually not elicited at all in eighth nerve disorders.

Figure 6-9 shows the relationship between hearing loss due to cochlear and eighth nerve disorder and acoustic reflex HTLs analyzed by Jerger and colleagues (1974). When hearing level is within normal limits, the likelihood of reflex absence in eighth nerve disorder is 30 percent. It increases disproportionately with hearing loss. A sensitivity loss of only 30 dB, for example, results in a 70 percent likelihood of absent acoustic reflexes.

Eighth Nerve: Reflex Decay

A second reflex abnormality associated with eighth nerve disorder is reflex decay. As shown in Figure 6-10, reflex decay is a remarkable phenomenon. When the reflex-eliciting signal is first turned on, the reflex appears normally. As the signal is sustained, however, the reflex amplitude gradually declines and eventually disappears altogether. Reflex decay may be observed for both crossed and uncrossed signal conditions.

Such reflex decay is common in many normal ears at 2000 Hz, and especially at 4000 Hz (Alberti, 1974; Habener and Synder, 1974; Cunningham, 1976; and Kaplan et al., 1976). Its presence in this frequency region, therefore, has no pathologic significance. At 500 and 1000 Hz, however, such decay is very rare in normal ears. Its appearance at either of these frequencies is strongly indicative of eighth nerve site. A useful test for reflex decay is to sustain a 500 or 1000 Hz test signal for 10 seconds at a reflex SL of 10 dB (i.e., 10 dB above reflex HTL at that frequency). If the reflex amplitude declines to less than one half of its initial value within the 10-second test period, abnormal decay is present. Some investigators (Hall, C., 1977) have proposed a time-limit of less than 10 seconds for the reflex decay test. This is based on the observation that in most cases of eighth nerve disorder, reflex decay is complete within

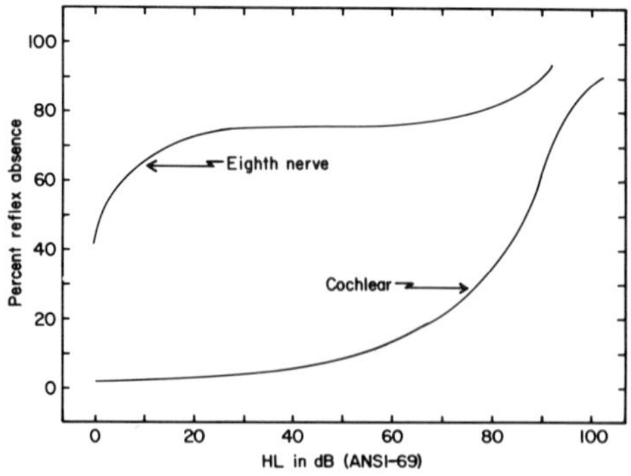

Figure 6-9 Relationship between degree of hearing loss and likelihood of reflex absence in cochlear and eighth nerve disorder.

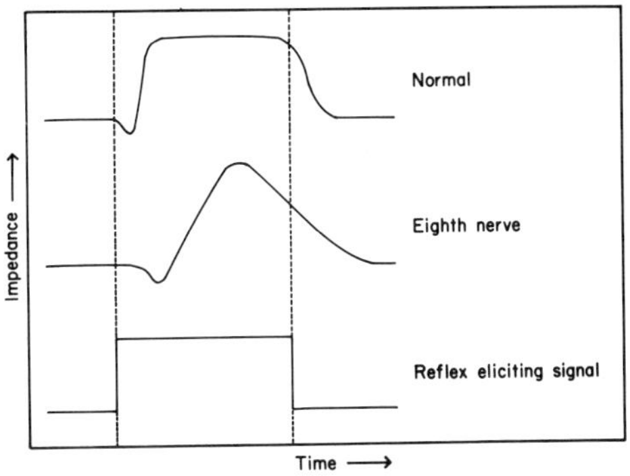

Figure 6-10 Time course of acoustic reflex in normal ear and in ear with eighth nerve disorder. Note that both show a normal amplitude deflection when reflex-eliciting signal is first turned on, but that eighth nerve reflex amplitude gradually declines and finally disappears altogether within a 10-second time period.

5 seconds (Anderson et al., 1969; Colletti, 1975; and Chiveralls et al., 1976). For practical purposes, however, we have found a reflex decay test of 10 seconds to be more clinically manageable. To carry out any reflex decay testing, some kind of strip-chart write-out of the reflex time course is virtually mandatory.

The combination of the acoustic reflex threshold test and the acoustic reflex decay test is exquisitely sensitive to eighth nerve disorders. Reports by Jerger and colleagues (1974), Olsen and colleagues (1975), Sheehy and Inzer (1976), Johnson (1977), and Hall (in press) indicate that the identification rate of eighth nerve disorders by both acoustic reflex tests ranges from 77 to 86 percent.

For such sensitivity, however, we must expect to pay a price. In the case of the acoustic reflex, the price is a high false-positive rate (Chiveralls et al., 1976; Chiveralls, 1977). In a survey of studies reporting reflex results in cochlear ears, Hall (in press) reported a false-positive rate in cochlear ears (either absent or decaying reflexes) ranging from 11 to 16 percent. The false-negative rate for ears with eighth nerve disorder (normal reflexes) was approximately 15 percent. These figures indicate that although acoustic reflex tests cannot replace the total "test battery" approach to the evaluation of sensorineural hearing loss (Thomsen and Terkildsen, 1975), these tests are among the most powerful for differentiating cochlear from eighth nerve disorders (Olsen et al., 1975; Sheehy and Inzer, 1976; and Johnson, 1977).

The fruitful diagnostic application of acoustic reflex tests lies in the clinician's ability to recognize the various relationships between crossed acoustic reflexes, uncrossed acoustic reflexes, and the pure-tone audiogram. It is essential, however, to remember that as in the case of conductive hearing loss and the total impedance picture, acoustic reflex results in sensorineural hearing loss cannot be analyzed in isolation.

OTHER DIAGNOSTIC APPLICATIONS OF THE ACOUSTIC REFLEX

Facial Nerve Disorder

The acoustic reflex test has become a valuable adjunct for localizing the site of a facial (seventh cranial) nerve disorder (Alford et al., 1973, 1974; Citron and Adour, 1978). In addition to ennervating the facial muscles, the facial nerve controls tearing, the stapedius muscle, salivation, and taste from the anterior two thirds of the tongue. The branch that controls tearing, the greater superficial petrosal nerve, branches proximal (above) the branching to the stapedius muscle. The branch controlling salivation and taste, the chorda tympani nerve, branches distal (below) the branch to the stapedius muscle. The acoustic reflex is helpful in determining if a facial nerve lesion is proximal or distal to the branching of the facial nerve to the stapedius muscle.

In general, three reflex patterns may emerge depending on the site of a facial nerve disorder. The first pattern is absence of the acoustic reflex whenever the probe is in the ear on the affected side. Regardless of whether the reflex-eliciting signal is delivered to the same (uncrossed condition) or opposite (crossed condition) ear, no contraction of the stapedius muscle is observed. This pattern may be seen when the facial nerve disorder is proximal to the branching to the stapedius muscle.

A second pattern that might be observed with a disorder in a proximal site is when acoustic reflexes are present but elevated. In this case, sound elicits the reflex contraction but only to abnormally loud signal levels (greater than 100 dB). This pattern may be observed in patients with recovering facial nerve function.

A third reflex pattern associated with facial nerve disorder is normal acoustic reflexes. In this pattern, all four reflexes (both crossed and both uncrossed) are present at normal reflex HTLs. This pattern is typically seen in patients with facial nerve disorder distal to the branching of the facial nerve to the stapedius muscle.

Acoustic reflex measures are helpful not only in localizing the site of a facial nerve disorder, but also in charting facial nerve recovery (Citron and Adour, 1978). In a subject with idiopathic facial nerve palsy, for example, reflex testing over the course of several days or weeks may show initially absent reflexes, then present but elevated reflexes, and finally normal reflexes as the disorder resolves from its initial, acute phase to complete recovery.

Neuromuscular Disorder

Recently, several investigators (Blom and Zakrisson, 1974; Morioka et al., 1976; Szmejz et al., 1976; and Warren et al., 1977) have advocated the diagnostic application of acoustic reflex measures in myasthenia gravis, a neuromuscular disorder. In general, findings in patients afflicted with this disorder are either absent or elevated reflexes, or reflex decay in the absence of any other retrocochlear sign. Following successful drug therapy, the reflex abnormality typically disappears altogether, or markedly improves. It appears, then, that the acoustic reflex might be useful not only in diagnosis but also in monitoring therapy for this disease.

The number of studies reporting acoustic reflex findings in neuromuscular disorder are, admittedly, small. Nonetheless, they represent a significant area for further investigation. Only the accumulation of more data will reveal whether acoustic reflex testing provides valuable diagnostic information in the evaluation of neuromuscular disease.

SUMMARY

Clinical experience with impedance audiometry leads to the seemingly contradictory conclusions that (1) no single impedance measure has much diagnostic value, but that (2) impedance audiometry is probably the most valuable contribution to the study of auditory disorder since the development of the standard blow for tuning forks.

The answer to this paradox lies in the essential difference between impedance measurement and impedance audiometry. Impedance measurement is the gathering of data (the tympanogram, the static compliance, and so on). Impedance audiometry, on the other hand, goes beyond mere measurement to include the skilled interpretation of the collective impedance measures in relation to other relevant audiometric data. With a minimum of training, almost anyone can carry out impedance measures, but only a person well trained in audiology can carry out meaningful impedance audiometry.

The difference is a critical one. As we have observed repeatedly in this chapter, the measures themselves are of little value. Tympanograms can delineate gross categories only. Maximum static compliance is so variable that a substantial percentage of otosclerotics show higher compliance than 50 percent of normal subjects. The acoustic reflex can be totally ambiguous, since it involves, simultaneously, the adequate sensation of loudness to one ear, the status of the middle ear in both ears, and the integrity of the entire central and peripheral portions of the reflex arc.

In spite of these limitations, however, the overall pattern of results that emerges from the various measures, coupled with other basic audiometric data, can have extremely significant diagnostic value. Only when this interpretive step is taken, however, can we say that impedance audiometry has been carried out.

REFERENCES

Alberti, P.: The stapedius reflex and otoneurological diagnosis. Paper presented at the Seventh Ibero-American Symposium of Otoneurology, Sao Paulo, Brazil, November, 1974.

Alberti, P. and Jerger, J.: Probe-tone frequency and the diagnostic value of tympanometry. *Arch. Otolaryngol.* 99:206, 1974.

Alberti, P. and Kristensen, R.: The clinical application of impedance audiometry: a preliminary appraisal of an electroacoustic impedance bridge. *Laryngoscope* 80:735, 1970.

Alford, B., Jerger, J., Coats, A., Peterson, C. and Weber, S.: Neurophysiology of facial nerve testing. *Arch. Otolaryngol.* 97:214, 1973.

Alford, B., Jerger, J., Coats, A., Peterson, C. and Weber, S.: Diagnostic tests of facial nerve function. *Otolaryngol. Clin. North Am.* 7: , 1974.

Anderson, H., Barr, B. and Wedenberg, E.: Intra-aural reflexes in retrocochlear lesions. In Hamberger, C. and Wersall, J. (Eds): *Nobel Symposium 10: Disorders of the Skull Base Region.* Stockholm, Almquist and Wiskell, 1969, 49–55.

Beery, C., Andrus, W., Bluestone, C. and Cantekin, E.: Tympanometric pattern classification in relation to middle ear effusions. *Ann. Otol. Rhinol. Laryngol.* 84:56, 1975.

Bel, J., Causse, J., Michaux, P., Cezard, R., Canut, Y. and Tapon, J.: Mechanical explanation of on-off effect (diphasic impedance change) in otospongiosis. Paper presented at Twelfth International Congress of Audiology, Paris, France, 1974.

Bel, J., Causse, J. and Michaux, P.: Paradoxical compliances in otosclerosis. *Audiol.* 14:118, 1975.

Bicknell, M. and Morgan, N.: A clinical evaluation of the Zwislocki acoustic bridge. *J. Laryngol.* 82:673, 1968.

Blom, S. and Zakrisson, J.: The stapedius reflex in the diagnosis of myasthenia gravis. *J. Neurol. Sci.* 21:71, 1974.

Causse, J., Bel, J., Michaux, P. and Vernieres, J.: Attempted explanation of the on-off effect in otospongiosis. *Acta Otorhinolaryngol. (Belg.)* 28:473, 1974.

Chesnutt, B., Stream, R., Love, J. and McLarey, D.: Otoadmittance measurements in cases of dual ossicular disorders. *Arch. Otolaryngol.* 101:109, 1975.

Chiveralls, K., Fitzsimmons, R., Beck, G. and Kernohan, H.: The diagnostic significance of the stapedius reflex. *Brit. J. Audiol.* 10:122, 1976.

Chiveralls, K.: A further examination of the use of the stapedius reflex in the diagnosis of acoustic neuroma. *Audiol.* 16:331, 1977.

Citron, D. and Adour, K.: Acoustic reflex and loudness discomfort in acute facial paralysis. *Arch. Otolaryngol.* 104:303, 1978.

Colletti, V.: Stapedius reflex abnormalities in multiple sclerosis. *Audiol.* 14:63, 1975.

Cunningham, D.: Admittance values associated with the acoustic reflex and reflex decay. *J. Am. Audiol. Soc.* 1:197, 1976.

Dancer, J., Shiffman, F. and Hill, W.: Tympanometry in otosclerosis. *E.N.T.J.* 56:177, 1977.
Deutsch, L.: The threshold of the stapedius reflex for pure tone and noise stimuli. *Acta Otolaryngol.* 74:248, 1972.
Dieroff, H.: Differential diagnostic value of tympanometry in adhesive processes and otosclerosis. *Audiol.* 17:77, 1978.
Djupesland, G.: Use of impedance indicator in diagnosis of middle ear pathology. *Audiol.* 8:570, 1969.
Djupesland, G.: Middle ear muscle reflexes elicited by acoustic and non-acoustic stimulation. *Acta Otolaryngol. (Suppl.)* 188:287, 1963.
Feldman, A.: Eardrum abnormality and the measurement of middle ear function. *Arch Otolaryngol.* 99:211, 1974.
Flottorp, G., Djupesland, G. and Winther, F.: The acoustic stapedius reflex in relation to critical bandwidth. *J. Acoust. Soc. Amer.* 49:457, 1971.
Habener, S. and Snyder, J.: Stapedius reflex amplitude and decay in normal hearing ears. *Arch. Otolaryngol.* 100:294, 1974.
Hall, C.: Stapedial reflex decay in retrocochlear and cochlear lesions. *Ann. Otol.* 86:219, 1977.
Hall, J.: Diagnostic audiometry in sensori-neural hearing loss, a survey and critical review of the literature. *Monographs in Contemporary Audiol.* In press.
Haughton, P.: Validity of tympanometry for middle ear effusions. *Arch. Otolaryngol.* 103:505, 1977.
Hayes, D.: Audiology Quiz # 1. *Arch. Otolaryngol.* 103:502, 1977.
Jerger, J.: Clinical experience with impedance audiometry. *Arch. Otolaryngol.* 92:311, 1970.
Jerger, J.: Second international symposium on impedance measurement, Houston, Texas. *Audiol.* 13:271, 1974.
Jerger, J., Anthony, L., Jerger, S. and Mauldin, L.: Studies in impedance audiometry. III. Middle ear disorders. *Arch. Otolaryngol.* 99:165, 1974a.
Jerger, J., Harford, E., Clemis, J. and Alford, B.: The acoustic reflex in eighth nerve disorders. *Arch. Otolaryngol.* 99:409, 1974b.
Jerger, J., Hayes, D., Anthony, L. and Mauldin, L.: Factors influencing prediction of hearing level from the acoustic reflex. *Monographs in Contemporary Audiol.* 1: , 1978.
Jerger, J., Jerger, S. and Mauldin, L.: Studies in impedance audiometry. I. Normal and sensori-neural ears. *Arch. Otolaryngol.* 96:513, 1972.
Jerger, J. and Jerger, S.: Audiological comparison of cochlear and eighth nerve disorders. *Ann. Otol. Rhinol. Laryngol.* 83:275, 1974.
Jerger, S., Jerger, J. and Hall, J.: A new acoustic reflex pattern. *Arch. Otolaryngol.* 105:24, 1979.
Johnson, E.: An analysis of auditory test results in 500 cases of acoustic neuromas. *Audiol.* 11:80, 1972.
Johnson, E.: Auditory test results in 500 cases of acoustic neuroma. *Arch. Otolaryngol.* 103:152, 1977.
Kaplan, H., Gilman, S. and Dirks, D.: Dynamic properties of acoustic reflex adaptation. *Trans. Am. Acad. Ophthalmol. Otolaryngol.* 83:368, 1976.
Keller, A.: Ossicular discontinuity. *Laryngoscope* 86:1792, 1976.
Klockhoff, I.: Middle ear muscle reflexes in man: a clinical and experimental study with special reference to diagnostic problems in hearing impairment. *Acta Otolaryngol.* (Suppl.) 164:1, 1961.
Lidén, G.: Tests for stapes fixation. *Arch. Otolaryngol.* 89:399, 1969a.
Lidén, G.: The scope and application of current audiometric tests. *J. Laryngol. Otol.* 83:507, 1969b.
Lidén, G.: Application of tympanometry and acoustic reflex measurements. *Acta Otorhinolaryngol. (Belg.)* 29:802, 1975.
Lidén, G., Bjorkman, G., Nyman, H. and Kunov, H.: Tympanometry and acoustic impedance. *Acta Otolaryngol. (Stockh.)* 83:140, 1977.
Lidén, G., Harford, E. and Hallen, O.: Tympanometry for the diagnosis of ossicular disruption. *Arch. Otolaryngol.* 99:23, 1974.
Lidén, G., Peterson, J. and Bjorkman, G.: Tympanometry. *Arch. Otolaryngol.* 92:248, 1970.
Morioka, W., Neff, P., Boisseranc, T., Hartman, P. and Cantrell, R.: Audiotympanometric findings in myasthenia gravis. *Arch. Otolaryngol.* 102:211, 1976.
Olsen, W., Noffsinger, K. and Kurdziel, S.: Acoustic reflex and reflex decay. Occurrrence in patients with cochlear and eighth nerve lesions. *Arch. Otolaryngol.* 101:622, 1975.
Orchik, D., Dunn, M. and McNutt, L.: Tympanometry as a predictor of middle ear effusion. *Arch. Otolaryngol.* 104:4, 1978b.
Orchik, D., Morff, R. and Dunn, J.: Impedance audiometry in serous otitis media. *Arch. Otolaryngol.* 104: 409, 1978a.
Paradise, J., Smith, C. and Bluestone, C.: Tympanometric detection of middle ear effusion in infants and young children. *Pediatrics* 58:198, 1976.
Segers, J.: Measurement of impedance in otosclerosis. *Acta Otorhinolaryngol. (Belg.)* 28:329, 1974.
Sheehy, J. and Inzer, B.: Acoustic reflex test in neuro-otologic diagnosis: a review of 24 cases of acoustic tumors. *Arch. Otolaryngol.* 102:647, 1976.
Szmeja, Z., Murlarek, J. and Obrebowski, A.: Fatigability of stapedius muscle in myasthenia. *Neurol. Neurochir. (Pol.)* 10:469, 1976.
Terkildsen, K. and Nielsen, S.: An electroacoustic impedance measuring bridge for clinical use. *Arch. Otolaryngol.* 72:339, 1960.

Terkildsen, K., Osterhammel, P. and Bretlau, P.: Acoustic middle ear muscle reflexes in patients with otosclerosis. *Arch. Otolaryngol.* 98:152, 1973.

Thomsen, J. and Terkildsen, K.: Audiological findings in 125 cases of acoustic neuromas. *Acta Otolaryngol.* 80:353, 1975.

Warren, W., Gutmann, L., Cody, R., Flowers, P. and Segal, A.: Stapedius reflex decay in myasthenia gravis. *Arch. Neurol.* 34:496, 1977.

Chapter Seven

DIAGNOSTIC APPLICATION OF IMPEDANCE AUDIOMETRY IN CENTRAL AUDITORY DISORDERS

SUSAN JERGER, M.S.

INTRODUCTION

In the evaluation of central auditory disorder, the goal is to differentiate among three different sites: the eighth nerve, the brain stem, and the temporal lobe. In the application of impedance audiometry toward this goal, acoustic reflexes provide the primary basis for differential diagnosis. In this chapter there is an outline of the organization of the acoustic reflex arc and a discussion of the reflex patterns characteristic of central auditory disorders. A variety of central mechanisms that seem to influence reflex activity in animals and humans are also discussed.

CENTRAL REFLEX ARC

The pathways of the acoustic reflex arc are located in the lower brain stem. Figure 7-1 summarizes schematically the most direct stapedial reflex pathways as defined by Borg (1973) in the rabbit. More recently, Browner and Webster (1975) described similar uncrossed projections between the trapezoid body (TB), medial superior olive (MSO), and seventh nerve nucleus (Nu 7) in kangaroo rats. Figure 7-1 shows that the acoustic reflex pathway is basically a four-neuron chain: (1) primary auditory neuron to the ventral cochlear nucleus (VCN), (2) secondary neuron from the VCN to the

The preparation of this chapter was supported, in part, by Public Health Service research grant NS-10940 from the National Institute of Neurological Diseases and Stroke. Patient data presented in this chapter were obtained in the Audiology Laboratories, Baylor College of Medicine, and the Neurosensory Center, under the direction of James Jerger.

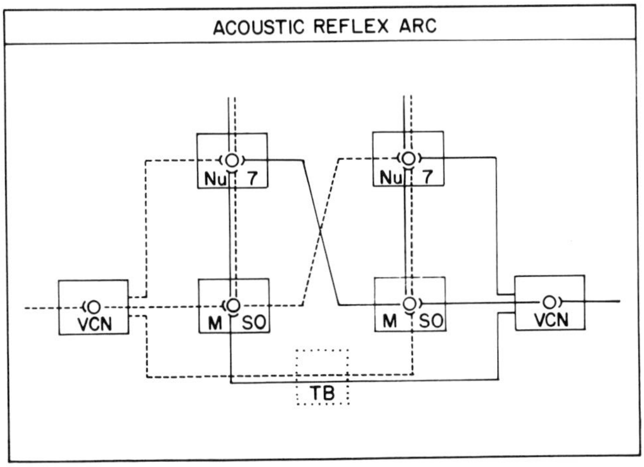

Figure 7-1 Schematic illustration of acoustic reflex arc. Reflex activation involves ventral cochlear nucleus (VCN), trapezoid body (TB), medial superior olive (MSO), and seventh nerve nucleus (Nu7). In this figure, notice that location of TB is indicated by dotted lines instead of solid lines. Dotted lines were selected as a reminder that TB is not a discrete, midline structure, but a strand of transverse fibers. Interposed in pathway are nuclei of TB.

MSO, (3) inter-neuron from the region of the MSO to the Nu7, and (4) motor neuron to the stapedial muscle. Parallel to these direct pathways, there exist slower, multisynaptic connections. For a more detailed description of the acoustic reflex arc, see Chapter 4.

One important distinction between uncrossed and crossed reflex pathways is that the uncrossed reflex pathway contains a direct connection from the VCN to the ipsilateral Nu 7 (a three-neuron chain) (Borg, 1976). In contrast, crossed reflexes do not have a direct collateral to the Nu 7 from a second-order neuron. Crossed reflexes are always activated through one additional relay in the region of the MSO.

A more complex neuronal organization for crossed than for uncrossed pathways has been repeatedly supported by pharmacologic studies demonstrating a greater susceptibility of crossed reflexes to some anesthetics. For example, Borg and Mϕller (1967, 1975) found that in rabbits and humans, barbiturates such as pentobarbitalsodium consistently depress crossed reflex thresholds more than uncrossed thresholds. Giacomelli and Mozzo (1964) and Bosatra and colleagues (Bosatra et al., 1975; Bosatra and Russolo, 1976; and Bosatra, 1977) described similar crossed reflex abnormalities in normal human subjects with temporary brain stem impairment due to barbiturates. Borg and Mϕller (1975) observed that the reflex abnormalities induced by barbiturates recover faster for uncrossed than for crossed pathways.

In addition to pharmacologic studies, investigations on unanesthetized animals and humans have consistently documented sensitivity differences between uncrossed and crossed paths. For example, at least nine previous studies (Mϕller, 1961, 1962; Borg and Mϕller, 1967, 1968, 1975; Borg, 1972a, 1972b; Reker, 1977; and Brask, 1978) have shown that in unanesthetized animals and humans, uncrossed reflexes can be elicited by lower sound intensities than crossed reflexes. In humans, uncrossed reflex thresholds are from 2 to 16 dB lower than corresponding crossed thresholds (Mϕller, 1961, 1962; Reker, 1977; and Brask, 1978). Borg and Mϕller (1975) attributed an uncrossed vs crossed sensitivity difference mainly to the presence of a direct connection from the VCN to the ipsilateral Nu 7 and the absence of any such connection with regard to the contralateral Nu 7.

HISTORICAL REVIEW

Interest in acoustic reflexes as an integral part of the central auditory system was initiated in 1935 by Lorente de Nó. However, approximately thirty years elapsed before the reflex abnormalities found in patients with retrocochlear disorders were described. Then, in Italy, Giacomelli and Mozzo (1964) reported crossed reflex threshold abnormalities in patients with toxic, vascular, and/or compressive brain stem disorders and in normal subjects with transient brain stem impairment due to barbiturates. Shortly thereafter, Anderson and his colleagues in Sweden (1969) described the phenomena of reflex threshold elevation and amplitude decay in seventeen patients with eighth nerve disorders. At approximately the same time in Denmark, Greisen and Rasmussen (1970) reported a discrepancy between uncrossed and crossed reflex thresholds in two patients with intra-axial brain stem disorders. In 1975, Jerger formally classified the uncrossed vs crossed reflex threshold patterns characteristic of eighth nerve or extra-axial brain stem and intra-axial brain stem sites.[1]

In the application of acoustic reflexes to the differential diagnosis of central auditory disorders, it's critical to remember that a reflex response depends on the physiologic functioning of the *entire* reflex arc. For example, in the clinical measurement of acoustic reflex thresholds, we are assessing, all at the same time, the functioning of a receptor-(middle ear and cochlea), an afferent neuron (eighth nerve), inter-neurons (brain stem), an efferent neuron (seventh nerve), and an effector organ (stapedial muscle). Localization of impairment within the reflex arc is effected primarily by comparing reflexes to uncrossed and crossed stimulation.

EIGHTH NERVE VS BRAIN STEM SITES

Uncrossed vs Crossed Reflex Threshold Patterns

The characteristic relation between uncrossed and crossed acoustic reflexes in eighth nerve and intra-axial brain stem auditory disorders is illustrated theoretically in Figure 7-2. Figure 7-2A illustrates the theoretic effect of an eighth nerve or extra-axial brain stem site; Figure 7-2B shows the theoretic effect of an intra-axial brain stem site. The upper half of Figure 7-2 A and B contains uncrossed and crossed reflex pathways. The crossed pathways are represented by solid lines and travel from the cochlea on one side to the stapedial muscle on the opposite side. The uncrossed pathways are represented by broken dashed lines and travel from the cochlea on one side to the stapedial muscle on the same side. The theoretic lesion is represented by a shaded area.

The lower halves of Figure 7-2A and B illustrate one method for visualizing the relation between crossed and uncrossed reflex threshold results. In this form, the four

[1]The adjectives extra-axial and intra-axial are radiographic terms referring to the origin of lesions in the area of the brain stem. Extra-axial refers to lesions arising on the outside of the brain stem; intra-axial refers to lesions located within the brain stem.

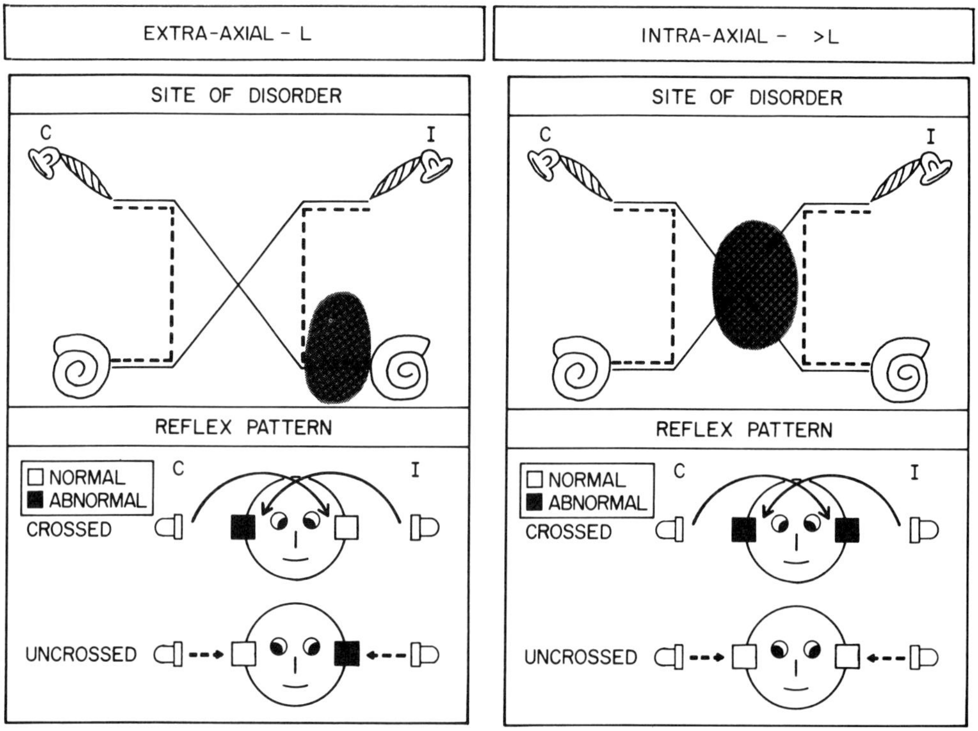

Figure 7-2 (A) Top: theoretic effect of left eighth nerve or extra-axial brain stem site of disorder (shaded area). Bottom: characteristic pattern of results for crossed and uncrossed acoustic reflexes. White box represents normal results; black box represents abnormal results. Reflexes are usually absent with sound to affected (ipsilateral or I) ear and usually present with sound to unaffected (contralateral or C) ear. Note diagonal configuration. (B) Top: theoretic effect of intra-axial brain stem site of disorder, eccentric to left (shaded area). Bottom: characteristic pattern of results for crossed and uncrossed acoustic reflexes. White box indicates normal results; black box indicates abnormal results. Reflexes are usually absent to crossed stimulation and usually present to uncrossed stimulation. Note horizontal configuration. (From Jerger, S. and Jerger, J.: Diagnostic value of crossed vs uncrossed acoustic reflexes. *Arch. Otolaryngol.* 103:445, 1977.)

boxes represent results on the probe ear for the two crossed and the two uncrossed reflex thresholds. A white box represents normal results; a black box represents abnormal results. Abnormal results may designate either elevated or absent acoustic reflex thresholds.

Figure 7-2A illustrates the theoretic site of disorder, and the pattern of crossed and uncrossed acoustic reflex results in a hypothetic patient with an eighth nerve (or extra-axial brain stem) disorder on the left. The disorder, indicated by the shaded area in the upper half of the figure, affects both the crossed and uncrossed reflex pathways when sound is presented to the left ear. The crossed and uncrossed pathways activated by sound to the right ear are not affected. The reflex pattern distinctive of eighth nerve disorders is characterized by a diagonal configuration (Jerger, 1975). Reflexes are absent with sound to the left ear and present with sound to the right ear. In patients with eighth nerve disorders, abnormal acoustic reflexes with sound to the affected ear have been extensively described and are detailed in Chapter 6.

Figure 7-2B shows the theoretic site of the disorder and the relation between crossed and uncrossed reflexes in a hypothetic patient with an intra-axial brain stem disorder eccentric to the left. The intra-axial disorder, represented by the shaded area, affects the crossed reflex pathways on both sides. The uncrossed pathways, however, are not involved on either side. The reflex pattern associated with an intra-axial brain stem disorder is characterized by a horizontal configuration (Jerger, 1975). On both ears, reflexes are typically abnormal to crossed stimulation and typically normal to uncrossed stimulation. Crossed acoustic reflex abnormalities in brain stem disorders have been reported previously in animals (Borg, 1971, 1977) and in humans (Greisen and Rasmussen, 1970; Steinberg and Lehnhardt, 1972; Lehnhardt, 1973; Lidén and Korsan-Bengtsen, 1973; Jerger and Jerger, 1974, 1975a, 1975b, 1977; Jerger et al., 1975; Coletti, 1975; McCandless and Harmer, 1975; Bosatra et al., 1975; Bosatra and Russolo, 1976; Bosatra, 1977; Stephens and Thornton, 1976; Alberti et al., 1977; and Brask, 1978).

Distribution of Reflex Patterns

Figure 7-3 summarizes five acoustic reflex patterns that may be found in patients with either eighth nerve or intra-axial brain stem disorders. The four boxes represent the probe ear for the two crossed (top row) and two uncrossed (bottom row) conditions. A white box indicates normal reflexes; a black box indicates abnormal reflexes. In the first pattern shown in Figure 7-3, the diagonal configuration, reflexes are abnormal with sound to the affected ear for both crossed and uncrossed conditions. In the second pattern, the horizontal configuration, reflexes to crossed stimulation are abnormal on both ears. Reflexes to uncrossed stimulation, however, are consistently observed at normal hearing levels (HLs) on each ear. In the third pattern, a normal configuration, reflexes are normal on both ears for both crossed and uncrossed conditions. In this circumstance, the eighth nerve or brain stem disorder does not produce any noticeable

REFLEX PATTERN	*DESCRIPTION* VISUAL	VERBAL
DIAGONAL	*C* ■ □ *UnCr* □ ■	Abnormal with sound to affected ear
HORIZONTAL	*C* ■ ■ *UnCr* □ □	Abnormal to crossed stimulaton on both ears
NORMAL	*C* □ □ *UnCr* □ □	Normal on both ears
INVERTED L SHAPE	*C* ■ ■ *UnCr* □ ■	Abnormal on both ears to crossed stimulation; abnormal on affected ear to uncrossed stimulation
UNI–BOX	*C* ■ □ *UnCr* □ □	Abnormal with sound to affected ear on crossed stimulation only

Figure 7-3 Description of five reflex patterns. For visual description, four boxes represent probe ear for two crossed (C) (top row) and two uncrossed (Un Cr) (bottom row) conditions. White box indicates normal reflexes; black box indicates abnormal reflexes. (From Jerger, S. and Jerger, J.: Diagnostic value of crossed vs uncrossed acoustic reflexes. *Arch. Otolaryngol.* 103:445, 1977.)

abnormality in threshold results on either ear. In the fourth pattern, an inverted L-shaped configuration, reflexes to crossed stimulation are abnormal on both ears. Reflexes to uncrossed stimulation are abnormal on the affected ear only. In the inverted L-shaped pattern, normal reflexes are observed only when the sound and the probe are both in the unaffected ear. For the final configuration, the uni-box pattern, reflexes are abnormal with sound to the affected ear on crossed stimulation only. This unusual reflex pattern, abnormal crossed reflexes and normal uncrossed reflexes with sound to the affected ear, is a relatively rare observation.

In 1977, Jerger and Jerger described the distribution of the five reflex patterns in a series of seventeen patients. Of these patients, eight had surgically confirmed eighth nerve lesions, six had radiographically confirmed intra-axial brain stem lesions, and three had radiographically confirmed eighth nerve and intra-axial brain stem disorders. In the latter three patients with combined extra-axial and intra-axial disorder, a primary intra-axial tumor mass exhibited an exophytic extension that invaded the cerebellopontine angle cistern as well as the brain stem pathways.

In the Jerger study, eleven of the seventeen patients (approximately 65 percent) showed the diagonal or horizontal reflex patterns. Of these patients, there were no false-positive findings in either the eighth nerve or intra-axial brain stem groups. None of the eighth nerve patients showed a horizontal (brain stem) configuration, and no patient in the brain stem group showed a diagonal (eighth nerve) pattern.

Of the remaining six patients, two had normal acoustic reflex thresholds. One of the patients had an intra-axial brain stem site; the other patient had an extra-axial brain stem disorder that involved the eighth nerve. Three other patients had the inverted L-shaped reflex pattern. The site of disorder in these three patients varied. One patient had an eighth nerve site; one had a brain stem site; and one had a combined eighth nerve and brain stem disorder. The remaining patient, a fifty three-year-old female with a large cerebellopontine angle neoplasm involving the eighth nerve and adjacent brain stem structures, showed the uni-box configuration.

Subsequent to the Jerger (1977) study, the unusual uni-box reflex pattern was reported in three additional patients (Jerger et al., 1979). A uni-box configuration, according to Borg's study (1973) of acoustic reflex pathways in the rabbit (Fig. 7-1), implies a lesion medial to the ventral cochlear nucleus at approximately the location of the medial superior olive. Clinically, however, the uni-box reflex pattern does not distinguish between eighth nerve and intra-axial brain stem sites. Of the four patients with uni-box configurations (Jerger and Jerger, 1977; Jerger et al., 1979), one had a surgically confirmed extra-axial brain stem disorder, one had a degenerative neural disorder, one had a viral disorder, and one had hydrocephalus.

An Unusual Variation

In 1975, Bosatra, Russolo, and Poli commented that some of their patients with brain stem disorders showed unusually sensitive, instead of normal or unusually poor acoustic reflex threshold HLs. Recently we observed this strange phenomenon in a sixteen-year-old male with a cerebellar medulloblastoma. At surgery, the tumor was noted to involve the brain stem, primarily on the left side, in the region of the fourth ventricle.

In this patient, audiologic test results were obtained ten days following surgery and at approximately weekly intervals thereafter for a period of forty one days. Figure 7-4 summarizes average pure-tone sensitivity (PTA) results for 500, 1000, and 2000 Hz

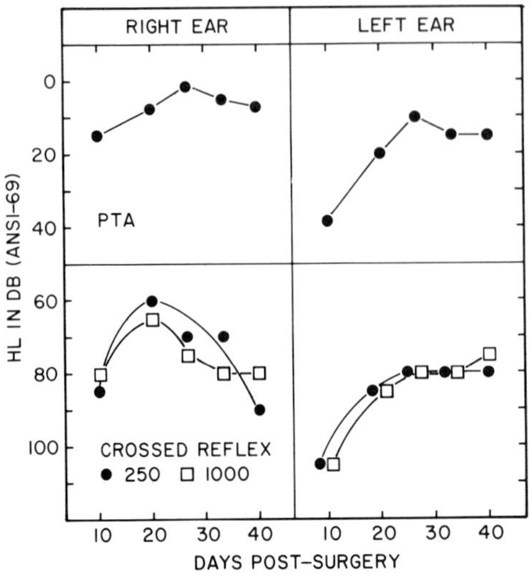

Figure 7-4 Average pure-tone sensitivity (PTA) results and crossed acoustic reflex thresholds (250 Hz and 1000 Hz) for right and left ears of sixteen-year-old male with surgically confirmed cerebellar medulloblastoma. Data are presented for ten to forty one days after surgery.

and crossed acoustic reflex thresholds for 250 and 1000 Hz. Data are presented for the right and left ears. Uncrossed reflex thresholds were the same as crossed reflex results and are not detailed in the figure.

As seen in Figure 7-4, serial hearing tests on the right ear during this time period consistently showed normal pure-tone sensitivity. Ten days postoperatively, the PTA was 15 dB; forty one days following surgery, the PTA was 8 dB. On the left ear, initial pure-tone sensitivity results showed a mild sensorineural loss. The PTA score was 38 dB. However, during the forty one postoperative days, pure-tone sensitivity on the left ear improved substantially. At forty one days after surgery, for example, the PTA score was 15 dB. On both ears, sensitivity measures seemed to stabilize about the twentieth day after surgery,

At the initial evaluation (ten days after surgery), crossed acoustic reflexes on the right ear were present at normal HLs, about 85 dB, at both 250 and 1000 Hz. However, between ten and twenty days postoperatively, reflex thresholds showed unusual improvement. For example, at twenty days postoperatively, reflex threshold HLs were 60 dB at 250 Hz and 65 dB at 1000 Hz. Subsequently, between twenty and forty one days postoperatively, reflex threshold HLs systematically declined to initial test levels (about 85 dB HL). On the left ear, crossed acoustic reflexes at the initial test session were elevated, 105 dB HL, at both 250 and 1000 Hz. However, between ten and twenty days postoperatively, crossed reflex thresholds improved from 105 dB HL to 85 dB HL. During the remaining sessions, crossed reflex thresholds on the left ear remained at about 80 dB HL.

In Figure 7-4, notice the unusually sensitive reflex threshold HLs that temporarily occurred on the right ear. In Jerger's series of about three hundred patients with normal hearing (Jerger et al., 1972), only 2.5 percent had reflex thresholds of less than 70 dB HL, and only 0.5 percent had thresholds of less than 65 dB HL. The abnormality of these unusually good threshold values is emphasized by the normal threshold HLs on the right ear at ten and forty one days postoperatively and by the normal values on the left ear between twenty and forty one days postoperatively.

In short, in a patient with a brain stem disorder primarily affecting the left side of the brain, uncrossed and crossed acoustic reflex thresholds with sound to the right ear were temporarily enhanced to HLs well outside the normal range. Uncrossed and crossed acoustic reflex thresholds with sound to the left ear did not show this unusual improvement. During part of the forty one day period that audiologic tests were administered, the patient received steroid and radiotherapy treatments. Perhaps, during this time, a normal inhibitory mechanism was temporarily changed by the effects of surgery, steroids, and/or radiotherapy.

In 1971, Borg reported intriguingly similar results in rabbits after transection of the crossed olivocochlear bundle. At 2000 Hz, for example, he found that reflex thresholds improved from about 72 dB sound pressure level (SPL) before sectioning to about 60 dB SPL after sectioning. Improvement was not observed for all frequencies, however. Further, lesions in the brain stem which did not interrupt the crossed olivocochlear bundle were not characterized by any improvement in reflex thresholds. In 1978, Igarashi and his coworkers tried to replicate Borg's findings in squirrel monkeys and failed. Igarashi attributed consistently negative results to a probable species difference between squirrel monkeys and rabbits. Observations in the present brain stem patient (Fig. 7-4), however, suggest an additional explanation. The present data suggest that acoustic reflex threshold improvements in brain stem disorders may be a transitory, rather than a permanent, observation. In this circumstance, negative findings may occur simply from a lack of sufficient sequential observations. Igarashi and his associates tested post-lesion animals on three different occasions, but they did not specify the time interval between test sessions.

Reflex Time Course

The reflex time course to sustained auditory signals has been evaluated in both humans and animals with eighth nerve and intra-axial brain stem disorders. Findings in patients with eighth nerve sites are detailed in Chapter 6. Results in intra-axial brain stem disorders may be grouped under two general observations. One observation is that in animals and humans with brain stem disorders, acoustic reflexes may show unusually reduced amplitude and/or amplitude decay. Since 1969, when the reflex amplitude decay phenomenon was initially described (Anderson et al., 1969), the reflex decay test has been viewed primarily as a diagnostic measure for eighth nerve or extra-axial brain stem disorders. Recently, however, at least three studies (Stephens and Thornton, 1976; Alberti and Kristensen, 1976; and Jerger and Jerger, 1977) have reported substantially reduced maximum amplitude or reflex amplitude decay in patients with pure intra-axial brain stem auditory disorders and no known abnormality of the eighth nerve per se.

It should be emphasized that broadening the possible sites of disorder associated with the reflex decay phenomenon does not weaken the diagnostic value of reflex decay measures. The primary basis for differentiating eighth nerve and intra-axial brain stem disorders is the diagonal vs horizontal reflex patterns of threshold results, not reflex decay testing. However, in both sites of disorder, reflex decay measures may offer valuable supplementary information to basic threshold data. For example, in patients with intra-axial brain stem sites, abnormal reflex decay on one ear may alert the clinician to the possibility that the lesion is eccentric to the side with the aberrant reflex amplitude time course.

The second general observation on the reflex time course concerns latency measures. Throughout the United States and Europe, numerous investigators (Borg, 1973, 1976; Borg and Møller, 1975; McCandless and Harmer, 1975; Coletti, 1975;

Bosatra et al., 1975; Bosatra and Russolo, 1976; and Bosatra, 1977) have shown that the reflex time course in animals and humans with brain stem disorders may show delayed onset latency and an unusually slow rise to maximum amplitude. These unusual latency and amplitude abnormalities of the reflex time course may show systematic recovery as auditory symptoms accompanying the brain stem disorder are reduced by radiotherapy, chemotherapy, and/or spontaneous remission (Noffsinger et al., 1975; Jerger and Jerger, 1977; and Bosatra, 1977).

CORTICAL AUDITORY DISORDERS

Reflex Thresholds

Acoustic reflexes in animals and humans with unilateral or bilateral cortical disorders have received limited attention to date. A lack of published data probably reflects the generally accepted clinical observation that patients with cortical auditory disorders have normal acoustic reflex thresholds. The data of Figure 7-5 support this viewpoint. This figure shows average pure-tone sensitivity results and crossed and uncrossed reflex thresholds in five patients with unilateral temporal lobe disorders. Patients were three females and two males ranging in age from sixteen to fifty seven years. The temporal lobe disorder was confirmed surgically or radiographically in all patients. Data in Figure 7-5 are presented in terms of the ear contralateral or ipsilateral to the affected side of the brain.

In Figure 7-5, the pure-tone audiogram shows normal, bilaterally symmetric, pure-tone sensitivity with the exception of a mild loss on the contralateral ear at 4000 Hz. The PTA scores are 13 dB on the contralateral ear and 14 dB on the ipsilateral ear. Crossed and uncrossed acoustic reflex thresholds are present at normal HLs at all frequencies on both ears. In particular, there is no difference between crossed and uncrossed reflex thresholds at 1000 Hz. Normal crossed acoustic reflex thresholds in patients with unilateral temporal lobe disorder have been reported previously (Jerger and Jerger, 1975a). However, to this author's knowledge, no one has previously documented the normal crossed vs uncrossed threshold pattern.

Figure 7-6 shows crossed acoustic reflex threshold results in a five-year-old girl with bilateral temporal lobe disorder and auditory agnosia. Auditory and medical findings in this patient have been described elsewhere (Jerger and Hayes, 1976). Electrophysiologic measures of hearing indicated normal peripheral pure-tone sensitivity bilaterally. However, during behavioral observation and structured audiologic testing, this patient did not appear to respond to any environmental sounds or auditory signals. In striking contrast to behavioral results, crossed acoustic reflex

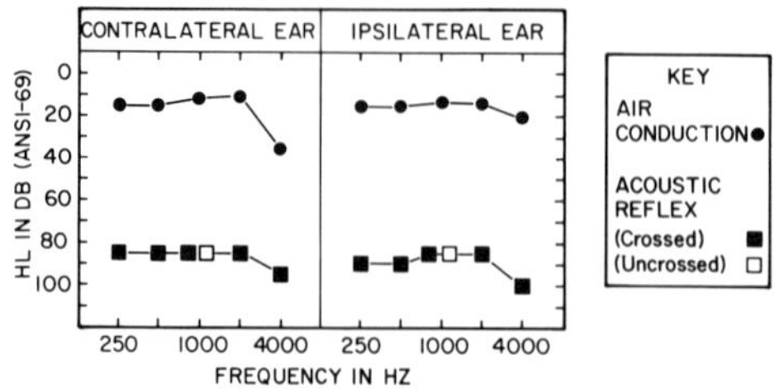

Figure 7-5 Average threshold hearing levels (HLs) and crossed acoustic reflex threshold HLs at octave frequencies between 250 Hz and 4000 Hz in five patients with unilateral temporal lobe disorders. Uncrossed acoustic reflex thresholds are shown at 1000 Hz. Data are presented in terms of ear contralateral or ipsilateral to affected side of brain.

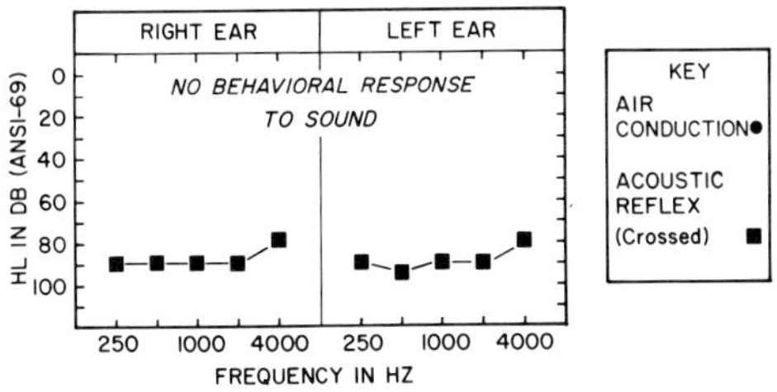

Figure 7-6 Behavioral pure-tone results and crossed acoustic reflex threshold HLs in a five-year-old girl with bilateral temporal lobe disorder and auditory agnosia.

thresholds were present at normal HLs at all frequencies on both ears.

Results in Figure 7-6 suggest that in humans, acoustic reflex thresholds are independent of cognitive awareness of sounds. This observation is supported by Bosatra's comment (1977) that drugs primarily influencing supra-brain stem structures did not affect acoustic reflex thresholds in his subjects. This observation is not, however, supported by previous findings in animals. Specifically, Baust and Berlucchi (1964) observed a striking reduction in the excitability of the tensor tympani reflex to clicks in cats with bilateral ablation of the acoustic cortex. Although Baust and Berlucchi's results certainly may not be applicable to the data in Figure 7-6 owing to differences between subjects (cats vs humans) and middle ear muscles (tensor tympani vs stapedial), their findings suggest that more information is necessary before we conclude that bilateral temporal lobe damage in humans does not influence acoustic reflex thresholds.

Reflex Amplitude vs Intensity Functions

In contrast to acoustic reflex thresholds, reflex amplitude vs intensity functions in patients with cortical disorders may be grossly abnormal. Unusually depressed amplitude growth functions in cortical lesions were first described by Peterson and Lidén (1972) in a patient with a tumor of the corpus callosum. Jerger and coworkers (1979) recently reported similar findings in a seventy-year-old female with nonspecific central auditory disorder. Figure 7-7 and 7-8 summarize pure-tone sensitivity results and acoustic reflex data on the Jerger patient. The audiogram, Figure 7-7, shows a mild sensorineural loss on both ears. The PTA scores are 26 dB on the right ear and 27

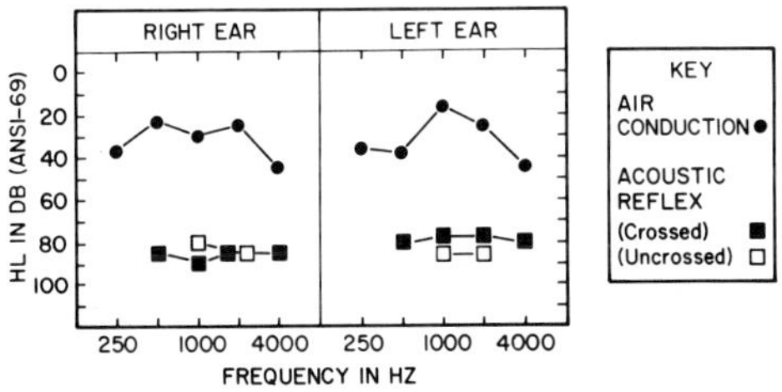

Figure 7-7 Audiogram and acoustic reflex results in seventy-year-old female with nonspecific central auditory disorder. (From Jerger, S., Jerger, J. and Hall, J.: A new acoustic reflex pattern. *Arch. Otolaryngol.* 105:24, 1979.)

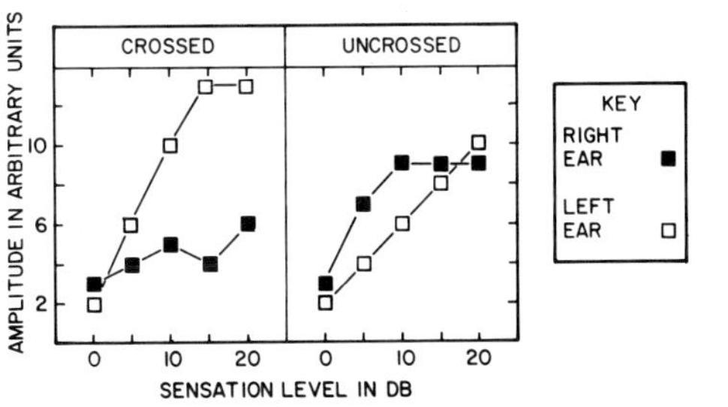

Figure 7-8 Crossed and uncrossed reflex amplitude functions at 1000 Hz for right and left ears. Notice large difference between crossed reflex amplitudes at suprathreshold levels. (From Jerger, S., Jerger, J. and Hall, J.: A new acoustic reflex pattern. *Arch. Otolaryngol.* 105:24, 1979.)

dB on the left ear. Crossed and uncrossed acoustic reflex thresholds, Fig. 7-7, are within the normal range at all frequencies on both ears.

Figure 7-8 presents crossed and uncrossed reflex amplitude functions at 1000 Hz for the right and left ears. Reflex amplitude functions for the crossed condition show a large difference between ears. With sound to the left ear, crossed reflex amplitude grows substantially with increasing loudness. With sound to the right ear, however, crossed reflex amplitude remains essentially unchanged as signal intensity increases. Reflex amplitude functions for the uncrossed condition do not show this unusual ear difference. On both ears, the amplitude of uncrossed reflexes increases as intensity increases in an orderly fashion.

Central Influences on Acoustic Reflexes

As discussed throughout this chapter, brain stem lesions, cortical lesions, and central nervous system (CNS) depressant drugs may alter the response of the stapedial muscle reflex to sound. In addition to these effects, middle ear muscle activity also seems to be influenced by a variety of complex central mechanisms. For example, previous studies have shown that middle ear muscle activity may be modified by the different physiologic stages of sleep (Baust and Berlucchi, 1964; Pessah and Roffwarg, 1972), by the descending auditory pathways (Borg, 1971), by intercollicular decerebration (Carmel and Starr, 1963; Baust and Berlucchi, 1964; and Salomon, 1966), by changing the significance of a sound (Carmel and Starr, 1963; Bench, 1971; and Yonovitz and Harris, 1972), and by a variety of motor activities such as vocalization, yawning, coughing, laughing, and swallowing (Carmel and Starr, 1963; Salomon and Starr, 1963; Simmons, 1964; and Borg and Zakrisson, 1975).

The above studies documenting central influences on middle ear muscle reflex activity have both theoretic and practical implications for clinicians. Theoretically, we are reminded that middle ear reflex activity is a complex sensorimotor mechanism related to the physical characteristics of sound stimuli, to the status of the peripheral and central auditory system, and to a variety of dynamic central nervous system processes.

Practically, we are reminded that our knowledge of acoustic reflex behavior in patients with CNS disorders is, to date, limited. For example, in the studies cited above, complex signal paradigms, such as preactivating acoustic signals and pulsed signal trains, were generally used to measure the effect of central processes on middle ear muscle activity. This observation suggests that in patients with CNS abnormalities, some interesting, and perhaps diagnostic, variations in reflex activity may be found with more sophisticated clinical methodologies. Attempts to apply pulsed signal trains, preactivating acoustic signals, and binaural vs monaural signal presentations have already been initiated (Sesterhenn and Breuninger, 1976; Brask, 1978). However, the applicability of complex signal paradigms and amplitude versus intensity growth functions to clinical audiologic evaluation has not been adequately investigated to date.

SUMMARY

The Following Points are Especially Important

The acoustic reflex arc is basically a three- or four-neuron chain.

The crossed reflex pathways are characterized by a more complex neuronal organization than uncrossed pathways.

A comparison of crossed vs uncrossed reflex thresholds is helpful in localizing disorders of the acoustic reflex arc.

Patients with eighth nerve disorders are usually characterized by abnormal reflex thresholds with sound to the affected ear for both crossed and uncrossed conditions (a diagonal pattern).

Patients with intra-axial brain stem disorders are usually characterized by abnormal reflex thresholds to crossed stimulation on both ears. Reflexes to uncrossed stimulation, however, are normal on both ears (a horizontal pattern).

Patients with temporal lobe disorders are usually characterized by normal crossed and uncrossed acoustic reflex thresholds.

The reflex time course and reflex amplitude growth functions may offer valuable supplementary information to threshold data. In particular, in some patients with central nervous system disorders, threshold data may be completely normal and the reflex time course or reflex amplitude vs intensity function may be grossly abnormal.

Middle ear muscle reflexes may be modified by complex dynamic central nervous system mechanisms that seem to influence a variety of motor behaviors.

REFERENCES

Alberti, P., Fria, T. and Cummings, F.: The clinical utility of ipsilateral stapedius reflex tests. *J. Otolaryngol.* 6:466, 1977.

Alberti, P. and Kristensen, R.: The clinical application of impedance audiometry. In Northern, J. (Ed.): *Selected Readings in Impedance Audiometry.* New York, American Electromedics Corp., 1976, 61-88.

Anderson, H., Barr, B. and Wedenberg, E.: Intra-aural reflexes in retrocochlear lesions. In Hamburger, C. and Wersall, J. (Eds.): *Nobel Symposium 10: Disorders of the Skull-Base Region.* Stockholm, Almquist and Wiskell, 1969, 49-55.

Baust, W. and Berlucchi, G: Reflex response to clicks of cat's tensor tympani during sleep and wakefulness and the influence thereon of the auditory cortex. *Arch. Ital. Biol.* 102:686, 1964.

Bench, J.: Anticipatory elicitation of the middle ear muscle reflex. *J. Laryngol. Otol.* 85:1161, 1971.

Borg, E.: Efferent inhibition of afferent acoustic activity in the unanesthetized rabbit. *Exper. Neurol.* 31:301, 1971.

Borg, E.: Acoustic middle ear reflexes. A sensory control system. *Acta Otolaryngol., (Suppl.)* 304:1, 1972a.

Borg, E.: Excitability of the acoustic muscle stapedius and muscle tensor tympani reflexes in the nonanesthetized rabbit. *Acta Physiol. Scand.* 85:374, 1972 b.

Borg, E.: On the neuronal organization of the acoustic middle ear reflex. A physiological and anatomical study. *Brain Res.* 49:101, 1973.

Borg, E.: Neurophysiology of the acoustic stapedius reflex. *Proceedings of Third International Symposium on Impedance Audiometry.* New York, American Electromedics Corp., 1976, 6-11.

Borg, E.: Dynamic characteristics of the intra-axial muscle reflex. In Feldman, A. and Wilbur, L. (Eds.): *Acoustic Admitance and Impedance—The Measurement of Middle Ear Function.* Baltimore, Williams & Wilkins, 1976, 236-299.

Borg, E. and Mϕller, A.: Effect of ethylalcohol and pentobarbital sodium on the acoustic middle ear reflex in man. *Acta Otolaryngol.* 64:415, 1967.

Borg, E. and Mϕller, A.: The acoustic middle ear reflex in unanesthetized rabbits. *Acta Otolaryngol.* 65:575, 1968.

Borg, E. and Mϕller, A.: Effect of central depressants on the acoustic middle ear reflex in rabbits. *Acta Physiol. Scand.* 94:327, 1975.

Borg, E. and Zakrisson, J.: The activity of the stapedius muscle in man during vocalization. *Acta Otolaryngol.* 79:325, 1975.

Bosatra, A.: Pathology of the nervous arc of the acoustic reflexes. *Audiol.* 16:307, 1977.

Bosatra, A., Russola, M. and Poli, P.: Modification of the stapedius muscle reflex under spontaneous and experimental brain stem impairment. *Acta Otolaryngol.* 80:61, 1975.

Bosatra, A. and Russolo, M.: Oscilloscopic analysis of the stapedius muscle reflex in brain stem lesions. *Arch. Otolaryngol.* 102:284, 1976.

Brask, T.: Extratympanic manometry in man. *Scand. Audiol.*, (Suppl.) 7:162, 1978.

Browner, R. and Webster, D.: Projections of the trapezoid body and the superior olivary complex of the kangaroo rat. *Brain Behav. Evol.* 11:322, 1975.

Carmel, P. and Starr, A.: Acoustic and nonacoustic factors modifying middle ear muscle activity in waking cats. *J. Neurophysiol.* 26:598, 1963.

Coletti, V.: Stapedius reflex abnormalities in multiple sclerosis. *Audiol.* 14:63, 1975.

Giacomelli, F. and Mozzo, W.: An experimental and clinical study on the influence of the brain stem reticular formation on the stapedial reflex. *Int. Audiol.*3:42, 1964.

Greisen, O. and Rasmussen, P.: Stapedius muscle reflexes and oto-neurological examinations in brain stem tumors. *Acta Otolaryngol.* 70:366, 1970.

Igarashi, M., Mauldin, L. and Jerger, J., Impedance audiometry in the squirrel monkey. Effect of transection of crossed olivo-cochlear bundle. *Arch. Otolaryngol.* 105:258, 1979.

Jerger, J.: Diagnostic use of impedance measures. In Jerger, J. (Ed.): *Handbook of Clinical Impedance Audiometry.* New York, American Electromedics Corp., 149-174, 1975.

Jerger, J. and Hayes, D.: The cross-check principle in pediatric audiometry. *Arch. Otolaryngol.* 102:614, 1976.

Jerger, S. and Jerger J.: Extra- and intra-axial brain stem auditory disorders. *Audiol.* 14:93, 1975b.

Jerger, S. and Jerger, J.: Diagnostic value of crossed vs uncrossed acoustic reflexes. Eighth nerve and brain stem disorders. *Arch. Otolaryngol.* 103:445, 1977.

Jerger, J. and Jerger, S.: Auditory findings in brain stem disorders. *Arch. Otolaryngol.* 99:342, 1974.

Jerger, J. and Jerger, S.: Clinical validity of central auditory tests. *Scand. Audiol.* 4:147, 1975a.

Jerger, J., Jerger, S. and Mauldin, L.: Studies in impedance audiometry. Normal and sensori-neural ears. *Arch. Otolaryngol.* 96:513, 1972.

Jerger, S., Neely, G. and Jerger, J.: Recovery of crossed acoustic reflexes in brain stem auditory disorder. *Arch. Otolaryngol.* 101:329, 1975.

Jerger, S., Jerger, J. and Hall, J.: A new acoustic reflex pattern. *Arch. Otolaryngol.* 105:24, 1979.

Lehnhardt, E: Audiometric localization of brain stem lesions. *Z. Laryngol. Rhinol. Otol.* 52:11, 1973.

Lidén, G. and Korsan-Bengtsen, M.: Audiometric manifestations of retrocochlear lesions. *Scand. Audiol.* 2:29, 1973.

Lorente de No, R.: The function of the central acoustic nuclei examined by means of the acoustic reflexes. *Laryngoscope* 45:573, 1935.

McCandless, G. and Harmer, D.: Abnormal intra-aural reflex in multiple sclerosis patients. *Impedance Newsletter* 4:16, 1975.

Møller, A: Bilateral contraction of the tympanic muscles in man, examined by measuring impedance change. *Ann. Otol.* 70:735, 1961.

Møller, A.: Acoustic reflex in man. *J. Acoust. Soc. Amer.* 34:1524, 1962.

Noffsinger, D., Kurdziel, S. and Applebaum, E.: Value of special auditory tests in the latero-medial inferior pontine syndrome. *Ann. Otol. Rhinol. Laryngol.* 84:384, 1975.

Pessah, M. and Roffwarg, H.: Spontaneous middle ear muscle activity in man. A rapid eye movement sleep phenomenon. *Science* 178:773, 1972.

Peterson, J. and Lidén, G.: Some static characteristics of the stapedial muscle reflex. *Audiol.* 11:97, 1972.

Reker, U.: Normal values of the ipsilateral acoustic stapedius reflex threshold. *Arch. Otorhinolaryngol.* 215:25, 1977.

Salomon, G.: Middle ear muscle activity. *Proceed. Royal Soc. Med.* 59:966, 1966.

Salomon, G. and Starr, A.: Electromyography of the middle ear muscles in man during motor activities. *Acta Neurol. Scand.* 39:161, 1963.

Sesterhenn, G. and Breuninger, H.: The acoustic reflex at low sensation levels. *Audiol.* 15:523, 1976.

Simmons, F.: Post-tetanic potentiation in the middle ear muscle acoustic response. *J. Acoust. Soc. Amer.* 32:1589, 1960.

Simmons, F.: Perceptual theories of middle ear muscle function. *Ann. Otol.* 73:724, 1964.

Steinberg, D. and Lehnhardt, E.: Impedance changes in central hearing disturbances. *Z. Laryngol. Rhinol. Otol.* 51:693, 1972.

Stephens, S. and Thornton, A.: Subjective and electrophysiologic tests in brain stem lesions. *Arch. Otolaryngol.* 102:608, 1976.

Yonovitz, A. and Harris, D.: Successful conditioning of the stapedius muscle. *Naval Submarine Medical Research Laboratory*, Report 730, 1972.

Chapter Eight

PREDICTING HEARING LOSS FROM THE ACOUSTIC REFLEX

JAMES W. HALL, Ph.D.

INTRODUCTION

In 1972, Niemeyer and Sesterhenn introduced the concept of hearing loss prediction from the acoustic reflex. The many published reports that followed, describing the use of various hearing prediction methods, provide ample evidence of the importance of the concept. The findings of numerous independent investigations, conducted in both laboratory and clinical settings, lead to a common conclusion—acoustic reflex measurements offer a rapid, objective, and reasonably accurate means of identifying hearing loss.

Initially, hearing loss identification, and estimation, from the acoustic reflex were studied primarily in adult populations (Niemeyer and Sesterhenn, 1974; Jerger et al., 1974a). More recently, however, hearing loss prediction from the acoustic reflex has been reported in children (Margolis and Popelka, 1975; Abahazi and Greenberg, 1977; and Margolis and Fox, 1977). Objective prediction of hearing loss in children has obvious clinical value. Recent reports of fruitful acoustic reflex measurements in children, including traditionally "difficult-to-test" children, are, therefore, highly encouraging (Popelka and Margolis, 1975; Jerger and Hayes, 1976; Keith, Murphey, Martin, 1976, 1977; and Niswander and Ruth, 1977).

The original concept of hearing loss prediction, as proposed by Niemeyer and Sesterhenn (1972, 1974) was based on the difference in acoustic reflex threshold levels for pure tone vs noise signals in normal ears. Subsequently, different methods of hearing loss prediction from the acoustic reflex have evolved and continue to be developed. The methods have in common the noise-tone reflex threshold difference. Yet they offer distinctively different approaches to hearing loss prediction.

Based on accumulated clinical experience with the prediction methods, investigators now report that hearing loss prediction methods may be influenced by chronologic age, minor tympanogram and middle ear abnormalities, and central auditory disorders (Handler and Margolis, 1977; Hall, 1978; Jerger et al., 1978a, b; and Hall and Weaver, 1979). While not detracting from the clinical usefulness of hearing loss prediction from the acoustic reflex, these factors are important for accurate interpretation of findings.

In this chapter, I will first present an overview of the basis for hearing loss prediction from the acoustic reflex, especially the critical band and the noise-tone threshold difference in acoustic reflexes. The major methods of hearing loss prediction will then be reviewed, and the advantages and disadvantages of each method noted. Next, the effects of the important factors influencing hearing loss prediction by the acoustic reflex will be described. Finally, based on current information on hearing loss prediction, I will offer suggestions for improved prediction methods.

BASIS OF HEARING LOSS PREDICTION BY THE ACOUSTIC REFLEX

In the normal ear, acoustic reflex thresholds for broad-band or white noise signals are 20 to 25 dB better than acoustic reflex thresholds for pure-tone signals. The noise-tone difference (NTD) in acoustic reflex thresholds, first reported in the 1960s (Møller, 1962; Dallos, 1964; Fisch and Schulthess, 1963; Lilly, 1964; and Djupesland, Flottorp, Winther, 1967), and carefully defined in the early 1970s (Deutsch, 1972; Peterson and Lidén, 1972) is the basis for hearing loss prediction from the acoustic reflex. These early investigations were conducted in adult populations. In children and infants, however, the NTD is comparable to, or may actually exceed the NTD in adults (Margolis and Popelka, 1975; Abahazi and Greenberg, 1977; and Hall and Weaver, 1979). In the normal ear, the acoustic reflex threshold level is related to signal bandwidth. Although expanding the bandwidth of a signal at first has no effect on threshold level, increasing the bandwidth beyond a "critical bandwidth" results in improved acoustic reflex threshold levels (Flottorp, Djupesland, Winther, 1971; Djupesland and Zwislocki, 1973; Popelka, Karlovich, Wiley, 1974; and Popelka, Margolis, Wiley, 1976). The width of the critical frequency band varies according to the center frequency. Generally, the higher the center frequency, the greater the "critical bandwidth."

The critical bandwidth effect was clearly demonstrated by Popelka, Margolis and Wiley (1976). In normal ears, acoustic reflexes were elicited by two tones. Separation of the two tones, a two-component tonal complex, beyond the critical bandwidth of the center tone produced an improvement in reflex threshold. Spectral density of the reflex-activating signal was then manipulated. Increasing the spectral density, that is, the number of tones or components within the initial two-tone bandwidth, further improved the reflex threshold. The greatest improvement in acoustic reflex threshold, from a very narrow bandwidth to a bandwidth exceeding the critical bandwidth, was approximately 20 dB. According to Popelka and colleagues (1976), this acoustic reflex threshold improvement was produced by "a tonal complex having approximately 5 to 9 components equally spaced in log frequency." The results were reflex thresholds comparable to those elicited by a Gaussian noise signal centered at 1000 Hz. This improvement in acoustic reflex threshold for the noise signal forms the basis of the NTD.

In sensorineural ears, there is usually little or no improvement in acoustic reflex threshold levels with an increase in signal bandwidth (Djupesland, Sundby, Hogstad, 1975; Popelka, Margolis, Wiley, 1976; Schwartz and Sanders, 1976; and Margolis and Fox, 1977). The normal advantage of the critical bandwidth in reflex thresholds for noise signals is diminished, or absent, in the sensorineural ears. Thus, the NTD is reduced in the sensorineural ear (Niemeyer and Sesterhenn, 1972, 1974; Jerger et al., 1974a; Djupesland, Sundby, Hogstad, 1975; Popelka et al., 1976; Schwartz and Sanders, 1976; Hall, 1978; Jerger et al., 1978a; and Hall and Weaver, 1979). Although there is general agreement that the NTD is useful in identifying sensorineural loss, the possible relationship of the magnitude of the NTD reduction to the degree of sensorineural loss is still unclear. A regular relationship between decrease in NTD and increase in sensorineural loss would seem to permit both identification of loss and reasonably accurate estimates of the amount of loss. The success of the Sensitivity Prediction from the Acoustic Reflex (SPAR) method based on the NTD lends support to this assumption (Jerger et al., 1974a; Keith, 1977; Tsappis, 1977; Van Wagoner and Goodwine, 1977; and Hall, 1978). However, consistent predictive error rates of 25 to 40 percent for the SPAR method argue for an incomplete correlation between changes in critical bandwidth and the degree of sensorineural loss (Schwartz and Sanders, 1976). The critical band phenomenon in the acoustic reflex, therefore, although fundamental to hearing loss prediction from the acoustic reflex, does not seem to explain fully the NTD prediction methods.

METHODS OF HEARING LOSS PREDICTION

Calculation of Hearing Threshold Level (HTL) from the Acoustic Reflex

Niemeyer and Sesterhenn Formula. In 1972, Niemeyer and Sesterhenn introduced the concept of hearing threshold prediction from the acoustic reflex. They developed a formula for relating hearing threshold level to the difference in reflex threshold for noise and pure-tone signals reported by previous investigators (Fisch and Schulthess, 1963; Dallos, 1964; and Peterson and Lidén, 1972). Their subjects were 50 normal-hearing young adults, 10 normal-hearing children, and 125 patients (223 ears) with sensorineural loss. The relatively consistent relationship between hearing level and the NTD in acoustic reflex thresholds for normal-hearing subjects led Niemeyer and Sesterhenn (1974) to suspect a similarly regular relationship in sensorineural ears. Indeed, there was an apparent relationship in sensorineural ears. They defined the relationship with the following equation:

$$\text{hearing threshold} = \text{ART tones} - 2.5\ \text{d}1\ 2,$$

where "hearing threshold" is the average pure-tone threshold for 500, 1000, 2000, and 4000 Hz, "ART" is the average acoustic reflex threshold for 500, 1000, 2000, and 4000 Hz, and "d1 2" is the difference between the average pure tone ART and the white noise ART. The product, "calculated hearing threshold," was within 4 dB of the "measured hearing threshold" in an illustrative case with a flat sensorineural loss attributed to Menière's disease. In cases with a sloping configuration, calculating hearing threshold with white noise ARTs was less accurate. Niemeyer and Sesterhenn (1974), therefore, modified their formula to include high-pass (1800 to 13500 Hz) and low-pass (100 to 1600 Hz) noise in place of white noise. Low-pass noise then would be used in calculating hearing threshold for lower frequencies (250 to 1000 Hz), while high-pass noise would be used in calculating hearing threshold for higher frequencies (2000 to 8000 Hz). In 223 ears with sensorineural loss, calculated hearing threshold and measured hearing threshold were within ± 10dB in 73 percent, ± 15dB in 17 percent, and ± 20dB in 10 percent.

Subsequent investigations of the original Niemeyer and Sesterhenn (1974) equation in populations of normal-hearing and sensorineural subjects have been reported (Miller, Davies, Gibson, 1976; Margolis and Fox, 1977; and Keith, 1977). Miller and colleagues (1976) studied forty-five subjects with normal hearing and thirty-nine with sensorineural loss. While 87 percent of the predictions were accurate to within −15 to +25 dB, their findings were characterized by a substantial proportion of false-positive predictions of loss in those with normal hearing (i.e., pure-tone average ≤ 20 dB for 500, 1000, 2000, and 3000 Hz). Keith's (1977) findings for twenty-six subjects with normal hearing and forty-eight sensorineural patients were marginally less accurate than those of Niemeyer and Sesterhenn (1974). Still, there was no prediction error in 35 percent of the subjects, and actual and predicted hearing level was accurate within ± 5 dB in 56 percent, ± 10 dB in 67 percent, ± 15 dB in 82 percent and ± 25 dB in 90 percent. Again, the predominant error was false-positive identification of loss in those with normal hearing, or overestimation of hearing loss. Mild-to-moderate and severe sensorineural losses were poorly differentiated. On one of the patients with a severe loss, normal hearing sensitivity was predicted. Margolis and Fox (1977) studied seventeen normal-hearing young adults (i.e., hearing level better than 15 dB at audiometric frequencies) and thirty-six sensorineural subjects (sixty ears). In those with normal hearing, hearing threshold predictions, on the average, exceeded the actual pure-tone average by 4.5 dB. The variability was sizeable, however, with an estimate of greater than a 25 dB hearing level in five of the seventeen subjects with normal hearing. In sensorineural subjects there was again the persistent problem of a high rate of false-positive results. As in Keith's (1977) study, the formula was least accurate in distinguishing mild-to-moderate and severe losses. Variability in the sensorineural group was greatest for subjects with sloping loss, a finding in agreement with Niemeyer and Sesterhenn (1974).

In summary, then, hearing level predictions with the Niemeyer-Sesterhenn formula are accurate to within ± 20 to 25 dB for 85 to 100 percent of all subjects. Serious errors in prediction are reported (Keith, 1977; Margolis and Fox, 1977). False identification of loss in those with normal hearing, or overestimation of mild-moderate loss, is a common problem.

Regression Equations. In 1976, Baker and Lilly reported a new method for estimating hearing threshold level (HTL) from the acoustic reflex. Using statistical regression techniques in a primarily adult, hearing-impaired population of one-hundred twenty-five subjects, they generated an equation for determining HTL from the acoustic reflex thresholds for broad-band noise (BBN) and pure tones of 500, 1000, 2000, and 4000 Hz. In the regression equation, the noise and tone signals are weighted differentially according to their contribution to the HTL prediction. The original Baker-Lilly formula is as follows:

$$\begin{aligned} \text{dB HTL} = {} & 1.11 \text{ ART BBN (SPL)} - 0.81 \text{ ART 500 Hz (HL)} \\ & + 0.85 \text{ ART 1000 Hz (HL)} - 0.43 \text{ ART 2000 Hz (HL)} \\ & + 0.25 \text{ ART 4000 Hz (HL)} - 64.7, \end{aligned}$$

where ART = acoustic reflex threshold, BBN = broad-band noise, SPL = sound pressure level, HTL = hearing threshold level, and HL = hearing level. The formula predicts hearing threshold level for pure-tone frequencies of 500, 1000, 2000, and 4000 Hz. We would expect that the acoustic reflex threshold for BBN would play an important role in the prediction equation, and, indeed, BBN is the best predictor variable, with a regression coefficient of 1.11. In contrast, the acoustic reflex threshold for 4000 Hz is a relatively poor predictor variable, with a regression coefficient of only 0.25. This original formula required computation of reflex threshold values for four pure-tone frequencies, plus BBN. Unfortunately, in some patients, acoustic reflex thresholds for one or more test frequencies are not available. In such cases, HTL could not be predicted with the original Baker-Lilly formula (Hall, 1978). Soon after the original formula was reported, Lilly (1977) introduced a set of predictive equations which permitted HTL prediction from the acoustic reflex threshold for a single signal (BBN) or combinations of BBN and 500 Hz, 500 and 1000 Hz, or 500, 1000, and 2000 Hz. In the interest of accuracy, however, Lilly advised using as many reflex threshold values as possible in HTL prediction. He also developed a separate set of equations for predicting the traditional pure-tone average of 500, 1000, and 2000 Hz.

Recently, regression equations have been developed by at least one additional investigating team. Rizzo and Greenberg (1979) developed a series of regression equations from acoustic reflex threshold data obtained in 158 normal-hearing and sensorineural children and adults. Two predictor variables, the reflex threshold for high-pass noise (1800 to 6000 Hz), and a 500 Hz pure tone, showed the highest correlation with a four-frequency (500, 1000, 2000, 4000 Hz) pure-tone average. As a result, the best equation for HTL prediction was as follows:

$$\text{dB HTL} = [0.216 \text{ ART HPN}_{(SPL)} - 0.078 \text{ ART 500 Hz}_{(HL)}2 - 7.515]^2,$$

where HPN = high-pass noise of 1800 to 6000 Hz, and ART = acoustic reflex threshold.

Both the Baker-Lilly and the Rizzo-Greenberg regression equations, in theory, offer a distinct clinical advantage: prediction of hearing threshold level in dB. For each equation, the product is a number that is supposed to correspond with the HTL for a specific pure-tone frequency, or the average of two to four test frequencies. The apparent precision of the regression equations in predicting HTL, then, is very attractive. For example, with the Baker-Lilly (1976) equation, the median error of prediction is slight. They reported a median error of 0 dB, while in Hall's (1978) study, the median error was only -3 dB. From 55 to 75 percent of all predictions were within $\pm$ 15 dB, and virtually all predictions (98 to 100 percent) were within $\pm$ 35 dB. A closer examination of the predictions of the Baker-Lilly (1976) regression equation, however, reveals some consistent inaccuracies. In subjects with normal hearing (e.g., PTA of better than 15 dB HTL), the predicted PTA routinely overestimates the actual PTA. In a substantial proportion of subjects with normal hearing, therefore, a mild hearing loss will be predicted. The problem of "false-positive" identification of hearing loss, so characteristic of the Niemeyer-Sesterhenn equation, seems to characterize the regression equations as well. With increased hearing loss, however, just the opposite is observed (Hall, 1978). That is, in general, actual hearing level exceeds predicted hearing level, and hearing loss is underestimated. As a result, there is a substantial proportion of false-negative predictions, in which a subject with a hearing loss is predicted to have hearing sensitivity within normal limits. The magnitude of the predictive errors seems to be directly related to the degree of loss. At the extreme, for example, in subjects with an actual PTA of 65 dB HTL, on the average, a hearing level of 30 dB HTL is predicted.

The source of these predictive errors is unclear. Unlike the Niemeyer-Sesterhenn (1974) equation and the SPAR methods, the regression equations are not based strictly on the NTD, or on the absolute levels of the acoustic reflex threshold. Therefore, the possible problem of a weak relationship between the size of the NTD and the degree of hearing loss would not be expected to influence seriously the predictive accuracy of the regression equations. However, there may be at least two fundamental problems in this approach to hearing level prediction.

First, hearing prediction by linear regression methods is, by definition, founded on the assumption that there is a linear relationship between hearing threshold levels and the relative acoustic reflex threshold levels for noise and tone signals. There is, however, no evidence to support this assumption. On the contrary, the effect of sensorineural loss on acoustic reflexes, while usually quite predictable, does not appear to be linear (Jerger et al., 1978a; Hall and Weaver, 1979). The effect of sensorineural loss on acoustic reflexes varies as a function of the degree of loss and the signal (Fig. 8–1). With increasing loss, the reflex threshold for the BBN signal worsens rather systematically. On the average, BBN reflex thresholds increase 3 to 5 dB for every 10 dB of loss. In contrast, reflex thresholds for pure-tone signals remain relatively constant or actually improve slightly with increasing hearing loss of up to 45 or 55 dB HTL. Then, with increasing loss, the reflex thresholds increase. The data in Figure 8–1 are based on 539 normal-hearing subjects and 132 sensorineural subjects having, for the most part, a sloping audiometric configuration. As a result, the acoustic reflex thresholds for 1000, 2000, and 4000 Hz are most influenced by the degree of sensorineural loss, while the reflex thresholds for the 500 Hz signal show relatively less effect. The differential effect of sensorineural loss on reflex thresholds for noise vs pure-tone signals produces irregular variations in the NTD as a function of the degree of loss. The initial effect of mild loss of 25 to 35 dB HL is to obliterate the NTD for all signals except 4000 Hz. With a 36 to 45 dB loss, the noise threshold exceeds all tone thresholds, producing a negative NTD. In the 46 to 55 dB range, there is a negative NTD relationship for noise and three of the pure-tone signals (500, 1000, and 4000 Hz). The threshold for the 2000 Hz signal increases to a level comparable to the noise threshold, producing essentially no NTD. With severe loss of 56 to 75 dB, there is essentially no difference between thresholds for the noise and higher frequency tone signals. The noise–500 Hz signal difference, however, increases slightly. In subjects with a loss of greater than 75 dB HL there is, again, a negative NTD difference.

These vagaries in the NTD are readily apparent when the NTD (average reflex threshold for 500, 1000, 2000 Hz minus reflex threshold for BBN) is plotted as a

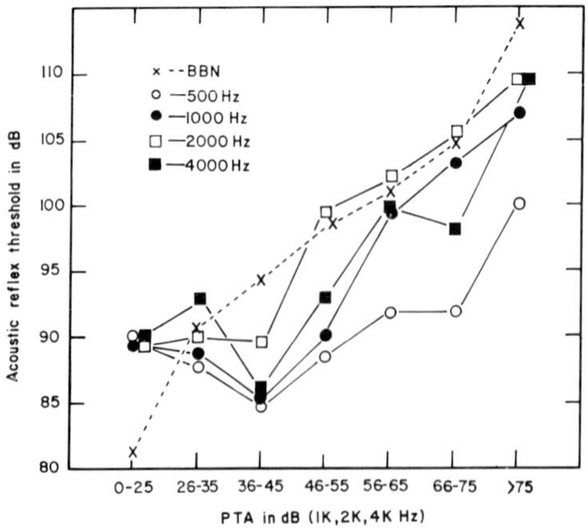

Figure 8–1 Effect of hearing loss on acoustic reflex thresholds of pure-tone and broad-band (BBN) signals (pure tones in dB HL, BBN in dB SPL). Results are for 539 normal-hearing and 132 sensorineural subjects, aged one through twenty years. (Reprinted by permission of the Journal of Otolaryngology from Hall, J.W. and Weaver, T.: Impedance audiometry in a young population: the effect of age, sex and tympanogram abnormalities. *J. Otolaryngol.* 8 (3):210-222, 1979.)

function of sensorineural loss (Fig. 8–2). Fitting a linear regression equation to acoustic reflex data in sensorineural loss, therefore, produces widely varying results depending upon the degree of loss. In addition, the primary effect of sensorineural loss is an increased BBN threshold, but the original regression equations included four pure tone factors and only one noise factor. Therefore, the influence of the BBN predictive factor, although weighted more than the other factors, seemed to be minimized.

Second, regression equations may be biased by the population on which they are developed. If a population is relatively homogeneous in degree of sensorineural loss or chronologic age, the predictive accuracy of the equation developed using it would probably vary in populations that are heterogeneous in sensorineural loss or age. For example, the predictive accuracy of a regression equation developed from a normal-hearing population would probably decrease substantially in a moderately to severely hearing-impaired population. Similarly, a regression equation developed in children would probably be less effective in predicting hearing level in adults.

Sensitivity Prediction from the Acoustic Reflex (SPAR). Two years after the original Niemeyer and Sesterhenn (1972) report, Jerger and colleagues (1974a) described the application of another method for predicting hearing level from the acoustic reflex. The efficiency of this new technique, now referred to as SPAR, was demonstrated in a clinical population of 1156 patients. Briefly, the acoustic reflex threshold (ART) for BBN is subtracted from the averaged ARTs for 500, 1000, and 2000 Hz. A correction factor, determined biologically for each impedance audiometer, is then added. This procedure yields a Noise Tone Difference (NTD). The SPAR-NTD is calculated with the following formula:

$$\text{NTD} = \frac{[\text{ART 500 Hz (HL)} + \text{ART 1000 Hz (HL)} + \text{ART 2000 Hz (HL)}]}{3} - \text{ART BBN (SPL)} + \text{correction factor.}$$

The result is the NTD, an arbitrary value (i.e., not HTL or SPL) in decibels. To facilitate relatively uniform clinical SPAR findings among various testers and

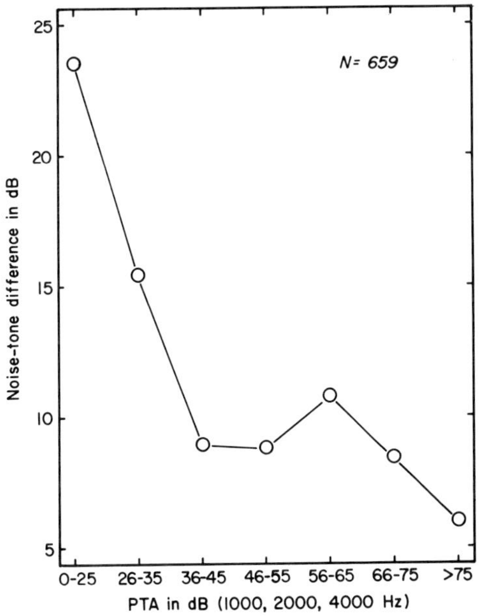

Figure 8–2 Effect of hearing loss on noise-tone difference (NTD). Results are for 527 normal-hearing and 132 sensorineural subjects aged one through twenty years. Mean age according to hearing loss group is as follows: 0 to 25 dB, 10 years; 26 to 35 dB, 12 years; 36 to 45 years, 10 years; 46 to 55 dB, 13 years; 56 to 65 dB, 12 years; 66 to 75 dB, 9 years; greater than 75 dB, 8 years.

impedance audiometers, Jerger and colleagues (1974a) recommend a biologic calibration of the impedance apparatus, rather than the traditional physical calibration. The calibration procedure is easily carried out with ten young (twenty to thirty year-old) subjects with normal hearing. The average reflex threshold of the group for BBN is subtracted from the average reflex threshold for the three pure-tone signals, 500, 1000 and 2000 Hz. The result is the normal NTD for the impedance apparatus. The original Jerger (1974a) norm was 25 dB. To permit comparison of SPAR findings according to the Jerger predictive criteria, the normal NTD from a particular impedance bridge is subtracted from the original norm of 25 dB. The difference, usually a value from 10 to 20 dB, is the correction factor for the impedance apparatus. Following calculation of the pure-tone–noise difference for each patient, the correction factor is added.

For determination of the SPAR, the corrected NTD is interpreted according to a set of criteria. The set of criteria originally described by Jerger and colleagues, (1974a) is shown in Table 8–1. The criteria are referred to as the 1974 SPAR. A corrected NTD of 20 or greater always predicts normal sensitivity. If the NTD is less than 20, a loss is predicted. Hearing loss prediction with the 1974 SPAR is thus a two-step process, involving both the corrected NTD and the absolute reflex threshold for BBN. To estimate the degree of loss, the NTD is first placed within one of three ranges: 15 to 19, 10 to 14, or less than 10. The reflex threshold for BBN is then considered (Table 8–1). As a result of this two-step process, hearing loss is predicted within one of three categories. (Table 8–2). If reflexes are not observed in a patient with otherwise normal impedance findings, a profound sensitivity loss is predicted.

Recently, a revised set of SPAR criteria referred to as the 1977 SPAR (Hall, 1978) were described. Although the 1977 SPAR criteria are simplified, they include an additional feature (Table 8–3). As with the 1974 SPAR, a loss is predicted if the corrected NTD is less than 20. No additional consideration of the NTD is required. With an NTD of less than 20, a reflex threshold for BBN of 95 dB SPL or less predicts a mild-moderate loss, while a BBN threshold of greater than 95 dB SPL predicts a severe loss. Uniquely, the 1977 SPAR takes into account the absolute reflex threshold for the 1000 Hz pure-tone signal. A threshold of more than 95 dB HL at 1000 Hz always predicts a loss, regardless of the BBN threshold. Thus, a prediction of normal hearing requires an NTD greater than 20, *and* a 1000 Hz reflex threshold of 95 dB SPL or less. If either or both of these requirements is not met, a loss is predicted and the BBN threshold is considered. Again, a BBN threshold of 95 dB SPL or better predicts a mild-moderate loss, and a BBN threshold of more than 95 dB SPL predicts a severe loss. The degree of loss predicted by the 1977 SPAR is categorized according to the same criteria

TABLE 8–1 THE 1974 SPAR CRITERIA FOR PREDICTION OF HEARING LOSS

NTD	BBN, dB SPL	Prediction
≥ 20	Anywhere	Normal
15 - 19	< 80	Normal
15 - 19	> 80	Mild-moderate
10 - 14	Anywhere	Mild-moderate
< 10	< 90	Mild-moderate
< 10	> 90	Severe
Reflexes not observed		Profound

From Jerger et al., 1974a
SPAR = Sensitivity Prediction from the Acoustic Reflex; NTD = noise-tone difference; BBN = broad-band noise

TABLE 8–2 CRITERIA FOR CATEGORIZING DEGREE OF LOSS ACCORDING TO THE SPAR METHODS

Category	Criteria
Normal	PTA less than 20 dB HL
Mild-Moderate	PTA 20 to 49 dB HL inclusive
Severe	PTA 50 to 84 dB HL inclusive
Profound	PTA 85 dB HL or more

Modified from Jerger et al., 1974a
SPAR = Sensitivity Prediction from Acoustic Reflex; PTA = pure-tone average for 1000, 2000, and 4000 Hz; HL = hearing level

for the three audiometric test frequencies (1000, 2000, 4000 Hz) described for the 1974 SPAR (Table 8–2).

The number of published reports of the SPAR technique reflects the clinical popularity of the method (Jerger et al., 1974a, 1978a, b; Schwartz and Sanders, 1976; Abahazi and Greenberg, 1977; Keith, 1977; Tsappis, 1977; Van Wagoner and Goodwine, 1977; and Hall, 1978). Since the original criteria and biologic calibration method of Jerger and colleagues (1974a) have been widely accepted, it is possible to compare the findings of most of these published studies. With the SPAR method, predicted hearing level is categorized as normal, a mild-moderate loss, or a severe loss (Table 8–2). An accurate prediction occurs when predicted hearing levels fall within the appropriate category for actual hearing loss—normal, mild-moderate loss or severe loss. For an accurate prediction of mild-moderate loss, the patient's actual average hearing threshold level for 1000 to 4000 Hz would be in the 20 to 49 dB range. Prediction errors, then, may be moderate or serious. In a moderate error, the hearing loss prediction differs from actual hearing level by one category. For example, a prediction of mild-to-moderate loss in a normal hearer is a moderate error. In a serious error, the hearing prediction differs from actual hearing by two categories. There are only two possibilities for serious error: a normal prediction in a patient with a severe loss or a prediction of severe loss in a person with normal hearing.

In general the 1974 SPAR method has a predictive accuracy rate of 60 to 75 percent (Hall, 1978). Moderate errors occur at a rate of 25 to 35 percent. In the remainder of the population (2 to 5 percent) there is a serious predictive error. Accuracy of the SPAR methods is influenced by a variety of factors, including degree of loss, the patient's age and minor middle ear abnormalities. The effect of these factors on the SPAR and other prediction methods will be discussed in a later section.

The SPAR method, like the Niemeyer-Sesterhenn equation and the regression equations, is characterized by false-positive prediction. That is, in most of the moderate errors and virtually all of the serious errors, actual hearing level is *better* than the predicted hearing level. Thus, for example in 10 to 20 percent of patients with normal hearing, a loss may be falsely predicted. Overestimation of hearing loss is the

TABLE 8–3 THE 1977 SPAR CRITERIA FOR PREDICTION OF HEARING LOSS

NTD	BBN	Prediction
$\geq$ 20 and 1000 Hz ART $\leq$ 95 dB HL	Anywhere	Normal
$<$ 20 or 1000 Hz ART $>$ 95 dB HL	$\geq$ 95 dB SPL	Mild-moderate
$<$ 20 or 1000 Hz ART $>$ 95 dB HL	$>$ 95 dB SPL	Severe

From Hall, 1978
SPAR = Sensitivity Prediction from Acoustic Reflex; NTD = noise-tone difference; BBN = broad-band noise; ART = acoustic reflex threshold; HL = hearing level; SPL = sound pressure level

common trend in prediction error, especially serious error. With the 1974 SPAR method, hearing loss rarely is seriously underestimated, i.e., there is rarely a prediction of normal hearing in severe loss. Moreover, inclusion of the 1000 Hz reflex threshold criterion in the 1977 SPAR virtually eliminates a serious underestimation of hearing loss (Hall, 1978). However, while the reduction of "false-negative" underestimation of loss has obvious clinical importance, the not uncommon problem of "false-positive" findings must not be dismissed as negligible.

Bivariate Plot Coordinate System. In 1976, Popelka, Margolis, and Wiley introduced an innovative method of hearing loss prediction from acoustic reflex thresholds for noise and pure-tone signals. These investigators were, in part, motivated by the clinical need for a method that would permit the prediction of hearing sensitivity in different frequency regions. Popelka and colleagues (1976) designed and subsequently, with other researchers. (Handler and Margolis, 1977; Margolis and Fox, 1977), refined a bivariate plot of acoustic reflex threshold data. Unlike the Niemeyer-Sesterhenn equation, the SPAR methods, or the regression equations, which are based on absolute or relative *differences* between acoustic reflex thresholds for tones vs noise, the bivariate plot system utilizes a noise/tone *ratio*. The bivariate plot system is described in detail by Popelka and colleagues (1976), in the later publications by Handler and Margolis (1977), and by Margolis and Fox (1977).

Briefly, the rationale for the system was generated by their appreciation of the documented finding that reflex thresholds in sensorineural ears differed from reflex thresholds in normal ears in two ways (Popelka et al., 1976). First, reflex thresholds tended to be elevated in the frequency region of the sensitivity loss. Second, increased signal bandwidth seemed to have relatively less effect on acoustic reflex thresholds in sensorineural ears. Uniquely, the bivariate plot system simultaneously incorporates *both* of these loss-related changes in reflex thresholds. In their coordinate system, the vertical axis (ordinate) represents the reflex threshold in SPL for a tone, while the horizontal axis (abscissa) represents 100 times the *ratio* of the reflex threshold (SPL) for a noise band to a reflex threshold (SPL) for a tone (Fig. 8–3). In plotting reflex threshold data for a sensorineural patient on the coordinate system, then, an elevated reflex threshold for the tone increases the data value plotted from the ordinate scale.

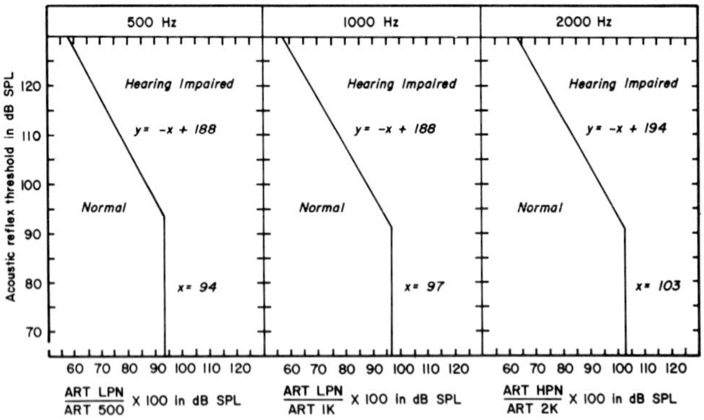

Figure 8–3 Bivariate plot system for identifying hearing loss. Acoustic reflex threshold data for pure-tone signals (500 Hz, 1000 Hz, and 2000 Hz) are represented on vertical axis. Ratios of acoustic reflex thresholds for pure-tone signals and noise signals (500 Hz/low-pass noise; 1000 Hz/low-pass noise; 2000 Hz/high-pass noise) are represented on horizontal axis. Normal and hearing-impaired regions for each pure-tone signal are separated by intersecting line segments defined by values for x and y shown in figure. (Modified from Popelka et al., 1976; Handler and Margolis, 1977; and Margolis and Fox, 1977.)

The relatively greater elevation of the noise reflex threshold vs tone reflex threshold increases the noise-tone ratio and shifts the reflex data value outward on the abscissa. As a result of this plotting procedure, sensorineural patients tend to cluster in the upper right portion of the graph, while normal-hearing subjects cluster in the lower left portion of the graph. As shown in Figure 8–3, the boundary separating the normal region from the sensorineural loss region may be defined by the intersection of two line segments. Handler and Margolis (1977) refer to the x-value as K_1 and the numerical value for the y-segment as K_2. These values were selected for each frequency on the basis of their efficiency in separating normal from sensorineural subjects. To increase predictive accuracy, a reflex threshold for low-pass noise (frequencies below 2600 Hz) is used in the noise-tone ratio for the 500 and 1000 Hz signals, while a reflex threshold for high-pass noise (frequencies above 2600 Hz) is used for 2000 Hz. According to Margolis and Fox (1977), a bivariate plot for 4000 Hz was not reported because reflex data for the 4000 Hz signal was relatively variable and did not contribute to the predictive efficiency of the technique.

The bivariate coordinate system identifies, but does not quantify, sensorineural loss. The patient's acoustic reflex threshold data for 500, 1000, and 2000 Hz are plotted on each of the three graphs. Margolis and colleagues (Handler and Margolis, 1977; Margolis and Fox, 1977) suggest that, as criteria for normal vs sensorineural prediction, a patient must fall within the appropriate region on the graphs for two of the three frequencies. Using these criteria, the accuracy of hearing categorization is 94 percent for normal-hearing subjects and 92 percent for patients with sensorineural loss greater than 32 dB.

The bivariate plot system, according to Margolis and colleagues, is designed to meet at least three objectives:

1. "To identify both normal hearing and clinically significant hearing loss with few errors" (Margolis and Fox, 1977, p. 247);
2. "To improve the frequency resolution" of hearing loss prediction" (Popelka, Margolis, Wiley, 1976, p. 158); and
3. "To minimize false positives" in hearing loss prediction (Margolis and Fox, 1977, p. 241).

From the review of the prediction methods currently available (Niemeyer-Sesterhenn equation, regression equation, and the SPAR method) and their limitations, the bivariate plot system seems well-motivated. Moreover, based on the bivariate plots of normal and sensorineural patients displayed in the published reports by Margolis and colleagues, and the conclusions of their studies, it would appear that this prediction method does indeed offer distinct clinical advantages over the previous methods.

Close examination of the bivariate plot theory and reported data, however, suggests that the method may not be clearly superior to previous methods. In fact, in some respects, the bivariate plot system presents unique limitations and inaccuracies in hearing loss prediction. First, as Margolis and Fox (1977) acknowledge, the bivariate plot system is designed to identify "significant hearing loss" rather than to estimate the magnitude of loss. This theoretic limitation in the designed objectives of the bivariate plot system has practical clinical consequences. The simple identification of sensorineural loss, while important, may provide inadequate information in clinical usage. For example, it would be difficult to develop a rational rehabilitation approach for an infant or young child with only the awareness of a hearing loss greater than 32 dB. Some estimation of the degree of loss would seem essential. Simple identification of a sensorineural loss in an adult with inconsistent behavioral audiometric findings and a possible functional hearing loss component provides inadequate evidence of the degree of actual sensorineural loss vs functional component. In some clinical cases, then, identification of loss alone contributes little to the description of auditory function. The bivariate plot system is designed to identify clinically significant loss. Yet the lower limit for the loss identified by the system is 32 dB, a hearing level typically regarded as creating little impairment. In contrast, the Niemeyer-Sesterhenn equation and the SPAR methods, as Margolis and Fox (1977) point out, "correctly identify moderate to severe hearing losses with high accuracy." Thus, the bivariate plot system seems to present a disadvantage in comparison with two previous methods in these not uncommon clinical entities.

Second, initially a stated objective of the bivariate plot system was to improve prediction of sensitivity loss in specific frequency regions (Popelka, Margolis, Wiley, 1976). According to clinical experience, sensorineural loss is, in most cases, not comparable for all test frequencies, but rather rising or sloping. Therefore, this objective has definite clinical value. Comparing high-pass vs low-pass noise bands to estimate hearing loss configuration is relatively inaccurate (Jerger et al., 1974a; Van Wagoner and Goodwine, 1977). The bivariate plot system, however, offers no apparent improvement in hearing loss prediction for specific frequency regions. Acoustic reflex threshold data for 4000 Hz, a common region for sensorineural loss, was not included in the most recent description of the bivariate plot system for reasons cited earlier. In fact, Margolis and Fox (1977) seem to abandon any attempt to estimate hearing loss by frequency region using the bivariate plot system. The three frequency plots are instead used jointly in their two out of three criteria for normal hearing vs sensorineural loss.

Finally, false-positive results present a recurring problem in the previously discussed prediction methods. With the bivariate plot system, the problem is reportedly minimized (Handler and Margolis, 1977; Margolis and Fox, 1977). Close assessment of the data presented by Margolis and colleagues and a consideration of the criteria for normal hearing and the data in normal hearers reported by different investigators, however, cast some doubt upon this benefit. Of the seventeen normal-hearing subjects in the Margolis and Fox (1977) study, 94 percent fell within the normal region. That is, the false-positive rate was only 6 percent. In contrast, for the SPAR method, the false-positive rate is usually 25 to 45 percent. A possible source of the inconsistencies in predictive accuracy between methods is the discrepancy in criteria for normal hearing in the Margolis and Fox (1977) study, and the studies reporting SPAR results according to the guidelines suggested by Jerger and colleagues (1974) (Table 8–2). The bivariate plot region for normal hearing has an upper average hearing threshold limit of 32 dB, while originally Jerger and colleagues (1974) used 20 dB HL as the upper limit of average hearing level for 500, 1000, and 2000 Hz. The high false-positive rate in normals for the SPAR method may, to some extent, be influenced by these differences in criteria for normal hearing.

The false-positive rate for the SPAR method vs. bivariate plot system may also be related to a difference in the noise signals. The SPAR method is based on the difference between reflex thresholds for pure tones and broad-band noise. In the bivariate plot system, low-pass noise is used in identifying loss for 500 and 1000 Hz, and high-pass noise is used in identifying loss for 2000 Hz. Johnsen and colleagues (1976) suggested that isolated, high-frequency sensorineural loss usually elevates the reflex threshold for white noise, even in patients with relatively normal hearing for the 500 to 2000 Hz

(PTA) region. According to the SPAR criteria for hearing loss (Table 8–2), these patients would have normal hearing. Yet the elevated BBN threshold for these patients would tend to produce a lower SPAR and predict a loss. The result would then be a false-positive prediction. In contrast, the isolated, high-frequency loss would exert a minor influence in the bivariate plot system. The bivariate plot for acoustic reflex thresholds for 2000 Hz and high-pass noise would probably be affected by the high-frequency loss. It is unlikely, however, that the high-frequency loss would affect the bivariate plot for acoustic reflex thresholds for 500 Hz, and 1000 Hz, and low-pass noise. The criteria for normal hearing, as recommended by Margolis and Fox (1977) are normal categorizations in two of the three bivariate plots. In the not uncommon patient with isolated high-frequency loss and normal PTA, therefore, the bivariate plot system probably yields a normal prediction, rather than a false-positive prediction.

The bivariate plot system, however, seems to be characterized by an unusually high rate of false-negative results. That is, normal hearing is frequently predicted in a patient with a sensorineural loss. Of those subjects (thirty-two) in the Margolis and Fox (1977) study who passed the criteria for normal hearing (i.e., falling within the normal region on two or three of the frequency plots), approximately 50 percent actually showed a sensitivity loss at one or more of the test frequencies from 500 to 4000 Hz. A sloping high-frequency loss, or a loss only at and above 4000 Hz, is a common configuration in a clinical population. In the Margolis and Fox (1977) study, these configurations account for 57 percent of the sensorineural group. Normal hearing was predicted in more than one-third of these subjects (35 percent). The bivariate plot fails to identify the loss.

The SPAR method, on the other hand, has a relatively low false-negative rate. In three out of four recent reports of the SPAR method in clinical populations (Keith, 1977; Tsappis, 1977; and Hall, 1978), 92 to 100 percent of the patients with a prediction of normal hearing actually had normal hearing. In the analysis of SPAR findings in the Margolis and Fox (1977) study, none of the subjects with sensorineural loss were predicted to have normal hearing. Only normal-hearing subjects received normal predictions. In these primarily adult populations, it seems natural first to determine audiometric hearing level, and then to assess the hearing loss predictive accuracy by acoustic reflexes. Viewing hearing prediction accuracy in this sequence emphasizes a problem with false-positive errors and actually minimizes false-negative errors. In a young population, however, a hearing loss prediction from the acoustic reflex may be the only viable measure of sensitivity. Without the benefit of valid behavioral results for comparison, then, a more pressing concern is this: The acoustic reflex data predicts normal sensitivity—what is the likelihood that a sensitivity loss is actually present? With the bivariate plot system, one out of every two such patients is likely to have a sensitivity loss. With the SPAR methods, there is relatively little likelihood of loss with a prediction of normal hearing. The benefit of the low false-positive rate attributed to the bivariate plot system, then, is obtained at the expense of a high false-negative result.

In summary, the bivariate plot system offers the advantage of identification of sensorineural loss with a minimal rate of predictive errors among those with normal hearing. The major disadvantages are a high rate of unidentified mild- and/or high-frequency sensorineural impairments, and the designed limitation of simple identification of loss without an estimate of the degree of loss. The value of the bivariate plot system, however, unlike the predictive methods, has not been assessed in a large clinical population.

FACTORS INFLUENCING HEARING LOSS PREDICTION

Hearing loss prediction from the acoustic reflex, although objective, may be influenced by a variety of factors. Recent investigations have shown that predictive accuracy is differentially affected by the degree of hearing loss, subject age, minor middle ear disorders, and central auditory disorder.

Effect of degree of loss. There is general agreement that the accuracy of hearing loss prediction by all methods varies as a function of degree of loss. The SPAR method has relatively greater accuracy in persons with normal hearing or those with severe or profound sensorineural loss; the greatest proportion of predictive errors occurs in persons with mild or moderate loss (Jerger et al., 1974a; Schwartz and Sanders, 1976; Keith, 1977; Tsappis, 1977; Van Wagoner and Goodwine, 1977; and Hall, 1978). The effect of magnitude of sensorineural loss on predictive accuracy of the Niemeyer-Sesterhenn equation is remarkably similar (Keith, 1977). Accuracy of the bivariate plot system in normal-hearing subjects has been discussed. Margolis and Fox (1977) also observed that the probability of a subject falling outside of the normal region increases with the severity of loss. In contrast to the findings of these three methods, the regression equation developed by Baker and Lilly (1976) most accurately predicted hearing in subjects with mild-to-moderate loss (Hall, 1978). Hearing level was usually overestimated in those with normal hearing. More importantly, in subjects with sensitivity loss the error of prediction (underestimation of hearing level) increased directly with the degree of loss.

The basis for these similarities and differences in the accuracy of the four types of prediction methods is unclear. As Schwartz and Sanders (1976) point out, if successful prediction of loss depends on an abnormal widening of the critical band in sensorineural ears, one would expect a rather direct relationship between degree of loss and abnormal width of the critical band for acoustic reflexes. However, these researchers found no consistent difference in abnormal widening of the critical band in subjects with mild-to-moderate loss vs severe loss. Abnormal widening of the critical band did separate those with normal hearing from those with sensorineural loss. With the exception of the bivariate plot system, the predictive methods attempt to differentiate degree of loss, at least partly, on the basis of the NTD, a critical band phenomenon. Therefore, the findings of Schwartz and Sanders (1976) may help to explain the inaccuracies that characterize these methods and the success of the bivariate plot system in separating normal-hearing patients from those with sensorineural loss.

Previously, in Figure 8–1, acoustic reflex thresholds for noise and tone signals were shown as a function of sensorineural loss. Reflex thresholds for the noise signal increase relatively systematically with loss, while reflex thresholds for tone signals improve slightly through the mild-to-moderate loss region (26 to 45 dB HL) and then, at different rates, increase with greater loss. The greatest critical band effect, it seems, occurs between the normal-hearing range and approximately 45 dB HL. The loss-related differences in thresholds for noise and tones are greatest in this region. From the mild-moderate to severe loss regions, reflex thresholds are elevated similarly for tone and noise signals, presumably owing to the effect of increased hearing level alone. Accurate differentiation of those with normal hearing vs those with sensorineural loss, then, is dependent primarily on the NTD, or a noise-tone ratio, a relative value. Above approximately 45 dB, therefore, accurate predictions must rely on the absolute level of the noise and/or tone reflex thresholds. Only two prediction methods incorporate criteria for both absolute and relative noise and tone reflex thresholds. One of them, the bivariate plot system, probably relies heavily on the noise-tone ratio to separate normal vs sensorineural subjects. The absolute tone threshold (the ordinate value) may account for the increased probability of a correct categorization as severity increases, since at higher tone threshold levels, the lines of intersect tend toward the ordinate (Fig. 8–3). The 1977 SPAR employs criteria for the noise-tone difference, as well as the absolute thresholds for both the noise and 1000 Hz tone signal. The NTD criteria primarily identify loss. The absolute noise and 1000 Hz criteria serve to estimate degree of loss. Based on the data in Figure 8–1, however, criteria for absolute thresholds for noise and 2000 Hz, rather than 1000 Hz, seem to be more directly related to degree of loss. This finding may be related to the predominantly sloping loss characterizing the population.

Effect of age. Chronologic age influences virtually every aspect of auditory function, including pure-tone sensitivity (Bunch, 1929; Goetzinger et al., 1961; and Hayes and Jerger, 1979a, b), speech understanding (Gaeth, 1948; Goetzinger et al., 1961; Pestalozza and Shore, 1955; Jerger, 1973; and Hayes and Jerger, 1979b), and the auditory brain stem response (ABR) (Beagley and Sheldrake, 1978; Rowe, 1978; Stockard, Stockard, Sharbrough, 1978; and Thomsen, Terkildsen, Osterhammel, 1978). The effect of age on acoustic impedance measures, therefore, is not unexpected. Static compliance changes as a function of age in adults (Jerger et al., 1972; Hall, 1979), and children (Hall and Weaver, 1979). Acoustic reflex thresholds are also affected by chronologic age in adults (Handler and Margolis, 1977; Jerger et al., 1978a) and in infants and children (Margolis and Popelka, 1975; Abahazi and Greenberg, 1977; Handler and Margolis, 1977; and Hall and Weaver, 1979). Age differentially affects thresholds for noise vs tone signals. In general, reflex thresholds for tone signals improve slightly in increasing age from infancy through adulthood. Reflex thresholds for noise signals, on the other hand, may increase slightly from infancy to adulthood. In adults, Handler and Margolis (1977) have reported increased reflex thresholds to noise signals in subjects greater than sixty years of age. Jerger and colleagues (1978a) found no age-related change in reflex thresholds to a noise signal in adults though fifty-nine years of age. Since Handler and Margolis (1977) did not systematically study reflex thresholds in subjects between approximately twenty and sixty years of age, and Jerger and colleagues (1978a) did not report data for subjects over sixty years old, the two sets of findings may not in fact be incompatible. In any event, the net result of the differential effect of age on reflex thresholds for tone and noise is a reduction in the NTD (Hall, 1978; Jerger et al., 1978a). This phenomenon is illustrated in Figure 8–4 for 539 normal-hearing subjects ages one to twenty years. Even in this young population, the NTD systematically decreases with age. The age effect is greater for males than females.

As a result of the effect of age on the NTD, the accuracy of hearing prediction methods based on the NTD, such as the SPAR technique, tends to diminish as a function of age (Hall, 1978; Jerger et al., 1978b). According to Hall (1978), the rate of accurate prediction for the 1974 SPAR, for example, decreased from 69 percent in the youngest age group (five to twenty years) to 52 percent in the forty-one- to sixty-year-old group. The rate of moderate predictive errors increased proportionately, while the rate of serious errors remained the same. The Baker-Lilly regression equation, as indicated previously, is not strictly based on the NTD. Consequently, a less pronounced age effect might be expected in predictive accuracy of the Baker-Lilly equation. However, this equation includes reflex data for four pure-tone frequencies as well as BBN. The effect of age seems to be greatest for pure-tone reflex thresholds. Accuracy of

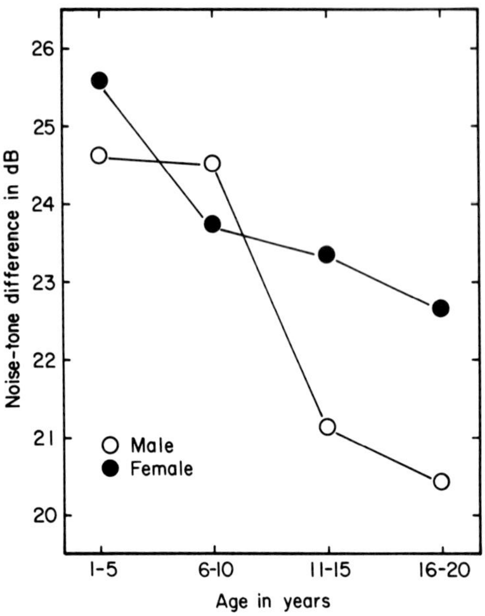

Figure 8-4 Effect of age on noise-tone difference (NTD). Results are for 539 normal-hearing subjects. Distribution of subjects according to age is as follows: 0 to 5 years, 123; 6 to 10 years, 220; 11 to 15 years, 108; 16 to 20 years, 88.

the Baker-Lilly equation, perhaps since it includes four tone factors to one noise factor, is noticeably influenced by age. In the Hall (1978) study, rate of accuracy decreased from 73 percent in the youngest group (five to twenty years) to fifty-six percent in the forty-one- to sixty-year-old group.

In contrast to these data, Handler and Margolis (1977) found no evidence of decreased reflex thresholds to pure-tone signals in eight subjects ages fifty-six and older. The mean age of these eight subjects was not provided. Using the bivariate plot system, accuracy of hearing loss identification in thirty-eight older subjects (mean age sixty-eight years) was comparable to previously reported identification rates in younger subjects. As noted above, noise reflex thresholds are relatively constant with age. The apparent heavy reliance of the bivariate plot system on the noise threshold, then, may explain the absence of an age-effect in predictive accuracy.

The greatest effect of age on the SPAR and Baker-Lilly prediction methods occurs between the youngest group (five to twenty years) and young adulthood (twenty-one to forty years) (Hall, 1978; Jerger et al., 1978b). It seemed reasonable, therefore, to suspect that accuracy of the SPAR method actually shows an age-effect within this young age range (zero to twenty years). To test this hypothesis, SPAR accuracy was assessed as a function of age in 537 subjects aged one to twenty years (Table 8–4). All subjects had normal hearing (hearing threshold levels of 25 dB or better for octave test frequencies from 250 through 4000 Hz) and normal middle ear function (normal type A tympanograms with peak at 0 to −50 mm H_2O pressure). Table 8–4 shows the error distribution of the 1974 and 1977 SPAR methods as a function of age in this young population. Each SPAR method is most accurate in the youngest (one- to five-year-old) group. Accuracy decreases through the eleven- to fifteen-year-old group for both methods, reaching a rate of accuracy that is comparable to that reported for adults in previous studies (Hall, 1978; Jerger et al., 1978b). As in adult populations, the rate of moderate predictive errors increases proportionately. Unlike previous findings in adults, however, the rate of serious errors in the young population also increases over the age range from one to fifteen years.

Effect of Minor Middle Ear Disorders. In 1970 and 1972, Jerger reported criteria

TABLE 8–4 ERROR DISTRIBUTION OF 1974 AND 1977 SPAR METHODS AS A FUNCTION OF AGE*

	Age In Years							
	1974				1977			
TYPE OF ERROR (%)	1–5	6–10	11–15	16–20	1–5	6–10	11–15	16–20
None	88	75	67	67	79	69	59	62
Moderate	12	23	29	28	20	29	34	32
Serious	0	2	5	6	1	2	6	6

*Data for 537 subjects with normal hearing sensitivity and normal middle ear function; distribution of subjects according to age: 0–5 years, 123; 6–10 years, 219; 11–15 years, 108; 16–20 years, 87
SPAR = Sensitivity Prediction by Acoustic Reflex

for normal middle ear function by impedance audiometry. These criteria, widely accepted clinically, were for tympanogram, static compliance, and acoustic reflex measurements. The normal, or type A, tympanogram has a distinct peak (point of maximum compliance) at or near normal atmospheric pressure, within the range of 0 to −100 mm water pressure. The type A is distinguished from two abnormal tympanogram types. One, the type B, has no distinct point of maximum compliance, appearing rounded or flattened. The other, the type C, has a distinct point of maximum compliance, but this peak occurs at a negative middle ear pressure exceeding −100 mm water pressure, relative to normal atmospheric pressure.

Static compliance, the second criteria for normal middle ear function, is an absolute value obtained by measuring the volume of air that is equivalent, in compliance, to the middle ear system. Static compliance is expressed as an equivalent volume of air in cm^3 (cc). Normal static compliance values range from about 0.30 to 1.60 cm^3 (Jerger et al. 1972). In normal ears, static compliance tends to increase with age from one to thirty-five years (Jerger et al., 1972; Hall, 1979; and Hall and Weaver, 1979). Above age thirty-five, static compliance gradually decreases (Jerger et al., 1972; Hall, 1979). At age seventy, the average static compliance value approaches the lower limit of the normal range (O.30 cm^3). In general, static compliance is greater in males than in females (Jerger et al., 1972; Hall, 1979; and Hall and Weaver, 1979).

Acoustic reflex thresholds are the third criteria for middle ear function. As indicated previously, in normal ears the acoustic reflex is elicited by pure-tone signals at 85 to 95 dB HL, and by broad-band noise at 65 to 85 dB SPL (Møller, 1962; Jerger et al., 1972, 1978a). With the impedance probe in an ear with middle ear disorder, acoustic reflexes are typically absent (Jerger et al., 1974b). There is a high likelihood of absent reflexes even if the air-bone gap is slight (5 to 10 dB). When sound is presented to the conductive ear, and the impedance change is measured in the opposite, normal ear (the contralateral reflex), there is a direct and predictable relationship between the reflex threshold level and the degree of conductive sensitivity loss. Acoustic reflex threshold is elevated by the degree of sensitivity loss. Elevated reflex thresholds (greater than 95 to 100 dB HL) are a sign of middle ear disorder. The pattern of impedance audiometry findings is most effective in detecting middle ear disorders. If one or more of the three impedance measures is abnormal, a middle ear disorder must be suspected. Since acoustic reflex thresholds are usually elevated or absent in middle ear disorders, even in the presence of relatively normal hearing sensitivity (Jerger et al., 1974 b), accurate prediction of hearing loss from the acoustic reflex is precluded by middle ear disorder. If any of the three criteria for normal middle ear function are not met, hearing loss prediction should not be attempted.

The effect of clinically significant middle ear disorder on acoustic reflex measurements was noted in the early reports of the clinical application of impedance audiometry (Jerger, 1970). Only recently, however, has there been an appreciation of the effect of minor middle disorders on reflex measurements. In patients meeting Jerger's (1970) three clinical criteria for normal middle ear function, there may still be spurious middle ear effects on hearing loss prediction from the acoustic reflex. Two not uncommon minor middle ear problems, realtively compliant tympanograms, and slight negative middle pressure (−50 to 100 mm water) may produce elevated reflex threshold for noise and tone signals. Hall and Weaver (1979) studied acoustic reflex thresholds in 212 subjects (average age ten years) with these two minor middle ear abnormalities. All subjects met clinical criteria for normal middle ear function (Jerger, 1970). In addition, all subjects had normal hearing sensitivity (no hearing threshold level greater than 25 dB for octave test frequencies of 250 to 4000 Hz). With the impedance probe in an ear with a high compliant middle ear system (type A-deep tympanogram) contralateral reflex thresholds for pure-tone signals were elevated from 3 to 5 dB. The reflex threshold for the BBN signal was elevated to 10 dB. With the impedance probe in an ear with slight negative pressure (−50 to −100 mm water), contralateral reflex thresholds were elevated from 2 to 5 dB for pure-tone and noise signals. These clinical findings, for pure-tone signals, were in close agreement with experimental results reported by Martin and Coombes (1974).

Probably as a result of the influence of minor middle ear disorders on reflex thresholds, and especially the NTD for reflex thresholds, predictive accuracy of the SPAR methods decreases in patients with these problems. Hall (1978) compared the error distribution of the 1974 and 1977 SPAR methods in 370 subjects with unequivocally normal middle ear function and in 36 subjects with tympanometric evidence of a highly compliant middle ear function. The rate of accurate prediction for both SPAR methods dropped from 55 to 60 percent in the normal group, to 20 to 23 percent in the group with A-deep tympanograms. The rate of moderate errors in prediction, as a consequence, increased from 38 to 42 percent and from 58 to 61 percent. More importantly, the proportion of serious predictive errors increased dramatically, from 2 to 3 percent and from 16 to 22 percent. Since the group with minor middle ear disorder had normal hearing, all serious errors were prediction of severe loss when, in fact, hearing sensitivity was normal.

A similar influence of minor middle ear disorders on SPAR accuracy is shown for 239 subjects aged one to twenty years in Table 8-5. Minor middle ear disorders for the

TABLE 8-5 COMPARISON OF ERROR DISTRIBUTION FOR THE 1974 AND 1977 SPAR METHODS*

	1974		1977	
Type of error (%)	**Normal**	**Middle ear disorder**	**Normal**	**Middle ear disorder**
None	70	59	69	42
Moderate				
Overestimate	22	33	26	39
Underestimate	05	03	02	02
Serious				
Overestimate	03	04	04	18
Underestimate	0.4	0.7	0.4	0

*Data for 670 subjects with normal middle ear function (average age 9.8 years) and 239 subjects (average age 9.5 years) with minor middle ear disorders; Ad tympanogram or negative middle ear pressure of from −50 to −100 mm H_2O in probe ear, or both ears
SPAR = Sensitivity Prediction by the Acoustic Reflex

239 subjects consisted of an A-deep tympanogram or negative middle ear pressure of from -50 to -100 mm water in the impedance probe ear or both ears. The middle ear findings in this group, then, are more varied than those of the group reported by Hall (1978). Also, average age in the group of 239 subjects was 9.5 years, while in the group of 36 subjects reported by Hall (1978), average age was approximately 40 years. Perhaps as a consequence of these two basic differences between the populations, the influence of minor middle ear disorders on the SPAR methods as shown in Table 8-5 is less pronounced than in the Hall (1978) study. Still, the rate of accurate prediction for the 1974 SPAR method drops 11 percent. For the 1977 SPAR method, the decreased rate of accurate predictions is greater—27 percent. The rate of moderate predictive errors increases proportionately for each SPAR method. For both methods, the moderate and serious errors are predominantly overestimations of loss, even though the population is composed of subjects with sensorineural loss as well as those with normal hearing. The greater influence of minor middle ear disorders on accuracy of the 1977 SPAR vs the 1974 SPAR in this population is probably related to the differences in predictive criteria for the two methods. Recall that the 1977 SPAR is calculated from the NTD, and the absolute reflex threshold for BBN *and* the 1000 Hz signal (Table 8-3). The 1974 SPAR, on the other hand, does not include criteria for the absolute threshold of 1000 Hz. Since minor middle ear disorders elevate pure-tone reflex thresholds as well as reducing the NTD, it seems likely that with the 1977 SPAR a proportion of normal-hearing subjects would pass the normal criteria for NTD ($\geq$ 20), yet fail the normal criteria for the 1000 Hz threshold ($>$ 95 dB HL) and, therefore, receive a prediction of mild loss. By the 1974 SPAR criteria, these subjects with an NTD of greater than 20 would receive a normal prediction.

In the Hall (1978) study, accuracy of the Baker-Lilly equation as compared with the SPAR methods seemed to be unaffected by minor middle ear disorder. The rate of accuracy in normal subjects (63 percent) was comparable to the middle ear group (67 percent). Moderate error rates were also comparable. Fortuitously, there were no serious predictive errors in either normal or middle ear group. A ready explanation for the success of the Baker-Lilly equation in spite of minor middle ear disorder is not available. However, the regression equation does not depend on either the strict NTD, or the absolute levels of any acoustic reflex threshold. Therefore, the effect of minor middle ear disorder in these two factors would probably not influence hearing loss prediction by the Baker-Lilly equation. The SPAR methods, especially the 1977 SPAR, which depends on both factors, are seriously influenced by middle ear disorder.

The possible effects of minor middle ear disorder on the Niemeyer-Sesterhenn equation and on the bivariate plot system have not been reported. In all likelihood, however, for reasons just cited, the NTD-based Niemeyer-Sesterhenn equation would be seriously influenced, while the bivariate plot system would be essentially unaffected.

In summary, minor middle ear problems may seriously reduce the accuracy of hearing loss prediction by the acoustic reflex. The clinical criteria for normal middle ear function do not rule out the possibility of a middle ear effect, at least in prediction methods based on the NTD and absolute reflex threshold levels. Accuracy of the Baker-Lilly regression equation is relatively unaffected by minor middle ear problems.

Central Auditory Disorder. In central auditory disorders at the brain stem level, contralateral acoustic reflex thresholds may be elevated or absent (Griesen and Rasmussen, 1970; Colletti, 1975; Bosatra, Russolo, Poli, 1976; Jerger and Jerger, 1977; and Jerger, Jerger, Hall, 1979). Borg (1973) demonstrated experimentally that the reflex threshold was impaired primarily by disorders affecting the lower brain stem auditory nuclei and pathways. Clinically, the abnormalities in reflex threshold level were reported in normal-hearing subjects with central auditory disorders (Jerger and Jerger, 1977; Jerger et al., 1979).

Elevation of reflex thresholds in central auditory disorders has obvious importance for hearing loss prediction. Prediction methods based in part on absolute reflex threshold level may tend to produce false-positive results in central auditory disorders (Margolis and Fox, 1977). For example, a patient with normal hearing sensitivity but with a central auditory disorder and, subsequently, and elevated reflex threshold for 1000 Hz would fail one of the 1977 SPAR criteria for a normal prediction (Table 8–3). The effect of central auditory disorder on acoustic reflex thresholds for tones vs noise is not known. It does not seem unreasonable, however, to hypothesize that acoustic reflex thresholds for complex auditory signals, such as noise, will be more sensitive to central auditory disorder than simpler signals, such as pure tones. If this hypothesis were correct, and reflex thresholds for noise signals were elevated relative to tone signals, the NTD would be reduced. The combination of a reduced NTD and elevated absolute reflex thresholds would contribute to a greater rate of predictive errors in patients with central auditory disorders. In adult patients with signs of central auditory disorders, or in children at risk for central auditory disorders, hearing loss prediction by the acoustic reflex must be interpreted cautiously.

DISCUSSION

In 1972, hearing loss prediction from the acoustic reflex was introduced with hopes that it would meet a long awaited clinical need—objective estimation of hearing sensitivity. Accumulated clinical experience with three general prediction methods has tempered this early optimism (Niemeyer and Sesterhenn, 1972, 1974; Jerger et al., 1974; Baker and Lilly, 1976; Popelka, Margolis, Wiley, 1976). As discussed in this chapter, each method seems to have distinct limitations. The original Niemeyer and Sesterhenn equation (1972, 1974) and Sensitivity Prediction by the Acoustic Reflex (SPAR) first described by Jerger et al. (1974) are usually characterized by a sizeable proportion of prediction errors (20 to 40 percent). Subsequent regression equations (Baker and Lilly, 1976: Lilly, 1977; Rizzo and Greenberg, 1979) tend to underestimate serious hearing loss (Hall, 1978). The bivariate plot system (Popelka et al., 1976; Handler and Margolis, 1977; Margolis and Fox, 1977) simply identifies either normal hearing or sensitivity loss greater than 32 dB HL, and seems to be relatively insensitive to mild and, especially, high frequency sensorineural loss. None of the methods, therefore, routinely identifies or estimates hearing loss accurately.

The outlook for hearing loss prediction, however, is good in spite of the limitation of the current methods. We are now learning about factors which influence acoustic reflex measurements and, consequently, hearing loss prediction. The principal factors appear to be age and minor middle ear disorders reflected by impedance audiometry. In adults, predictive accuracy decreases as a function of chronologic age (Hall, 1978; Jerger, Hayes, Anthony, 1978). Fortuitously, prediction methods are most accurate in children (Jerger, Hayes, Anthony, 1978; Hall and Weaver, 1979). The exact basis of the apparent age effect is still unclear. There is evidence, however, that age influences the relationship of reflex thresholds for pure tone and noise signals (Jerger et al., 1978; Hall and Weaver, 1978). Since this relationship is central to hearing loss prediction, the limitations of the methods may, in part, stem from the age effect. In both children and adults, minor impedance abnormalities may seriously influence hearing loss prediction (Hall, 1978; Jerger et al., 1978; Hall and Weaver, 1978). Impedance audiometry findings in these patients meet accepted clinical criteria for normal middle ear function (Jerger, 1970). There is no concommitant hearing sensitivity loss or audiometric evidence of a conductive disorder. Yet, close examination of impedance audiometry findings typically reveals subtle aberrations, such as slight negative pressure in the middle ear (e.g., − 50 to − 100 water pressure), or an unusually deep or unusually shallow tympanogram. Reflex thresholds, although usually present, tend to be slightly elevated (4 to 10 dB) for pure tone and/or noise signals. By clinical standards, these findings are not significant. Perhaps for this reason minor impedance abnormalities were not recognized until recently. Their deleterious effect on hearing loss prediction, however, is dramatic. Predictive accuracy may decrease by as much as 40 to 50 percent (Hall, 1978). Minor impedance audiometry abnormalities, then, probably contribute to the limitations of current prediction methods.

Although the initial expectations for hearing loss prediction were not borne out by clinical experience, there is reason for optimism about the potential of the concept. In very young children, acoustic reflex prediction methods clearly offer the most rapid and viable objective measure of hearing sensitivity. Even in the "difficult-to-test" child, the nemesis of traditional behavioral techniques, reflex measurements permit a reasonably accurate estimate of hearing level. In addition, since hearing loss prediction methods have assumed a preeminent role in audiology, we now are able to exploit accumulated clinical experience in developing improved techniques. Examination of the strengths and weaknesses of the methods presented in this chapter, for example, suggests a general principle for the design of improved techniques. Consistently accurate prediction of hearing, it seems, requires a combination of both relative and absolute measures of reflex thresholds for pure tone and noise signals. With an integration of our accumulated knowledge of individual prediction methods, and an appreciation of the factors influencing these methods, the probabilities of generating an algorithm suitable for hearing loss prediction seem quite high.

REFERENCES

Abahazi, D.A. and Greenberg, H.J.: Clinical acoustic reflex threshold measurement in infants. *J. Speech Hear. Dis.* 42: 514, 1977.

Baker, S.R. and Lilly, D.J.: Prediction of hearing level from acoustic reflex data. Read before the American Speech and Hearing Convention, Houston, Texas, November 20, 1976.

Beagley, H.A. and Sheldrake, J.B.: Differences in brainstem response latency with age and sex. *Brit. J. Audiol.* 12:69, 1978.

Borg, E.: On the neuronal organization of the acoustic middle ear reflex. *Brain Res.* 49:101, 1973.

Bosatra, A., Russolo, M. and Poli, P.: Oscilloscope analysis of the stapedius muscle reflex in brainstem lesions. *Arch. Otolaryngol.* 102:284, 1976.

Bunch, C.C.: Age variations in auditory acuity. *Arch. Otolaryngol.* 9:625, 1929.

Colletti, V.: Stapedius reflex abnormalities in multiple sclerosis. *Audiol.* 14:63, 1975.

Dallos, P.J.: Dynamics of the acoustic reflex: phenomenological aspects. *J. Acoust. Soc. Amer.* 36:2175, 1964.

Deutsch, L.: The threshold of the stapedial reflex for pure tone and noise stimuli. *Acta Otolaryngol.* 74:248, 1972.

Djupesland, G., Flottorp, G. and Winther, F.O.: Size and duration of acoustical elicited impedance changes in man. *Acta Otolaryngol. (Suppl.)* 244:220, 1967.

Djupesland, G., Sundby, A. and Hogstad, K.: A study of critical bandwidth in Meniére's syndrome using the acoustic stapedial reflex. *Scand. Audiol.* 4:127, 1975.

Djupesland, G. and Zwislocki, J.: On the critical band in the acoustic stapedius reflex. *J. Acoust. Soc. Amer.* 54:1157, 1973.
Fisch, U. and Von Schulthess, G.: Electromyographic studies on the human stapedial muscle. *Acta Otolaryngol.* 56:287, 1963.
Fitton, R.A.: Sensitivity prediction using acoustic reflex threshold measures in children. Unpublished doctoral dissertation, Wayne State University School of Medicine, Detroit, Michigan, 1979.
Flottorp, G., Djupesland, G. and Winther, F.: The acoustic stapedius reflex in relation to critical bandwidth. *J. Acoust. Soc. Amer.* 49:457, 1971.
Gaeth, J.H.: A study of phonemic regression in relation to hearing loss. Unpublished doctoral dissertation, Northwestern University, 1948.
Gersdorff, M. C.: Comparative study between the normally hearing child and the hard of hearing child, by acoustic impedance measurements of the ear. *Arch. Otol., Rhinol., Laryngol. (Berlin)* 217:13, 1977.
Gersdorff, M.C.: Modificatione du reflexe acoustico-facial chez l'homme en fonction de l'age, par etude impedancemetrique. *Audiol.* 17:260, 1978.
Goetzinger, C.P., Proud, G.O., Dirks, D. and Embrey, J.A.: Study of hearing in advanced age. *Arch. Otolaryngol.* 73:662, 1961.
Griesen, D. and Rasmussen, P.E.: Stapedius muscle reflexes and otoneurological examination in brainstem tumors. *Acta Otolaryngol.* 70:366, 1970.
Hall, J.W.: Predicting hearing level from the acoustic reflex: a comparison of three methods. *Arch. Otolaryngol.* 104:601, 1978.
Hall, J.W.: Effects of age and sex on static compliance. *Arch. Otolaryngol.* 105:153, 1979.
Hall, J.W. and Weaver, T.: Impedance audiometry in a young population: the effect of age, sex and tympanogram abnormalities. *J. Otolaryngol. (Toronto)* 8 (3):210-222, 1979.
Handler, S.D. and Margolis, R.H.: Predicting hearing loss from stapedial reflex thresholds in patients with sensorineural impairment. *Trans. Am. Acad. Ophthalmol. Otolaryngol.* 84:425, 1977.
Hayes, D. and Jerger, J.: Aging and hearing aid use. *Scand. Audiol.* 8:33, 1979a.
Hayes, D. and Jerger, J.: Low-frequency hearing loss in presbycusis: a central interpretation. *Arch. Otolaryngol.* 105:9, 1979b.
Jerger, J.F.: Clinical experience with impedance audiometry. *Arch. Otolaryngol.* 92:311, 1970.
Jerger, J.F.: Diagnostic use of impedance measures. In Jerger, J. (Ed.): *Handbook of Clinical Impedance Audiometry.* Dobbs Ferry, New York, American Electromedics Corporation, 1975, 149–174.
Jerger, J., Jerger, S. and Mauldin, L.: Studies in impedance audiometry: I. Normal and sensorineural ears. *Arch. Otolaryngol.* 96:513, 1972.
Jerger, J.: Audiologic findings in aging. *Adv. Otorhinolaryngol.* 20:115, 1973.
Jerger, J., Burney, P., Mauldin, L. and Crump, B.: Predicting hearing loss from the acoustic reflex. *J. Speech Hear. Dis.* 39:11, 1974a.
Jerger, J., Anthony, L., Jerger, S. and Mauldin, L.: Studies in impedance audiometry III. Middle ear disorders. *Arch. Otolaryngol.* 99:165, 1974b.
Jerger, J. and Hayes, D.: The cross-check principle in pediatric audiometry. *Arch. Otolaryngol.* 102:614, 1976.
Jerger, S. and Jerger, J.: Diagnostic value of crossed vs uncrossed acoustic reflexes. *Arch. Otolaryngol.* 103:445, 1977.
Jerger, J., Hayes, D., Anthony, L. and Mauldin, L.: Factors influencing prediction of hearing level from the acoustic reflex. *Contemp. Mon. Audiol. (Maico)* 1 (1):1, 1978a.
Jerger, J., Hayes, D. and Anthony, L.: Effect of age on prediction of sensorineural hearing level from the acoustic reflex. *Arch. Otolaryngol.* 104:393, 1978b.
Jerger, S., Jerger, J. and Hall, J.W.: A new acoustic reflex pattern. *Arch. Otolaryngol.* 105:24, 1979.
Johnsen, N.J., Osterhammel, D., Terkildsen, K., Osterhammel, P. and Huis in't Veld, F.: The white noise middle ear muscle reflex threshold in patients with sensorineural hearing impairment. *Scand. Audiol.* 5:131, 1976.
Keith, R.W.: An evaluation of predicting hearing loss from the acoustic reflex. *Arch. Otolaryngol.* 103:419, 1977.
Keith, R.W., Murphey, K.P. and Martin, F.: Acoustic impedance measurement in the otological assessment of multiply handicapped children. *Clin. Otolaryngol.* 1:221, 1976.
Keith, R.W., Murphey, K.P. and Martin, F.: Acoustic reflex measurements in children with cerebral palsy. *Folia Phoniatrica (Basel)* 29:311, 1977.
Lamb, L.E. and Norris, T.W.: Relative acoustic impedance measurement with mentally retarded children. *Am. J. Ment. Defic.* 75:51, 1970.
Lilly, D.J.: Some properties of the acoustic reflex in man. *J. Acoust. Soc. Amer.* 36:2007, 1964.
Lilly, D.J.: Prediction of points on the audiogram from acoustic reflex data. Read before the American Speech and Hearing Association Convention, Chicago, Illinois, November 4, 1977.
Margolis, R.H. and Fox, C.M.: A comparison of three methods for predicting hearing loss from acoustic reflex thresholds. *J. Speech Hear. Res.* 20:241, 1977.
Margolis, R.H. and Popelka, G.R.: Static and dynamic acoustic impedance measurements in infant ears. *J. Speech Hear. Res.* 18:435, 1975.

Martin, F.N. and Coombes, S.: Effects of external ear canal pressure on the middle ear muscle reflex threshold. *J. Speech Hear. Res.* 17:526, 1974.
Miller, R., Davies, C.B. and Gibson, W.P.R.: Using the acoustic reflex to predict the pure tone threshold. *Brit. J. Audiol.* 10:51, 1976.
MØller, A.R.: Acoustic reflex in man. *J. Acoust. Soc. Amer.* 34:1524, 1962.
Niemeyer, W. and Sesterhenn, G.: Calculating the hearing threshold from the stapedius reflex threshold for different sound stimuli. Read before the Eleventh International Congress of Audiology, Budapest, October 5, 1972.
Niemeyer, W. and Sesterhenn, G.: Calculating the hearing threshold from the stapedius reflex threshold for different sound stimuli. *Audiol.* 13:421, 1974.
Niswander, P.S. and Ruth, R.A.: Prediction of hearing sensitivity from acoustic reflexes in mentally retarded persons. *Am. J. Ment. Defic.* 81:474, 1977.
Pestalozza, G. and Shore, I.: Clinical evaluation of presbycusis on the basis of different tests of auditory function. *Laryngoscope* 65:1136, 1955.
Peterson, J.L. and Lidén, G.: Some static characteristics of the stapedial muscle reflex. *Audiol.* 11:97, 1972.
Popelka, G.R., Karlovich, R.S. and Wiley, T.L.: Acoustic reflex and critical bandwidth. *J. Acoust. Soc. Amer.* 55:883, 1974.
Popelka, G.R., Margolis, R.H. and Wiley, T.L.: Effect of activating signal bandwidth on acoustic reflex thresholds. *J. Accoust. Soc. Amer.* 59:153, 1976.
Ransome, J.: Impedance measurements: some recent developments. *J. Laryngol. Otol.* 91:655, 1977.
Rizzo, S., Jr. and Greenberg, H.J.: Predicting hearing loss from the acoustic reflex. Paper presented before Fiftieth Meeting of the Acoustical Society of America, Boston, Massachusetts, June 12, 1979.
Rowe, M.J., III: Normal variability of the brainstem auditory evoked response in young and old adult subjects. *Electroencephal. Clin. Neurophysiol.* 44:459, 1978.
Schwartz, D.M. and Sanders, J.W.: Critical bandwidth and sensitivity prediction in the acoustic stapedial reflex. *J. Speech Hear. Dis.* 41:244, 1976.
Sesterhenn, G. and Breuninger, H.: Determination of hearing threshold for single frequencies from the acoustic reflex. *Audiol.* 16:201, 1977.
Stockard, J.J., Stockard, J.E. and Sharbrough, F.W.: Nonpathologic factors influencing brainstem auditory evoked potentials. *Am. J. EEG Technol.* 18:177, 1978.
Suria, D., and Serra-Raventos, W.: Acoustic impedance measurement and autistic children. *Folia Phoniatrica (Basel)* 27:387, 1975.
Thomsen, J., Terkildsen, K. and Osterhammel, P.: Auditory brainstem responses in patients with acoustic neuromas. *Scand. Audiol.* 7:197, 1978.
Tsappis, A.: Prediction of auditory sensitivity: small sample confirmation using acoustic reflex thresholds. *Arch. Otolaryngol.* 103:322, 1977.
Van Wagoner, R.S. and Goodwine, S.: Clinical impressions of acoustic reflex measures in an adult population. *Arch. Otolaryngol.* 103:582, 1977.

Chapter Nine

IMPEDANCE IN SCREENING

DENZIL N. BROOKS, M.Sc.

INTRODUCTION

Responsibility of the state for the health and well-being of schoolchildren was initiated in 1883 when Frankfurt-am-Main appointed the first school doctor. Other European countries rapidly followed suit and by the turn of the century medical inspection of schoolchildren was becoming the rule rather than the exception.

Testing of hearing was normally carried out by using conversational speech (Wolf, 1899) or the whispered voice produced after complete exhalation (Bezold, 1896); the latter technique was more consistent and reliable. Studies around this period in Germany (Von Hartmann, 1905) suggested that approximately 27 percent of the school population were partially hard of hearing owing essentially to middle ear malfunction. Von Hartmann stressed the need to identify these handicapped children at the earliest possible opportunity so that "the curable could be cured and the incurably deaf might be educated to be worthy citizens."

The high prevalence of hearing loss in schoolchildren was confirmed by Van Den Borg (1942), who suggested that between 20 and 35 percent of schoolchildren showed impaired hearing by means of whispered-voice testing at 8 meters. He drew attention to the fact that slight losses of hearing would be undetected by this technique, which is roughly equivalent to a pure-tone screening test at a level of 20 to 25 dB HL.

The imperfections of whispered-voice testing were noted in the Board of Education report (1931), and the comment was added that "the need for a more scientific method has now been met by the introduction of the audiometer." Some of the earliest audiometric studies were carried out in the United States. Watson and Tolan (1949) reported on the use of the Seashore audiometer in Chicago schools in the early years of the twentieth century. In Germany also experimental studies had been carried out using the Hartmann Acoumeter (1878) and the Otaudion. All the early instruments tended to be complex in operation and suffered from the major limitation of having no uniform zero reference level. By 1930 audiometers were being produced on a commercial basis and their use was rapidly expanding. In 1938 to 1939 standards were formulated not only for threshold, but also for accuracy of attenuation, tonal purity, freedom from extraneous noise, and so on.

At about this time also the audiometer was making a real impact on school screening, and in the United Kingdom the Education Act of 1944 gave local education authorities the duty of ascertaining children with handicaps, including those with defective hearing. Nowadays most countries in the Western hemisphere have adopted hearing screening as a routine procedure for schoolchildren, and indeed many countries employ some method of assessing hearing ability much earlier in life.

HEARING SCREENING—THE CURRENT SITUATION

Although many efforts have been made to assess hearing of neonates and hence identify all profoundly deaf children at the earliest possible opportunity (Downs and Hemenway, 1969; Mencher, 1974; and Barr et al.; 1978) the more conventional and practicable age for infant screening is at around nine months. The Ewings (1944) pioneered the use of health visitors in testing the hearing of babies by simple distraction techniques that operate at a level of approximately 35 to 50 dB HL. As Herer (1977) indicates, the purpose of screening at this early age is to determine which children have moderate-to-profound sensorineural hearing losses in order that amplification and appropriate remedial action can be instituted at the earliest possible opportunity.

In some communities a second screening may be made at around the age of two to three years, again with the principal goal of identifying children with moderate-to-severe sensorineural losses that may not have been established at an earlier age. Fortuitously, some children with conductive deafness may also be identified, but this is not normally the prime objective even though conductive hearing losses may considerably outweigh sensorineural losses numerically in this population (Kessner et al., 1973; Borkowska-Gaertig, 1976). The next major hearing screen as usually in the first year at school. Pure tones are now the accepted stimuli, and intensity levels of between 20 dB HL and 30 dB HL provide the accepted criteria for passing or failing.

However, the purpose of hearing screening in schoolchildren is, perhaps, less clearly defined and accepted than the purpose of screening infants. The Joint Committee on Health Problems in Education of the NEA and AMA (Wilson, 1964) stated, "From the point of view of school health services, primary responsibilities are an awareness of the importance of early recognition of suspected hearing loss, especially in the primary grades; intelligent observation of pupils for signs indicative of hearing difficulty; organization and conduct of an audiometric screening survey; and a counselling and followup program to help children with hearing difficulties obtain diagnostic examinations, needed treatment, and such adaptations of their school program as their hearing condition dictates." In essence the need expressed here is for hearing to be the principal concern—hearing on the day of test. Undoubtedly, the commonest cause of auditory impairment in children in their first years at school is conductive in type and predominantly secondary to middle ear dysfunction.

Harvey and Wilmot (1969) reviewed the records of all children reported as having a hearing deficiency "sufficient to handicap them in any way" arising from a population of approximately 125,000 over a ten- to fourteen-year period. Ninety-two percent of the childen were diagnosed as having a conductive hearing loss. Of the sensorineural hearing losses at least 60 percent were congenital in origin and should, in consequence, have been detected by the infant screen, or failing that, by the parents, long before the children reached school age. A substantial proportion of the children with acquired sensorineural hearing loss should also have been detected prior to their entry into full-time education. Hence, it is to be expected that 98 to 99 percent of all hearing losses discovered in school screening audiometry should be of a conductive nature. Support for this supposition comes from some unpublished data arising from the screening of children in the Holland County of Lincolnshire, England, where there are good preschool services. One thousand five hundred eighty new school entrants were screened and 357 failed to pass at the 25 dB HL criterion. Of the first-time failures only two were discovered to have sensorineural hearing losses that had previously been undetected. Additionally, three children were found with total or almost total unilateral losses. Similarly, Cooper and colleagues (1975), in a study of 2712 children where pure-tone audiometry was backed up with an abbreviated form of impedance audiometry, found one child with a flat bilateral sensorineural hearing loss of about 50 dB,all the other failures being of a conductive type.

Unfortunately, pure-tone audiometry is of very limited efficiency in detecting mild middle ear dysfunction. Eagles (1972), after an extensive study in which both pure-tone testing and otology were employed, stated "An unpredicted and startling 61 percent of the otoscopically abnormal children had hearing sensitivity in the normal range." Cohen and Sadé (1972) found that 50 percent of children with confirmed secretory otitis media demonstrated hearing threshold levels within the "normal" range when tested at a screening level of 25 dB HL.

In the study of Beery and colleagues (1975), 47 percent of children with tympanometrically determined effusion or tympanic membrane perforation passed the hearing screening test employing a pass-fail criterion of 25 dB HL at two or more frequencies. An even higher "miss-rate" by pure-tone screening was reported by Cody and colleagues (1975). Tympanometric and audiometric testing was performed on 2144 children. Two hundred eighty-two children failed one or other test and some 94 percent were found to have an otologic problem felt by the ENT physician to be in need of attention. Pure-tone andiometry identified only 38 percent of these children.

The situation, then, appears to be that pure-tone audiometry is the conventional technique employed in school screening and that hearing level is, by inference, regarded as the criterion established and accepted for determining the child's need for further evaluation and possible assistance. In consequence, a substantial proportion (probably around 50 percent) of children with middle ear disorders are classified as within normal limits, and hence not in need of further evaluation or treatment.

This poses the question, is it important to detect and treat mild middle ear conditions that do not depress the hearing level below the arbitrarily determined level regarded as "normal" for screening purposes? To answer this question, the causes and possible long-term consequences of conductive deafness should be considered.

CONDUCTIVE LOSS IN CHILDREN

Fabritius (1968) reporting on more than fifty thousand hearing tests carried out on schoolchildren over a nine-year period, attributed no less than 70 percent of the detected losses to otitis media. Among children seen in hospitals with conductive hearing loss, the percentage with secretory otitis media is even higher. Robertson (1966) suggests 80 percent, Carter (1963) puts the figure at 90 percent and Wehrs and Proud (1958) at virtually 100 percent.

The conclusion to be drawn from these figures is that otitis media with effusion is responsible for the majority of conductive impairments in schoolchildren. What are the possible consequences of failure to detect and treat this condition? First, there are potential medical consequences. These have been succinctly summarized by Proud and Duff (1976), who list the following possibilities: "Ossicular fixation through fibrosis, severe conductive hearing loss, myringosclerosis, retraction pocket formation, tympanic membrane perforation, appearance of cholesteatoma, ossicular necrosis and mastoid process destruction, the last of which carries its own list of complications." To this can be added the very real possibility of sensorineural hearing loss secondary to the effusion (Paparella and Brady, 1970; Brooks et al., 1972; English, Northern, Fria, 1973; and Ganzer and Arnold, 1977), and the equally real possibility of vertigo (Stell, 1978).

Second, there are possible educational consequences for some children. Some twenty years ago the hypothesis was advanced (Ling, 1959) that there was a relationship between mild hearing loss due to middle ear malfunction and educational retardation in fundamental subjects. Support for this hypothesis has been found in studies of Holm and Kunze (1969), Quigley and Thomure (1970), Hamilton (1973), and Lewis (1976) and may be summarized in a quote from Hamilton's paper. He states, "The evidence leads to the conclusion that the children with relatively minor impairments show considerable retardation as a group. Even when compared with children who are, when measured by a widely used and respected test of non-verbal abilities, of apparent inferior ability and from the same educational, social and cultural backgrounds, the hearing impaired children show that they have significant difficulties in subjects fundamental to educational progress."

Third, the studies of Holm and Kunze (1969), Lewis (1976), and Needleman and Menyuk (1977) point to the possibility of deleterious effects on the development of speech and language in children who have episodic or persistent otitis media.

Fourth, the suggestion has been advanced that mild hearing loss, especially when fluctuant, may lead to emotional or psychological disturbance or both. This has been observed in children with mild degrees of hearing loss who were attending normal schools (Fisher, 1965) and has been supported by the comments of an educational psychologist who wrote, "Fluctuating hearing impairment not infrequently produces emotionally disturbed children and distraught, stressed parents and families" (Struggles, 1975).

Fifth, studies at the Manchester Audiology Clinic relating to the ages of individuals applying for hearing aids under the provisions of the National Health Service have suggested that subjects who have had even quite mild conductive impairments in and from childhood seek amplification at a significantly earlier age than do those patients in whom the loss is attributable to presbycusis alone.

In the total therefore, there is much evidence to support the hypothesis that middle ear effusion in childhood, if undetected and untreated, may lead to any of a number of uncomfortable or even disabling conditions, and we may answer the question posed earlier, "Is it important to detect and treat middle ear conditions that do not depress the hearing level below the arbitrarily determined level regarded as normal for screening purposes?" with a very vehement affirmative.

Recall that approximately 50 percent of middle ear effusions are not detected by conventional screening audiometry. Consequently, we need to devise more efficient means of detecting this condition. It is unlikely for a number of reasons that pure-tone screening can be refined to improve its sensitivity and selectivity. Environmental noise is one limiting factor. A study carried out in England on ambient noise levels in thirteen schools indicated a median noise level of 44 dB HL with frequent peak levels exceeding 60 dB HL (Harrison, 1971). A more recent study by Bryan (1977) on noise in open-plan schools demonstrated that noise levels frequently exceeded 70 dB HL. It is obvious that such high levels of background noise have a very detrimental effect on the accuracy of screening tests. The skill of the tester and the accuracy of calibration and stability of the audiometer have been factors that in the past have tended to reduce the accuracy of pure-tone screening. These problems might be overcome by ensuring high standards of competence in those administering the tests and by regular checking on the performance of the equipment employed. However, there are still other factors involved in pure-tone screening which make it most improbable if not impossible for all middle ear dysfunction to be identified by this process.

One of these factors is the very nature of the test itself. In determining pure-tone threshold the subject must discriminate and accurately report the presence of a minimally perceptible acoustic stimulus. Even for adults this is frequently a difficult task involving, as it does, many nonauditory factors such as motivation, attention, and intellectual maturity. The interest of the subject must be sufficiently aroused in the test to concentrate on what may appear, especially for a child, to be a meaningless stimulus. The subjects must be intelligent enough to understand what response is required of them and to make that response. Their attention span must be sufficient for the maintenance of concentrated listening and swift and accurate responses throughout the whole test. The presence of this minimal stimulus has to be judged against a background of, at best, normal physiologic noise, but more generally in schools against a background of school activity noise.

Furthermore, normal-hearing children in their first year or two at school do not have a median hearing threshold at 0 dB HL (re ISO 1964). For five-year-old children the median hearing threshold is much nearer 10 dB HL, and the range of "normality" is wider in children of tender years than in adults. Whereas the 95 percentile range for adults spans only some 20 dB, for children it may span 35 to 40 dB.

The second major factor militating against the use of pure-tone screening, however refined, is the small degree of hearing impairment that may be associated with middle ear effusion in its early stages. Eagles and colleagues (1963) found that in children whose eardrums showed clinical signs of middle ear effusion described as "impaired mobility, discolouration and retraction of the tympanic membrane," the hearing loss was only of the order of 13 dB by air conduction. Kearsley and Wickham (1966) measured the changes in hearing threshold following myringotomy and paracentesis the day after the operation. This was on average 18.8 dB, falling to 15.4 dB ten days afer the operation. The standard deviation in this measurement was about 10 dB. A different approach was that of Harbert and colleagues (1970), who measured the airbone gap change brought about by paracentesis. This again was fairly flat over the range 250 to 4,000 Hz and averaged 17.8 dB with a standard deviation of 9.8 dB. In a clinical trial of the effectiveness of grommets in the treatment of middle ear effusion, Richards and colleagues (1971) found that the change brought about in hearing level by grommets alone was 15.1 dB and by myringotomy alone 13.4 dB. The difference between the two was not significant and averages 14.3 dB. Another study suggesting a similar degree of hearing loss is that of Cohen and Sadé (1972). The hearing thresholds of 408 children with middle ear effusion were measured. The average was approximately 25 dB HL. Assuming the children to be about six years of age, the "normal" threshold would be about 6 dB. Consequently, the hearing loss attributable to middle ear effusion is of the order of 19 dB. The author measured the hearing of 199 children aged three to ten immediately before and within seven days after treatment for middle ear effusion. The changes were: at 250 Hz, 14 dB; at 1000 Hz, 14 dB; and at

4000 Hz, 16 dB, the average change being 14.7 dB (SD = 8 dB; range 5 to 37 dB). From these six studies it may reasonably be concluded that the hearing loss secondary to effusion in the middle ear averages only 15 to 20 dB with a standard deviation of about 10 dB. Hence, even if the screening level is reduced from 25 dB HL to 20 dB HL a substantial proportion of children with middle ear dysfunction will be passed as within normal limits. At the same time there will be a rising rate of false-positive results. The situation becomes even worse if the threshold is further lowered to 15 dB HL, where possibly 90 percent of middle ear effusion may be detected, but at the price of a 25 percent false-positive rate among normal-hearing children.

Hence it can be concluded that however one seeks to refine pure-tone audiometric screening, it cannot be made adequately sensitive and at the same time reasonably selective. The need therefore is for a more efficient alternative means of testing for those children who have middle ear effusion that may lead to serious consequences.

ALTERNATIVES TO PURE-TONE SCREENING

The deficiencies of pure-tone screening in identifying children with otoscopic abnormalities were highlighted by the studies of Eagles and colleagues (1963), and it was this group of workers who suggested that the remedy was the addition of otologic input to the screening program. However, the time of the physician is limited and the skills of such highly trained individuals are inevitably expensive. Few communities can employ an otologist on a screening team on a regular, as opposed to a research, basis.

Hildyard, Stool, and Valentine (1963) suggested a method for overcoming this difficulty—using tuning fork tests alone as an addition to the pure-tone screen. In their study 920 children were evaluated, and of those who passed the hearing screen 9 percent were found who had a negative Rinne, possibly indicative of a conductive impairment. However, the tuning fork tests in this study were performed by skilled otologic staff, and the results would most probably have been very different if relatively unskilled screeners had administered the tuning fork tests. Application and interpretation of tuning fork tests requires a high degree of skill, especially for testing young children, a skill that comes only from extensive clinical experience.

Another proposition advanced for improving the efficiency of hearing screening is the use of bone conduction testing in addition to the air conduction tests (Osborn, 1971; Kelly and Denniston, 1976; and Harford, 1977). This is the audiometric equivalent of the tuning fork test, and the air-bone gap may be equated with the negative Rinne response. However, in view of the already noted difficulties in testing air conduction in young children in noisy schools, and the wide span of threshold intensities given by normal-hearing children, it seems improbable that substantially more information might be obtained by assessing bone conduction, which has always proved to be more difficult to test than air conduction. As König has demonstrated (1955), variation of the pressure of the bone vibrator in contact with the skull can introduce considerable variations in threshold. The variations are largest in the lower frequencies, but it is in this region that the air-bone gap is most significent from a diagnostic standpoint. With children, low contact pressures are likely to arise when vibrators are mounted on headbands designed to fit the larger heads of adults. Overall, there appear to be as many drawbacks to air-bone gap measurements as potential advantages in identifying children with mild middle ear dysfunction.

Quite recently whispered-voice testing was reassessed and compared with conventional pure-tone screening (Groen, 1973). Despite the obvious limitations of a test that employs a poorly controlled stimulus, results comparable with pure-tone screening audiometry were obtained, indicating that the efficiency of whispered-voice testing—or rather the inefficiency of this type of testing—was of the same order as pure-tone testing. However, in these days of precise scientific measurement, few authorities would accept a return to such subjective methods as live-voice testing, where equally good or better alternatives exist.

Van Den Borg (1942) tested 500 schoolchildren with the Van Dishoek pneumophone (1938). With the active cooperation of the child being tested, middle ear pressure and hence the function of the Eustachian tube were assessed with this instrument, but because of its cumbersome nature and the need for subject participation in the test, the pneumophone could not be regarded as a suitable instrument for mass screening. However, its descendant, the impedance bridge, appears to be the most likely alternative or addition to pure tone screening for rapid and simple detection of children with middle ear dysfunction.

Impedance Screening

The appeal of impedance measurement as a technique for screening lies first in the physical basis of operation. In essence, impedance instruments assess the flow of acoustic energy through the tympanic membrane. Where middle ear dysfunction exists the normal flow pattern is disrupted, and this is particularly evident when the middle ear is filled with fluid.

Additionally, impedance measurement has proven to be very practicable with young children. It is simple to perform, has high sensitivity and selectivity, and suffers from few of the drawbacks of pure-tone screening.

Consideration will now be given to some of these features.

Acceptability/Practicability. In a study performed on 1026 children aged from four to eleven years in two schools for children with normal hearing (Brooks, 1969) not one child was encountered who could not be tested. Admittedly, the fact that a piece of candy was given on successful completion of the test may have been a significant factor, but this experience does demonstrate that with perseverence the great majority of children will accept impedance testing. In the study reported by Walton (1975), only 5 children proved to be untestable out of over 8000 reviewed, a success rate of 99.94 percent. Harker and Van Wagoner (1974) tested 710 children, 35 of whom were under 2 years of age. Only 9 of the total number proved to be untestable compared with 211 who could not be tested by pure-tone audiometry.

Fulton and Lamb (1972) demonstrated the practicability of impedance testing in a mentally retarded population. They examined 100 children aged from 7 to 21 years with I.Q.s ranging from 21 to 87. Many of these would be classified as difficult to test by normal audiometric precedures, but all were satisfactorily tested with impedance measurement. Givens and Seidemann (1977) similarly carried out assessment on 38 mentally retarded subjects, all with I.Q.s of less than 35. Only four of these (10.5 percent) proved to be untestable owing to behavioral problems.

Another population in which audiometric testing may frequently prove to be difficult is children classified as "developmentally disabled." Bashore (1976) tested 340 children so classified, aged between 5 and 21 years. There were no children who would not allow the test to proceed, but almost 5 percent did render test results invalid because of crying or physical movement. A further 4 percent could not be tested completely owing to failure to obtain or maintain an adequate air seal. Overall, acceptable information was obtained in 91 percent of children tested.

The newcomer to impedance testing may find such high levels of acceptability and successful test results surprising, as most novices find some difficulty in obtaining the essential airtight seal in the ear canal. Many operators can testify, however, that with experience the obtaining of a complete seal becomes easier, ultimately becoming a matter of simplicity and facility.

Another valuable feature of impedance testing is that, unlike pure-tone audiometry, it is virtually unaffected by background noise, even of the levels cited previously (Bryan, 1977) as occurring in some open-plan schools.

Reliability. McCandless and Thomas (1974) examined 730 children using impedance and otoscopy, the latter being performed by a senior resident in otolaryngology using a battery-powered pneumatic otoscope. Ears with old scarring and small monomeric areas were passed otoscopically as normal, the criterion for failure being that in the judgment of the examiner the ear was in need of medical or surgical treatment. Failure in the impedance test was established as a middle ear pressure more negative than -100mm H_2O and the absence of an acoustic reflex. Concordance between the two forms of examination ranged from 89 percent in the 3 to 5-year age range to 100 percent in the 12 to 15-year-old children. Overall the agreement was 93 percent. Agreement of a slightly higher degree (96 percent) was obtained by Schwartz and Redfield (1976) in a study of fifty-three subjects (fifty-three ears) selected from patients being seen for otologic examination. If absence of reflexes was taken as the impedance criterion, agreement rose to 98 percent. Slightly lower correlations between otologic examination and impedance screening were obtained in the studies of Urban (1977) and Findlay and colleagues (1977). Urban examined 510 students using an American Electromedics AE 85R tympanometer. Of those failing the test and followed up by otologists, 87 percent have been confirmed as having a middle ear dysfunction. In the study of Findlay and colleagues fifty-one deaf children were evaluated by both tympanometry and otologic examination on two occasions two months apart. Forty-five of the children were re-examined after a further interval of three months. Overall agreement between the two modes of testing was 85 percent. In eighteen subjects there was disagreement between the two methods of testing on the first occasion. At the follow-up tests approximately half of these disagreements were resolved in harmony with the original otologic diagnosis and the other half in harmony with the original tympanometric findings. It may reasonably be concluded from this observation that neither impedance testing nor otology is infallible, but that in the majority of subjects there is a substantial measure of agreement. Roeser and colleagues (1977) confirmed the fallibility of otologic examination in two studies where, first, impedance tests and pneumatic otoscopy were compared, and, second, otoscopic diagnoses by two physicians were compared. The agreement between tympanometry and otoscopy ranged between 73 and 79 percent depending on the criterion adopted for the boundary between normal and abnormal middle ear pressure. The agreement between otologist's was stated as "generally poor" and from the data appears to have been approximately 55 percent. In other studies in which otoscopy and impedance have been compared, the percentage agreement has been 87 percent (Randolph, 1975); 75 percent (Cooper et al., 1975); 75 to 79 percent (Fernandes et al., 1978); and 81 percent (Bashore, 1976).

Taken together these data suggest that impedance testing will agree with otologic examination in about 80 to 90 percent of children screened. This compares very favorably with the figures for agreement between pure-tone audiometric screening and otologic examination, these being at best 78 percent (Randolph, 1975) but more commonly around 50 to 60 percent (McCandless and Thomas, 1974; Cooper et al., 1975; and Roeser et al., 1977).

However, is agreement between otoscopy and impedance the most appropriate factor to be considered in evaluating impedance as a diagnostic tool? It is perhaps at least as important to consider the agreement between impedance and the confirmed findings in the middle ear at surgery.

Brooks (1968) employing measurements of the compliance, gradient, and middle ear pressure in 120 children, attained a predictive accuracy of 87 percent relative to findings at surgery. In a further 8 percent of the subjects, tympanometry suggested the presence of fluid in the middle ear, but at surgery no fluid was discovered. Other authors since this time (Grimaldi, 1976; Haughton, 1977) have commented on the "dry tap" and suggested that the impedance indications may well be correct, the surgical findings being distorted by changes brought about in the middle ear by the anesthetic.

The correlation between impedance measurement and middle ear effusion appears to be approximately 85 to 95 percent, depending somewhat on the criteria adopted for classifying the information derived from impedance measurement. However, we have not so far considered the many different possible parameters of impedance measurement which have been employed by the different researchers. Consideration will be given to some of these that appear to have practical application in the screening for middle ear effusion.

POSSIBLE CRITERIA FOR IMPEDANCE SCREENING

Tympanometric pattern: Jerger (1970) suggested that pressure-compliance functions might be categorized by three basic patterns. Such a concept has the appeal of simplicity if it can be substantiated. The type A curve is stated to be characterized by a "relatively sharp maximum at or near 0 mm H_2O." Type B shows "little or no maximum," and type C has a "maximum shifted to the left of zero by negative pressure in the middle ear." The degree of negativity to qualify as a type C is suggested as -100 mm H_2O or greater. Unfortunately, such terms as "relatively sharp maximum" and "little or no maximum" leave room for individual difference in interpretation of curve types, which is undesirable in a screening procedure. An approach to resolving this ambiguity was made by Fiellau-Nikolajsen and colleagues (1977) in testing over 500 three-year-old children. The definition they adopted for a type A curve was that it should have a gradient (see definition below) in excess of 0.1 ml and a negative pressure not more negative than -100 mm H_2O. A type B curve was defined as having a gradient equal to or less than 0.1 ml regardless of middle ear pressure; and type C as having a middle ear pressure more negative than -100 mm H_2O and a gradient greater than 0.1 ml.

A somewhat more complex pattern classification was advocated by Beery and colleagues (1975) based on otoadmittance measurements at two probe tone frequencies. In this study an accuracy of prediction of middle ear effusion of 93 percent was achieved. Recall that we are seeking to find a screening technique, not a research protocol. In consequence, the test should be simple to execute and to classify. The two classifications mentioned above may perhaps demand too high a level of operating and interpretive skill from the operators than is reasonable to expect. Furthermore, Renvall and colleagues (1975) in a temporal bone study demonstrated that relatively normal tympanograms might be obtained from middle ears containing small amounts of fluid. Possibly then, tympanometry alone may not be completely satisfactory if we require that every ear with effusion be detected. This aspect of screening will be considered further in a later section.

Absolute compliance measurements. Even in ears regarded as clinically normal, the range of absolute compliance is wide, the lower limit of normality being around 0.35 ml and the upper limit around 1.4 ml. It is possible for an ear to have quite gross physical changes and still remain within the bounds of normality. For example, the tympanic membrane may have areas of thinning such that the compliance tends to rise toward the upper limit of normality. At the same time there may be adhesions within the middle ear that reduce its mobility and would, in the absence of the tympanic membrane abnormality, reduce the compliance to below 0.35 ml. The effect of the two conditions combined may result in a compliance close to the median value for normal subjects. Absolute compliance measurements cannot in consequence be considered as a practical method for screening.

Gradient or curve steepness. In the majority of cases of middle ear effusion the tympanogram is flat, whereas with the normal middle ear and most other pathologic abnormalities of the conductive system, the curve has a very definite peak. The "peakiness" of the curve can be quantified by measuring the change in compliance that is brought about by reducing or increasing the pressure by a predetermined amount from the ambient middle ear pressure. Brooks (1968) suggested a change of ± 50 mm as a suitable range and coined the term "gradient" for the average compliance change in the positive and negative directions. A high correlation was obtained between low gradient and the presence of effusion in the middle ear.

As a screening measure, gradient may require a higher degree of skill in application than is reasonable to expect from the testers. Small errors in the pressure shift may result in disproportionately large errors of gradient, as may lack of care in measuring the compliance at exactly the point of middle ear pressure. Undoubtedly instruments could be designed to perform this function automatically and accurately, but until that time measurement of gradient is unlikely to be adopted in routine screening.

Middle ear pressure. One function of the Eustachian tube is to maintain pressure equality between the middle ear and the atmosphere. Normally this task is performed efficiently, and the middle ear pressure does not depart by more than a few mm H_2O or a fraction of 1 percent from the atmospheric pressure. Dysfunction of the middle ear in children is almost always associated with reduced middle ear pressure brought about by temporary or more longstanding Eustachian tube incompetancy. The difficulty in employing measurement of the middle ear pressure as a criterion for screening is the uncertainty that exists as to how negative that pressure must be before it may be regarded either as clinically significant or in need of intervention. Jerger (1970), in defining his three suggested basic tympanometric shapes, took the boundry value as -100 mm H_2O on the basis that "when the maximum (of the pressure compliance curve) equals or exceeds approximately 100 mm (water) significant negative pressure in the middle ear may be presumed." Many clinicians and research workers have followed this lead and adopted -100 mm H_2O as the boundary value between normality and abnormality, but complete unanimity has not yet been achieved.

Renvall and colleagues (1975) felt that -100 mm H_2O was a little too severe and wrote, "We suggest a pressure level around -150 mm H_2O as a borderline for referral to an otologist." However, even with this amended pressure level, some ears with effusion are inevitably over-looked on the basis of pressure measurement alone, and a large number of ears without effusion are referred for suspicion of effusion. Renvall and colleagues (1978) found that four of twenty-seven ears with surgically verified effusion had pressures less negative than -150 mm H_2O, and twenty of twenty-eight ears without effusion had pressures more negative than -150 mm H_2O.

The cut-off pressure might be regarded as a function of age. In a study of over one thousand children aged four to eleven years (Brooks, 1969), 697 were classified as having "normal" middle ear function on the basis of the presence of bilateral stapedial reflexes to tones of 2000 Hz presented at a level of 95 dB HL. In the subgroup of children aged four to seven years, only 59 percent had middle ear pressures in the range 0 to -50 mm H_2O; 77 percent were within the range from 0 to -100 mm H_2O, and 95 percent within the range 0 to -170 mm H_2O. There was a notable difference in older children. In the nine to eleven-year age group the corresponding figures were: in the 0 to -50 mm H_2O range 78 percent; in the 0 to -100 mm H_2O range, 89 percent; and the 95 percent boundary value was -135 mm H_2O. With adult subjects pressures more negative than -50 mm H_2O might well be regarded as significant.

Possibly then, different degrees of negativity might have to be adopted for screening, depending on the ages of children being screened. The use of -100 mm H_2O with children in the age range of four to six years would result in a failure rate of 23 percent of children who were otherwise sympton free, with consequent overload of the otologic services. Adopting Renvall's suggestion of -150 mm H_2O would reduce the number of false-positives to 10 percent. Even with this criterion, many children would be screened out with only negative middle ear pressure and without middle ear effusion. Before advocating otologic referral for this condition, the significance of negative middle ear pressure in the absence of other pathologic factors should be considered. There are, perhaps, three possibilities. The negative pressure may be the precursor of middle ear effusion. Second, it may be the remaining sign of a recovering middle ear effusion. Third, there appear to be some children who maintain relatively high negative middle ear pressures over quite long periods, apparently without untoward effects. In the first instance there may or may not be a need to intervene, depending on whether the effusion is persistent or transient. More will be said about this in a later section.

In the second instance intervention would serve no useful purpose, although there might be some merit in monitoring recovery from the (assumed) effusion. In the third instance, where the threshold of Eustachian tube function appears to be high, there would be little merit in intevening if there are no apparent untoward effects.

Presence or absence of middle ear muscle reflexes. The concept of reflex screening is based on the premise that the presence of a reflex response to a pure-tone stimulus in the mid-frequency range having an intensity of approximately 100 dB HL indicates a middle ear that, for all clinical and practical purposes, is within normal limits. Klockoff (1961) stated that the presence of a stapedial reflex to such an acoustic stimulation ruled out the possibility of a conductive lesion of any significance with a very high degree of certainty, and although one might quibble over fine details, the statement essentially sums up the situation. Although presence of a reflex clears the ear of conductive dysfunction, absence of the reflex does not necessarily indicate a middle ear condition that requires intevention. Some individuals with perfectly normal middle ear and auditory function do not produce stapedial muscle responses to any type of stimulation. Absence of reflex response does, however, alert the tester to the possibility of aural pathologic factors.

The attraction of reflex testing is first its simplicity, and second the go/no-go nature of the test. For a school screening test to be effective and efficient it must be simple, quick, reliable, and preferably not demanding with regard to resources. Reflex screening meets these criteria. The major limitation at first sight is that of over-referral. Renvall and colleagues (1973) tested 206 randomly selected ten-year-old children. Eight percent were regarded as having a disorder on otoscopy and 12 percent on tympanometry, but 35 percent failed the reflex test. (Incidentally, pure-tone audiometry only identified 1.5 percent of the total as having a hearing deficit.)

Brooks (1973) tested 543 children using the presence of an ipsilateral reflex to a tone of 2000 Hz as the pass/fail criterion. Almost 31 percent of the children failed the test. Somewhat over half of these appeared, by tympanometry, to have middle ear effusion. A further quarter had middle ear pressures more negative than -100 mm H_2O. Even if only the children with apparent middle ear fluid were referred on to otology clinics, this would pose a subtantial problem for the diagnostic and treatment services, since these children represent almost 20 percent of those screened in the latter study. A further question may then be posed as to whether it is essential that every child indicated by screening as possibly having an effusion be referred immediately for otologic examination. To answer this, more information is required about the natural course of otitis media in children. One study that throws some light on this has been undertaken by the author over the last ten years.

MIDDLE EAR FUNCTION, LONG TERM STUDIES

In September 1968, thirty-eight four- and five-year-old children commencing full-time education were tested with an acoustic impedance instrument. A further forty-two entered the study in September 1969. During their first year at school impedance tests were performed at approximately two-week intervals. In the second school year the intervals were widened slightly, and as the children have grown up the intervals have lengthened to annual tests. Records exist therefore for the middle ear function of these children over a ten-year span, defined in terms of middle ear pressure, compliance, gradient, and reflex thresholds.

Three basic patterns of middle ear behavior have emerged in the course of this study. Forty-one of the children have maintained very stable, normal middle ear function as illustrated in Figure 9-1. Within the limits of repeatability and accuracy of measurement of the impedance instruments employed (and three different models have been used over the course of this study), the compliance and gradient have remained remarkably stable. There have been minor variations in middle ear pressure in many of the children, sometimes to -200 mm H_2O, but very rarely with the extinction of the reflexes. Reflex threshold has generally remained very stable.

Twenty-six children exhibited a clearly different pattern. This is illustrated with the record of one ear (for clarity) of a child who entered school in September 1968, at which time all the parameters were within normal limits (Figure 9-2). With the exception of a slightly negative pressure, the test three weeks later was similar. However, after a further interval of some three weeks the compliance and gradient dropped sharply, as did the middle ear pressure. The tympanogram at this time was typical of

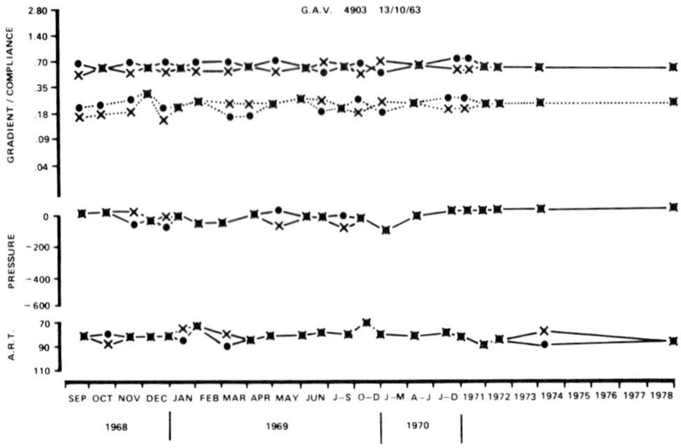

Figure 9-1 Ten-year record of impedance data for child with stable middle ear function.

middle ear effusion; note that the reflexes were absent. Recovery to normal function took place over a period of a few weeks without any intervention. The largest number of effusion episodes occurred some six to eight weeks after entering school, eleven children having this single, isolated bout of effusion. Five children passed through this period without apparent middle ear dysfunction but then had a single episode of effusion in the spring. Ten children had effusion both in the initial period and in the spring period, but then recovered and have since not exhibited any signs of further middle ear malfunction.

Finally, there are thirteen children in the third category. These are children who have shown either persistent or repeated bouts of middle ear effusion by tympanometry. Within this small group two distinct patterns may be seen. The majority (nine) entered school with, at the first test, normal middle ear function (Figure 9-3). They then had multiple episodes of effusion over a period of some two years or so, after which, without treatment, they returned to normal middle ear function complete with normal muscle reflexes. The second subgroup consists of four children who have, over the whole period of observation, shown very poor middle ear function and who have rarely, if ever, produced reflex responses to acoustic stimulation (Figure 9-4). (For further details see Brooks, 1976.)

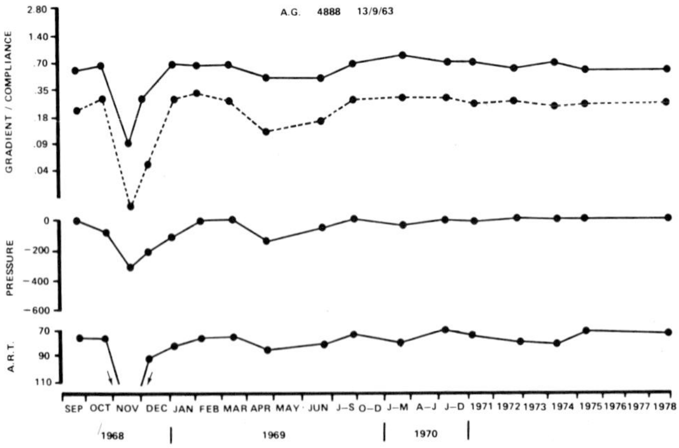

Figure 9-2 Data as Figure 9-1 for child (right ear only) showing development of spontaneous recovery from single episode of middle ear effusion.

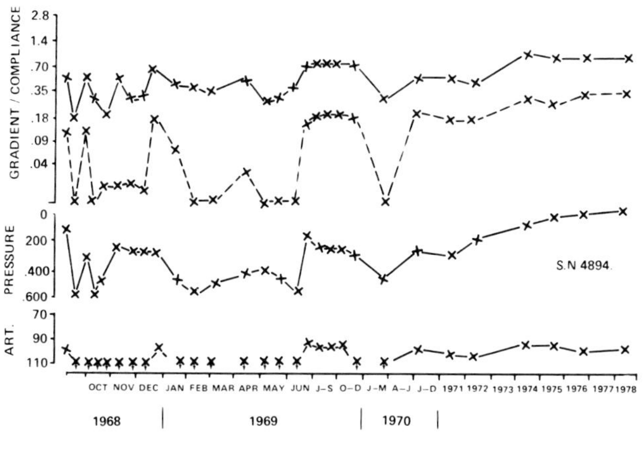

Figure 9-3 Data as Figure 9-1 for child (left ear only) showing early episodic middle ear effusion and return to normal function after one to two years.

The children in the first category would have passed an impedance screen employing any of the suggested criteria at any time during the the years of observation. The children in the second category would also have passed, except during the one or two short periods during which they had effusion. There would seem to be little merit in referring these children for otologic examination, since recovery took place quite spontaneously. Probably this would have taken place between the time the child was referred for examination and the actual examination. The likely outcome of the otologist seeing substantial numbers of children without effusion would be to bring the test procedure into disrepute and perhaps more seriously delay the examination of children in real need of help.

The children in the third category are those who are in greatest need of detection and, where appropriate, treatment.

Fundamental requirements for a screening test of middle ear function

A test is required that identifies every child with chronic or potentially disabling

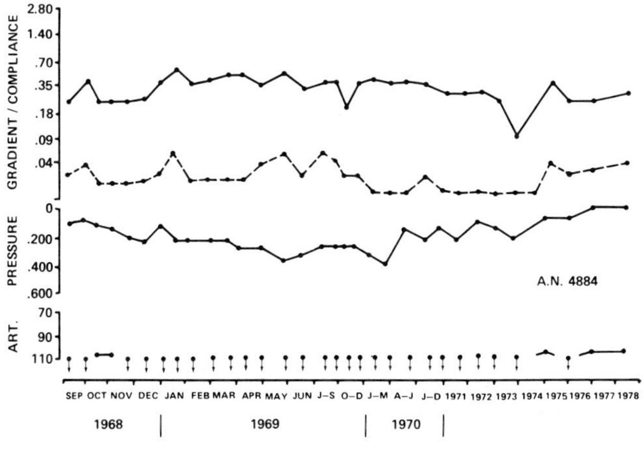

Figure 9-4 Data as Figure 9-1 for child (right ear only) showing long-term persistent middle ear effusion. Note particularly absence of muscle reflexes.

middle ear dysfunction but that does not overload the diagnostic and treatment services with minor middle ear conditions that are self-correcting or transient. In the present state of knowledge there does not appear to be a single one-stage test that meets this objective. Tympanometry, even with quite complex curve definitions, still has an unacceptable degree of ambiguity, plus the problem of fluid in ears with normal tympanograms. Absolute compliance is much less satisfactory and no simpler. Gradient correlates well with effusion, but again there is the problem of the ear with effusion that produces a normally peaked tympanogram. Measurement of middle ear pressure alone, though simple in execution, also produces a degree of ambiguity. Absence of middle ear muscle response to acoustic stimulation produces an unacceptably high rate of referral

Time alone appears to be the crucial factor in differentiating between transient and chronic middle ear dysfunction, and herein lies a possible solution to the problem—the performance of repeated tests at carefully chosen time intervals. Lewis and colleagues (1975) suggested daily tests until the situation resolved either to normality or to such a condition as was deemed to require otologic examination and treatment. However, this technique is demanding of staff and resources, and a simpler alternative might be that of performing two tests at a somewhat wider time interval. This time interval should be long enough to allow for the recovery from transient effusion to take place, but otherwise as short as possible so that treatment for chronic conditions is not delayed.

Edström and colleagues (1977) carried out a double-blind study on children diagnosed as having secretory otitis media, some being treated with mucolytic agents, some with decongestants, and some with placebo. About 60 percent recovered normal function over a period of six weeks, and only 6 percent thereafter, there being no significant difference according to the type of treatment received. In the study already referred to (Brooks, 1976), the children with transient episodes of effusion usually went through the complete cycle of development, effusion, and recovery of normal function in a period not greater than six weeks. Six weeks, then, appear to be about the optimal period for the two-part screen test.

In the two-stage procedure, not every child would require two tests. If the first test indicated normal middle ear function, that child would be regarded as having passed the screen—as is currently the situation with pure-tone audiometric screening. Unless the tests had been performed during the first few days after beginning full-time education, few, if any, children with middle ear dysfunction or even potential middle ear dysfunction should be missed. Six weeks later a second test would be performed on those failing the first screen. Those passing would be regarded as normal, or if one wishes to be ultra-cautious, might be retested after a further interval. Those failing would proceed to the next stage of evaluation—perhaps a full clinical work-up with pure-tone threshold testing and full impedance studies—before referral, where deemed necessary, to an otology clinic.

With the safeguards of a second screen for the first-time failures and an audiologic check before referral to an otologist, a high rate of first test over-referrals can be tolerated.

Reviewing our possible screening methods, curve types may now be considered, only type A being regarded as a pass and all others as reason for review. (The rare middle ear effusion in the presence of a type A tympanogram would, admittedly, be passed as normal.) Absolute compliance, because of its insensitivity to pathologic factors, remains impracticable. So, perhaps, does gradient measurement, but for reasons of technical measurement and not insensitivity. Negative pressure may at first sight appear suitable, but a drawback to this as a sole criterion is that middle ear effusion may occasionally exist in an ear with normal pressure. However, in that one has to effectively perform tympanometry to determine the middle ear pressure, the combination of tympanogram and pressure measurement would appear to be a suitable screening procedure for identifyıng middle ear dysfunction, albeit with the same reservation as for tympanometry alone.

Middle ear muscle reflex observations, while being too sensitive for a single stage screen, meet the requirements of simplicity, speed, practicability, and high accuracy when employed in the two-stage precedure.

A reservation regarding the use of a simple impedance screen is that, although it might be effective in identifying all middle ear dysfunctions of consequence, it would fail to pick up children with sensorineural losses, especially those with hearing loss for the high tones only (Brooks, 1973, Orchik and Herdman, 1974; and Cooper et al., 1975). First, most of the children with sensorineural losses have been identified long before they began full-time education, this being the primary purpose of infant and preschool screening. Second, it is not necessarily true that all sensorineural losses will pass in impedance screen. If the reflex technique is employed and the eliciting tone is of fairly high frequency, for example, 3000 Hz, most children with hearing losses in the high frequencies only will fail to produce a response to that stimulus. In children with moderate or severe sensorineural losses, the reflex threshold may well be depressed to a level such that there is no response to the stimulus. Third, although sensorineural loss is generally regarded as a more severe disability than conductive hearing loss, because of its permanence, the latter greatly exceeds the former in frequency of occurrence. The incidence of sensorineural loss in children is measured in tenths of a percentage; the prevalence of conductive loss may exceed 20 percent in some groups of children. It is not being advocated that the rare sensorineural loss be casually disregarded because it is rare, but that due regard should be paid to the many children with conductive loss. Until recently, the moderate conductive hearing loss has been underrated and consequently underdetected. The emphasis has been entirely on the detection of the child with sensorineural loss, and a more balanced point of view is now desirable.

If it is still maintained that every case of sensorineural hearing loss must be detected (and does this happen at present with pure-tone audiometry?), then to the simple impedance reflex screen a subjective pure-tone test may be added such as a warbled tone of 3000 Hz.

IMPEDANCE SCREENING COSTS

In advocating a change from one type of screening to another, or the addition of fresh methods of screening, cost must obviously play a great part. Increased expenditure can be justified only in terms of increased efficiency. However, with regard to impedance screening it is conceivable that costs might be reduced relative to pure-tone audiometric screening, while at the same time efficiency is improved. Cooper and colleagues (1975) suggested a formula for estimating the costs of a screening program. The cost per child was given as $\frac{S}{R} + \frac{C + (M \times L)}{N \times L}$. S = the salary of the screening assistant in dollars per hour, R = screening rate at which children can be tested per hour, C = initial cost of the equipment, M = annual maintenance cost, L = estimate life time of the equipment, and N = total number of children screened per annum. Cooper and his colleagues proposed an impedance test rate of twenty-one per hour, which is a very reasonable value. It is certain that much higher rates can be achieved over small periods. However, to be sustained over the working hours of a school, twenty-one per hour seems very realistic. The cost of a simple impedance screener may now be approximately $1500 for commercially available equipment. Eight years is a reasonable life span for equipment that takes such heavy usage, and maintenance costs over that period should not exceed half the initial cost of the instrument. The salary assigned to the screener has been generously allowed as $5 per hour. It is quite evident that salary is the dominating factor in screening costs (and the same applies for pure-tone audiometry). If only 3000 children are screened per annum, the cost is 35 cents per test. As the number screened increases the cost falls toward a value of 25 cents per test. Pure-tone audiometry probably costs about 40 cents per test for large numbers.

SUMMARY

Impedance measurement is a reliable, cost-effective, acceptable method of testing middle ear function in children. It appears to be technically suited to employment as a screening procedure, provided a measure of agreement can be reached on criteria for referral for otologic evaluation. A correct balance must be achieved between detection of apparent dysfunction in the middle ear and referral. Under-referral may lead to preventable damage to the auditory system and the general health and well-being of the child. Over-referral may lead to overload of the otologic services with consequent delays for essential treatment. Alternatively it could lead to unnecessary treatment in some children.

As advocated by the Task Force at the Nashville Symposium on Impedance Screening for Children (Harford et al., 1978) further research is needed in the epidemiology, natural history, and optimal clinical management of middle ear disease before impedance screening can be advocated for general adoption. At present it is a most valuable research tool, the use of which, in carefully designed and monitored studies, is highly recommended.

REFERENCES

Barr, B., Stensland Junker, K. and Svard, M.: Early discovery of hearing impairment. A critical evaluation of the BOEL test. *Audiol.* 17:62, 1978.

Bashore, S.R.: The use of tympanometry for screening developmentally disturbed children. *Audiol. Hear. Educ.* 6(2):35, 1976.

Beery, Q.C., Andrus, W.S., Bluestone, C.D. and Cantekin, E.: Tympanometric pattern classification in relation to middle ear effusions. *Ann. Otol.* 84:56, 1975.

Beery, Q.C., Bluestone, C.D. and Cantekin, E.I.: Otologic history, audiometry and tympanometry as a case finding procedure school screening. *Laryngoscopy* 85:1976, 1975

Bezold, F.: Ueber den gegenwärtigen Stand der Horprufund. *Zeitschrift. Ohrenheilkunde* 29:1, 1896.

Board of Education: Annual Report. Published by H.M. Stationery Office, P20, 1931.

Borkowska-Gaertig, D.: Communication for hearing handicapped people in Poland. In Oyer, H.J. (Ed.): *Communication for the Hearing Handicapped—an International* perspective. Pub.U.P.P., 1976.

Brooks, D.N.: An objective method of detecting fluid in the middle ear. *Int. Audiol.* 7:280, 1968.

Brooks, D.N.: The use of the electro-acoustic impedance bridge in the assessment of middle ear function. *Int. Audiol.* 8:563, 1969.

Brooks, D.N.: Hearing screening—a comparative study of an impedance method and pure tone screening. *Scan. Audiol.* 2:67 1973.
Brooks, D.N.: School screening for middle ear effusions. *Ann. Otol. Rhinol. Laryngol. (Suppl.)* 25:223, 1976.
Brooks, D.N., Wooley H. and Kanjilal, G.C.: Hearing loss and middle ear disorders in patients with Down's syndrome. *J. Ment. Defic. Res.* 16:21, 1972.
Bryan, M.E.: Personal communication, 1977.
Carter, B.S.: Secretory otitis as a cause of conductive deafness in children. *Proc. Roy. Soc. Med.* 56:699, 1963.
Cody, R.C., Studley, A., Knicely, C., Moran, L. and Sumpter, D.: Tympano-audiometric hearing screening in the Harrison County Schools. *J. West Virginia Speech Hear. Assn.* 1:21, 1975.
Cohen, D. and Sadé, J.: Hearing in secretory otitis media. *Canad. J. Otolaryngol.* 1:27, 1972.
Cooper, J.C., Gates, G.A., Owen, J.H. and Dickson, H.D.: An abbreviated impedance bridge technique for school screening. *J. Speech. Hear. Dis.*40:260, 1975.
Downs, M.P. and Hemenway, W.G.: Report on the hearing screening of 17,000 neonates, *Int. Audiol.* 8:72, 1969.
Eagles, E.L.: Selected findings from the Pittsburg study. *Trans. Am. Acad. Opthalmol. Otolaryngol.* 76:343, 1972.
Eagles, E.L., Wishik, S.M., Doerfler, L.G., Melnick, W. and Levine, H.S.: Hearing sensitivity and related factors in children. *Laryngol. Suppl.*, 114, 1963
Edstrom, S., Lundin, K. and Jeppson, P.: Secretory otitis media. Aspects on treatment and control. *O.R.L.* 39:68, 1977.
English, G.M., Northern, J.L. and Fria, T.J.: Chronic otitis media as a cause of sensorineural hearing loss. *Arch. Otolaryngol.* 98:18, 1973.
Ewing, I.R. and Ewing, A.W.G.: The ascertainment of deafness in infancy and early childhood. *J. Laryngol. Otol.* 59:309, 1944.
Fabritius, H.F.: Hearing investigations of school children in North Trondelag County. *J. Oslo City Hosp.* 18:3, 1968.
Fernandes, D., Gupta, S., Sly, R.M. and Frazer, M.: Tympanometry in children with allergic respiratory disease. *Ann. Allergy* 40:181, 1978.
Fiellau-Nikolajsen, M., Lous,J.,Vang Pedersen, S. and Schousboe, H.H.: Tympanometry in three year old children. *Scand. Audiol.* 6:199, 1977.
Findlay, R.C., Stool, S.E. and Svitko, M.S.: Tympanometric and otoscopic evaluations of a school-age deaf population: a longitudinal study.*A.A.D.* 122:407, 1977.
Fisher, B.: The social and emotional adjustment of children with impaired hearing attending ordinary classes. Dissertation for Master of Education, University of Manchester, 1965.
Fulton, R.T. and Lamb, L.E.: Acoustic impedence and tympanometry with the retarded: a normative study. *Audiol.* II:199, 1972.
Ganzer, U. and Arnold, W.: Das Innerohrhörvermogen beim chronischen SeroMukotympanon. *Larynol. Rhinol.* 56:850, 1977.
Givens, G.D. and Seidemann, M.F.: Middle ear measurements in a difficult to test mentally retarded population. *Ment. Retard.* 15:40, 1977.
Grimaldi, P.M.G.B.: The value of impedance testing in diagnosis of middle ear effusion. *J.L.O.*90:141, 1976.
Groen, J.J.: Pure tone audiometry and whispered voice test. *O.R.L.* 35:65, 1973.
Hamilton, P.: Reading and language skills in children with impaired hearing in normal schools. Some recent research findings and discussion of educational provision. Occasional Paper No. 6. North Regional Association for the Deaf, 1973.
Harbert, F.,Young, I.M. and Menduke, H.: Audiological findings in serous otitis media. *EENT Monthly*, September, 1970.
Harford, E.R.: Paper presented Symposium on Impedance Screening for Children, Nashville, 1977.
Harford, E.R., Bess, F.H., Bluestone, C.D. and Klein, J.O.: *Impedance Screening for Middle Ear Disease in Children* New York, Grune & Stratton, Inc., 1978.
Harker, L.A. and Van Wagoner, R.S.: Application of impedance audiometry as a screening instrument. *Acta. Otolaryngol.* 77:198, 1974.
Harrison, D.R.: An investigation into the effects of ambient noise on pure tone screening tests. Sound 5:94, 1976.
Hartmann, A.: Ueber eine neue Methode der Hörprüfung mit Hülfe elektrischer Ströme. *Arch. Anat. (Physiol. Abat.)* 155, 1878.
Harvey, R.M. and Wilmot, T.J.: The incidence of deafness in childhood. *J.L.O.* 83:449, 1969.
Haughton, P.M.: Validity of tympanometry for middle ear effusions. *Arch. Otol.* 103:505, 1977.
Herber, G.: Early recognition of hearing loss in children. *E.N.T.J.* 56:5, 1977.
Hildyard, V.H., Stool, S.E. and Valentine, M.A.: Tuning fork tests as aid to screening audiometry. *Arch. Otolaryngol.* 78:151, 1963.
Holm, V.A. and Kunze, L.H.: Effects of chronic otitis media on language and speech development. *Pediatrics* 43:833, 1969.

Jerger, J.: Clinical experience with impedance audiometry. *Arch. Otolaryngol.* 92:311, 1970.
Kearsley, J.A. and Wickham, H.: Exudative otitis media in children. *J.L.O.* 80:26, 1966.
Kelly, B.R. and Denniston, G.L.: Unoccluded bone conduction screening as an alternative to impedance screening. *J. Amer. Aud. Soc.* 2:83, 1976.
Kessner, D.M., Snow, C.K. and Singer, J.: Assessments of Medical Care in Children, Contrasts in Health Status. Vol. 3, Natural Academy of Sciences, Washington, D.C., 1973.
Klockhoff, I.: Middle ear muscle reflexes in man. *Acta. Otolaryngol.* Suppl. 164: 1961.
König, E.: Variations in bone conduction as related to the force of pressure exerted on the vibrator. *Translations of The Beltone Institute For Hearing Research*, No. 6, 1957.
Lewis, N.: Otitis media and linguistic incompetence. *Arch. Otolaryngol.* 102:387, 1976.
Lewis, N., Dugdale, A., Canty, A. and Jerger, J.: Open ended tympanometric screening: a new concept. *Arch. Otolaryngol.* 101:722, 1975.
Ling, D.: The education and general background of children with defective hearing. Unpublished PhD. Thesis, Cambridge University Institute of Education, 1959.
McCandless, G.A. and Thomas, G.K.: Impedance audiometry as a screening procedure for middle ear disease. *Trans. Amer. Acad. Opthalmol. Otolaryngol.* 78:2, 1971.
Mencher, G.T.: A program for neonatal screening. *Audiol.* 13:495, 1974.
Needleman, H. and Menyuk, P.: Effects of hearing loss from recurrent otitis media on speech and language development. In Jaffee B. (Ed.): *Hearing Loss in Children*, Baltimore, University Park Press, 1977, 642—649.
Orchik, D.J. and Herdman, S.: Impedance audiometry as a screening device with school children. *J. Aud. Res.* 14:283, 1974.
Osborn, C.D.: Air-bone gap measurement in identification audiometry. Maico Library 9:2, 1971.
Paparella, M.M. and Brady, D.R.: Sensorineural hearing loss in chronic otitis media and mastoiditis. *Trans. Am. Acad. Opthalmol, Otolaryngol.* 74:108, 1970.
Proud, G.O. and Duff, W.E.: Mastoidectomy and epitympanotomy. *Ann. Otol. Rhinol. Laryngol. (Suppl.)*25:289, 1976.
Quigley, S.P. and Thomure, F.E.: Some effects of hearing impairment upon school performance. Division of Special Education Services, Springfield, Ill., 1970.
Randolph, K.: Application of impedance audiometry to the identification of hearing problems in schoolchildren. Proceedings of special study institute on impedance auditometry. (Ed.) Rosica, S.J., Buffalo, N.Y., 1975.
Renvall, U., Lidén, G., Jungert, S., and Nilsson, E.: Impedance audiometry as screening method in schoolchildren. *Scand. Audiol.* 2:133, 1973.
Renvall, U., Lidén, G., Jungert, S. and Nilsson, E.: Impedence audiometry in the detection of secretory otitis media. *Scand. Audiol.* 4:119, 1975.
Renvall, U., Lidén, G., Jungert, S. and Nilsson, E.: Long term observation of ears with reduced middle ear pressure. *Acta Otolaryngol.* 86:104, 1978.
Richards, S.H., Kilby, D., Shaw, J.D. and Campbell, H.: Grommets and glue ears: a clinical trial. *J. Laryngol. Otol.* 85:17, 1971.
Robertson, M.S.: Conductive deafness in children. *New Zealand Med. J.* 65:118, 1966.
Roeser, R.J., Soh, J., Dunckel, D.C. and Adams, R.: Comparison of tympanometry and otoscopy in establishing pass/fail referral criteria. *J. Am. Aud. Soc.* 3:20, 1977.
Schwartz, D.M. and Redfield, N.P.: Evaluation of automatic screening tympanometry in the identification of middle ear pathology. *J. Am. Audiol. Soc.* 1:276, 1976.
Stell, P.M. (Ed): Vertigo and glue ear in children (Editorial). *Clin. Otolaryngol.* 3:198, 1978.
Struggles, D.E.: Personal communication, 1975.
Urban, B.: Impedance in a school screening programme. Paper presented at Symposium on Impedance Screening, Nashville, 1977.
Van Den Borg, R.E.: An investigation about the pressure in the tympanic cavity in schoolchildren and the consequences of an abnormal pressure for hearing. *Acta Otolaryngol.* 30: 500, 1942.
Van Dishoeck, H.A.E.: De Pneumofoon. *Ned. Tijdschr. v. geneesk.* 82:00, 1938.
Von Hartmann: Die Schwehörigen in der Schule. Paper given to German Otological Society, Hamburg, June, 1905.
Walton, W.K.: A Tympanometry-ASHA model for identification of hearing impaired. (Project TAMI) Capitol Region Education Council, Windsor, Conn., 1975.
Watson, L.A. and Tolan, T.: *Hearing Tests and Hearing Instruments.* Baltimore, Williams & Wilkins, 1949.
Wehrs, R.E. and Proud, G.O.: Conductive deafness in children. *Arch. Otolaryngol.* 67:16, 1958.
Wilson, C.C.: School Health Services. Publication Joint Committee on Health Problems in Education of the NEA and AMA, 1964.
Wolf, O.: Die Hörprüfung mittelst der Sprache. *Zeitschrift. Ohrenheilkunde* 34:289, 1899.

Chapter Ten

IMPEDANCE MEASUREMENTS WITH DISTINCTIVE GROUPS

JERRY L. NORTHERN, Ph.D.

INTRODUCTION

Impedance audiometry is especially valuable in the auditory evaluation of distinctive patient groups such as various disadvantaged children. In this chapter information and literature review related to impedance measurements in infants and difficult-to-test children including the retarded, developmentally delayed, deaf-blind, and multiply handicapped are provided. Impedance audiometry has been advocated as a high-priority test in special populations in whom a high incidence of middle ear disorder may be expected, for example, children with cleft lip and palate and Down's syndrome, and children with craniofacial anomalies. Information is also presented for larger special populations such as the native Americans (Indians and Eskimos) and deaf students enrolled in residential schools. Finally, recent literature has also shown impedance measurements to be of potential value in patients with myasthenia gravis and in those with nonfluent speech.

DIFFICULT-TO-TEST CHILDREN

The Mentally Retarded

The evaluation of hearing in the mentally retarded population presents a most difficult task. Many retarded children do not condition well to pure-tone play audiometry. They may not have sufficient neurologic maturation to perform reflexive auditory awareness or localization tasks. They may be too hyperactive to cooperate or too lethargic to respond. Brain damage in these children often makes physiologic auditory responses unreliable. Yet accurate assessment of hearing function or middle ear status of these children may be critical for educational placement or medical/surgical treatment. Sometimes even a tympanogram or acoustic reflex measure can be a valuable result, since the clinician can then make reasonably accurate assumptions regarding the presence or absence of middle ear problems and the need for medical referral. Impedance audiometry is also valuable in the evaluation of the severely mentally retarded "mattress care" children, who are virtually impossible to test with any other procedure. These institutionalized youngsters are certainly at high risk for developing chronic middle ear disease.

The earliest acoustic impedance studies with retarded children were published by Lamb and Norris (1969, 1970). They compared acoustic reflex thresholds in fifteen mentally retarded children and fifteen children of normal intelligence. All subjects had normal hearing, and the acoustic reflex thresholds for both groups were at similar levels. Although it was reported that considerable variability in reflex thresholds was noted among the mentally retarded subjects, the authors note that the retarded subjects were easily tested, and they recommended that the impedance technique be included as a part of the audiometric test battery. Fulton and Lamb (1972) reported normative results from a retarded population with tympanometry, and demonstrated that tympanometry can be of use to help differentiate etiologic factors in hearing loss.

Borus (1972) used impedance measurements in a group of twenty-three young retarded children to establish the value of impedance audiometry in determining the nature of hearing loss. She concluded that impedance measurements "offer great promise" in quickly determining normal hearing in a retarded, difficult-to-test child, identifying cases where there is clearly a conductive component, and singling out retarded children who do have some auditory anomaly requiring further evaluation.

A rather comprehensive report on tympanometry in "developmentally disturbed" children was recently published by Bashore (1976). Developmentally disturbed children are described as youngsters with mental deficiency or severe physical disabilities who are not testable under Pennsylvania mandate, which requires pure-tone evaluation. Some 1.4 million children are given annual pure-tone hearing tests in Pennsylvania, and an estimated 50,000 are classified as "developmentally disabled." The Bashore study reported otoscopic findings and tympanometric results in 340 such children, comprising 308 trainable retarded children, 31 physically handicapped children, and one profound mental retardate. The study was conducted to evaluate six tympanometry failure criteria: (1) no well-defined maximum compliance peaks; (2) compliance greater than normal; (3) maximum compliance worse than 100 mm H_20; (4) less than normal compliance; (5) inability to secure and maintain seal; and (6) untestable children.

Bashore found 97 percent of the population to be testable; only five children could not be tested because of too much crying, and five children could not be sealed with an airtight probe cuff. An agreement of only 62 percent was found between results of otoscopy and tympanometry, although it should be pointed out that the article specifically stated that the "otologic examination did not have the benefit of a pneumatic otoscope," and tympanograms were considered abnormal when middle ear pressures were worse than -100 mm H_20—a rather rigid failure criterion. Almost certainly, better correlation would have been achieved between tympanometry and otoscopy if pneumatic otoscopy had been employed and if the failure criterion for tympanometry been established at -150 mm H_20 or even -200 mm H_20. Other disagreements between otoscopy and tympanometry were due to the utilization of "less than normal" compliance (type A_s) tympanograms. The most effective criteria for tympanometric failure in the Bashore study proved to be nonmobile tympanograms (type B) and negative middle ear pressure tympanograms.

The incidence of defective hearing in the mentally retarded is several times greater than in the normal population (Lloyd and Reid, 1966; Rittmanic, 1971). Jordan (1972) points out that even a mild degree of hearing loss may have a disproportionate impact on the mental retardate because he is less capable of compensating cerebrally with the aid of his other senses. Mentally retarded children now considered to be educable were "mattress cases" ten or twenty years ago. Standards set forth by the Accreditation Council for Facilities for the Mentally Retarded in 1971 require that all new residents of institutions and all other residents at regular intervals be given audiometric screening. Audiologists in such facilities find themselves faced with great numbers of retarded patients of all ages and functioning levels for auditory screening. I can see no alternative for auditory evaluation of such patients without impedance audiometry.

The Deaf-Blind Child

Evaluation of hearing in deaf-blind children is one of the most difficult tasks faced by the audiologist. The task is even more formidable when mental retardation accompanies the deaf-blind handicap. Audiometrically we are limited to observation of basic behavioral auditory orientation responses, the acoustic startle reflex, and quieting behavior to brief introduction of various interesting sound stimuli. When severe visual, motor, or other neurologic deficits are present, the primitive reflexive auditory behavior responses may be inhibited or absent. The audiologist is often left with little upon which to base the hearing evaluation.

It is the audiologist's responsibility to make the decision about the blind child's hearing ability. Little textbook information and few standardized developmental scales are available regarding techniques for evaluating the hearing response in these children. It is often useful to the audiologist to discuss the hearing potential of deaf-blind children with the parents and or teachers who are with the child for long periods of time. Sometimes the peripheral reflexive hearing mechanism seems within normal limits but the child is "functionally deaf," since sounds are seldom imitated, little vocalization occurs, and response to verbal cues is inconsistent (Fig. 10-1).

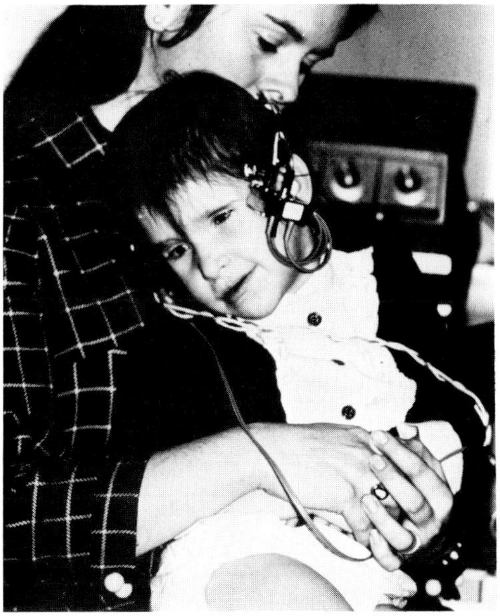

Figure 10-1 Acoustic impedance measurements are especially valuable in the auditory evaluation of deaf-blind children.

We routinely use impedance measurements in the auditory evaluation of deaf-blind children. The tympanogram information helps us identify those who are in need of medical evaluation. The presence of acoustic reflexes confirms the child's ability to hear. We recently attempted to utilize Jerger's SPAR test with twelve deaf-blind, retarded institutionalized children, aged four to fourteen (Zarnoch and Northern, 1977). Unfortunately, tympanometry revealed a high incidence of conductive problems that prohibited the measurement of acoustic reflexes. In our sample of twenty-four ears, we found eleven type A tympanograms, four type B tympanograms, and nine severe negative middle ear pressure type C tympanograms. In only eight out of the twenty-four ears of these deaf-blind retarded children were we able to elicit contralateral acoustic reflex thresholds. Many of the children had severe neurologic motor problems, so that absence of the acoustic reflex in ears with a type A tympanogram did not necessarily indicate profound sensorineural deafness. Utilizing a previously established biologic calibration for pure tones and broad band noise on normal-hearing listeners, prediction of hearing sensitivity with the SPAR technique was in good agreement with the teachers' impression of the child's auditory ability in seven out of eight cases. Medical treatment of the conductive loss may allow emergence of acoustic reflexes which can be used for SPAR during our next routine assessment of these multiply handicapped youngsters.

Children with Cerebral Palsy

Two groups of seven children with cerebral palsy and normal hearing were evaluated to examine acoustic reflex differences related to spasticity and hypotonia (Snow and McCandless, 1975). The study concluded that both spasticity and hypotonia differentially alter the acoustic reflex pattern in terms of latency and reflex release times. Both groups demonstrated elevated reflex thresholds as compared with normal subjects. Keith, Murphy, and Martin (1976) found 42 percent of multiply handicapped spastic children to have some type of middle ear problems.

HIGH-INCIDENCE GROUPS

Children with Cleft Lip and Palate

Deformities of the lip and palate are among the most common major congenital malformations, occurring in one out of nine hundred newborns. The incidence of recurrent otitis media in children with oral clefts has been reported in various studies as between 10 and 90 percent, depending on the criteria selected for definition of hearing impairment (Northern and Downs, 1978). Children with cleft palate are noted to have a higher incidence of hearing loss than normal children (Paradise and Bluestone, 1974).

The diagnosis of ear disease and hearing loss in the infant with cleft palate is difficult because of the small structure of the external ear and the infant's neurologic immaturity (Stool, 1971). Bluestone and colleagues (1972) found that 100 percent of their infants and young children with unrepaired cleft palate had abnormal Eustachian tube function. Numerous authors have shown that the incidence and severity of middle ear problems related to the cleft palate decrease as the patient grows older. Evaluation of a group of fifty-eight patients with submucous cleft palate showed an incidence of 39 percent with recurrent or chronic disease of the middle ear ranging from serous otitis media to cholesteatoma.

A few articles dealing with impedance evaluations of children with cleft palate have appeared in the recent literature. Billings and Lowry (1974) attempted to examine 107 children with cleft palates with the impedance test battery. They reported that 60 percent of their sample could not be evaluated with impedance because of "excessive cerumen, perforations or myringotomy tubes." In addition, 28 percent of the ears of children with cleft palates which were evaluated with impedance yielded data that were contrary to otologic findings. These authors concluded that impedance measurements were not appropriate in children with cleft palates in screening for middle ear pathologic factors.

In an excellent summary of hearing problems in 350 children with cleft palate, Jarvis (1976) states that the overall picture is that the incidence of hearing loss in children with cleft palate rises steadily to a peak at six years and then declines somewhat and levels off at about age nine. Half the children in his review had hearing loss in at least one ear worse than 20 dB at some time, and 35 percent of his case sample had recurrent hearing loss. It is readily apparent that impedance audiometry contributes substantially to the total management and evaluation of these children.

Two articles by Bess on acoustic impedance measurements in children with cleft palate are considerably more positive about impedance screening in such children. These researchers made clinical impedance measurements in a group of forty children with cleft lip or palate (1975). Although they reported an inability to evaluate 17 percent of the group, the authors noted that impedance measurements identified middle ear pathologic factors even when the audiogram revealed near-normal hearing levels. These authors described a typical impedance audiometry profile for children with cleft palate as negative middle ear pressure (usually greater than -100 mm H_2O), a type B or C tympanogram, low static compliance, and elevated or absent acoustic reflexes. Bess and colleagues (1976) evaluated a group of thirty-four children with cleft palate using pure-tone audiometry, pneumatic otoscopy, and the impedance test battery. The overall incidence of hearing loss and/or otitic problems ranged from 57 to 68 percent depending on which mode of evaluation was considered. Pure-tone hearing tests exhibited the poorest diagnostic efficiency. The authors concluded that with awareness of the poor sensitivity of pure-tone audiometry to otologic pathologic factors and when otoscopic examination is not routinely available, their results support the use of impedance studies in children with cleft palate (Fig. 10-2).

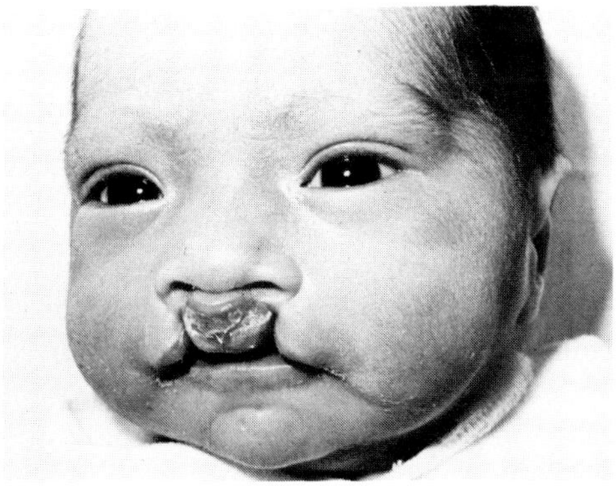

Figure 10–2 Cleft plate children require routine evaluation with impedance audiometry.

We recently reviewed the medical records of eighty-seven children with cleft palate between the ages of one year and seventeen years (average age 7.3 years) seen at least once at the Otolaryngology Clinic at the University of Colorado Medical Center. These children came to our clinic for routine well-child visits as well as when they had ear trouble. There was no way to determine if these children had all of their ear, nose, and throat problems treated only at our facility. Our sample composed of fifty-seven males and thirty females, nine of whom had only cleft lip, and ten others of whom had only submucous cleft palate. Multiple congenital problems, in addition to the cleft lip or palate, were noted in sixteen of the eighty-seven children, including mental retardation, Moebius, Klippel-Feil, Down's, Pierre-Robin, and Rubinstein-Taybi syndromes, cerebral palsy, and microtias and atresias of the external ear and ear canal. Although the findings in our group of children with cleft palate are not intended for generalization to the cleft-palate population in general, the eighty-seven children had an accumulated total of 991 ENT visits! It would be meaningless to attempt to determine an average number of visits per child because of the range of medical problems represented in the group. However, some illustrative cases include forty visits for one six-year-old, forty-two visits for one nine-year-old, and fifty-six visits for one of our ten-year-olds! Six other children between five and nine years of age had between twenty-three and forty clinic visits each. Although these visit frequency figures are not intended to be conclusive in themselves, these statistics do confirm the fact that children with cleft palates can expect to spend considerable time in otolaryngology offices because of numerous episodes of ear disease.

Children with Down's Syndrome

Down's syndrome, or mongolism, is the result of chromosomal abnormality, either as a twenty-one trisomy, a translocation trisomy, or as mosaicism with a high incidence of occurrence—1 in 770. The clinical findings include a list of nearly fifty features with varying penetrance. Mental retardation is almost universal in children with Down's syndrome, as is a characteristic personality that is warm, friendly, and affectionate. Ear symptoms commonly associated with Down's syndrome include small pinnae, narrow external auditory canals, abnormal external ear configuration, and a strong tendency for otitis media. The child with Down's syndrome may be more susceptible to upper respiratory tract infection than the normal child because of abnormal skull development that can adversely affect proper drainage of sinuses and middle ear cavities (Fig. 10-3).

It has been suggested in the literature that children with Down's syndrome have a higher than normal incidence of hearing loss, but little unanimity exists regarding the incidence or nature of the hearing problem. Figures for incidence of hearing loss in this special population range from 8 to 85 percent (Northern and Downs, 1978). Glovsky (1966) reported that only two out of thirty-eight children with Down's syndrome had "normal hearing"—an incidence of hearing impairment of 95 percent. Fulton and Lloyd (1968) reported the incidence of hearing loss in Down's syndrome to be the same as in the retarded population in general. The Glovsky study found the prevalent type of hearing loss in Down's syndrome to be sensorineural, while Fulton and Lloyd reported conductive-type hearing impairment to be dominant. No doubt much of this confusion in the literature regarding the incidence and type of Down's syndrome hearing loss is due to the difficulty of evaluating hearing in this population.

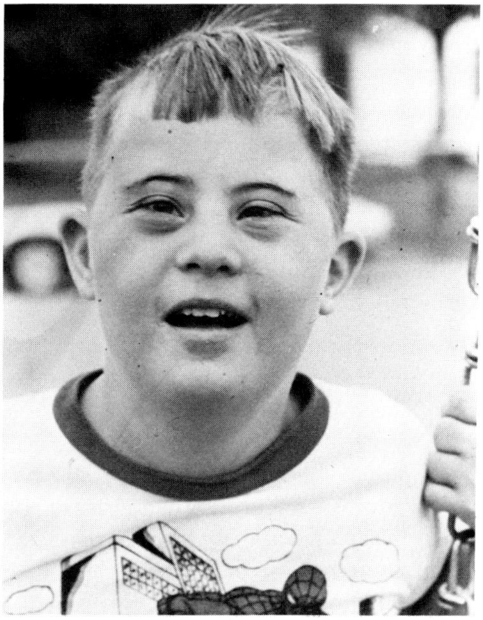

Figure 10–3 Children with Down's syndrome have an extremely high incidence of middle ear effusions.

Brooks (1972) reported impedance findings in a population of 100 children with Down's syndrome. He evaluated these children with audiometry and tympanometry and compared results with a matched control group of 100 retarded children. His results indicated that middle ear conductive loss problems existed in 60 percent of those with Down's syndrome and in only 17 percent of the control group; that 36 percent of the Down's group showed some element of sensorineural hearing loss compared with 11 percent in the control group; and finally, that only 23 percent of the children with Down's syndrome had normal auditory function as compared with 74 percent in the control group. Brooks reported the conductive loss in Down's syndrome to be due primarily to otitis media. Schwartz and Schwartz (1977) examined 39 noninstitutionalized children with Down's syndrome using impedance audiometry and otoscopy. Nearly 70 percent of their sample population demonstrated evidence of ear disorders.

An extensive research effort has been continuing at the University of Colorado Medical Center to evaluate the incidence and type of hearing problem in 100 children with Down's syndrome. Previous hearing studies of this particular population have been without contribution of otologic evaluation. Our project, under the direction of Marion Downs, M.A. and Marilyn Krajicek, R.N., resulted in reliable pure-tone and speech audiometry in 90 percent of the Down's syndrome group older than five years of age. The findings indicate that only 15 percent of the group has bilaterally normal hearing, while 50 percent have significant bilateral conductive loss, 15 percent have sensorineural hearing loss, and 9 percent show mixed-type hearing impairment. A number of the conductive hearing impairments are of such a degree as to not be commensurate with otitis media. Approximately one half of the group has normal type A tympanograms, while one fourth has type B tympanograms and one fourth has type C tympanograms. Acoustic reflexes were also evaluated in these children.

All the children with Down's syndrome in our study had thorough otoscopic evaluation, and some were treated with ventilation tubes. A number of children had persistent conductive-type hearing impairment despite placement of tubes and improvement in the condition of their middle ears. Four children suffering from Down's syndrome, carefully selected from the study, had exploratory tympanotomy. An additional middle ear was viewed by microscope through a 90 percent tympanic membrane perforation. All five of these ears showed congenital abnormalities of the middle ear ossicles. Two cases were observed to have abnormally shaped incudi, and three cases had a congenitally fixed stapedial footplate. We also have a temporal bone in our laboratory from a Down's syndrome patient which shows middle ear ossicular deformity. The results confirmed an 85 percent incidence of hearing impairment in Down's syndrome and suggest that middle ear anomalies may be a relatively common clinical feature.

Children with Craniofacial/Skeletal Disorders

Middle ear anomalies are of major importance because they are frequently correctable by modern otomicrosurgical procedures. Accurate diagnosis of the particular middle ear problem can minimize surgical misadventures. There is a tendency for middle ear anomalies to occur together, such as branchial arch abnormalities that involve the external ear and ear canal in cases of microtia and/or atresia. Since the mandible shares a common embryonic origin with the middle ear ossicles, malformation of the lower jaw may be accompanied by congenital conductive hearing impairment (Sando and Wood, 1971). Multiple congenital malformations frequently "run together" in syndromes. Children with craniofacial and/or skeletal disorders may also have congenital conductive or sensorineural hearing loss. Although audiometry in older children can be used to describe the nature of the hearing impairment, impedance audiometry has an important contribution to make in the overall diagnosis of the auditory defect. Sample patients are presented below, selected from our Birth Defects Clinic, to illustrate the value of impedance measurements in children with various craniofacial disorders.

Apert's Syndrome. (acrocephalosyndactyly). M.T. was noted at birth to have syndactyly (fused fingers and toes) and a "gargoyle-type" face. He was diagnosed as having Apert's syndrome within 25 hours. However, the initial otolaryngologic-audiologic evaluation was not conducted until age two and one-half years. At that time his tympanic membranes were intact, with normal appearance and normal mobility bilaterally. Audiologic findings were indicative of mild conductive hearing loss. By age three, a bilateral conductive loss of approximately 50 dB was confirmed. M.T. was fitted with a bone-conduction hearing aid. Acoustic impedance findings showed bilateral normal tympanograms, normal static compliance, and absent acoustic reflexes. Following some six hospital admissions for surgical procedures related to his head, hands, and toes, M.T.'s left ear was explored at age eight years, and an abnormal incus was found to be in continuity with a nonmobile stapes footplate. A stapedectomy was performed and the hearing improved to 15 dB. Three years later a similarly successful stapedectomy was performed on the right ear. Interpretation of the impedance findings and conductive hearing loss were consistent with bilateral middle ear fixation (Fig. 10-4).

W.G. is a black female with Apert's syndrome who also has acrocephaly and syndactyly. She has been known for several years to have a bilateral maximum conductive hearing impairment. Her impedance findings differ somewhat from M.T., described above. W.G.'s tympanograms are bilaterally type B (flat), although the

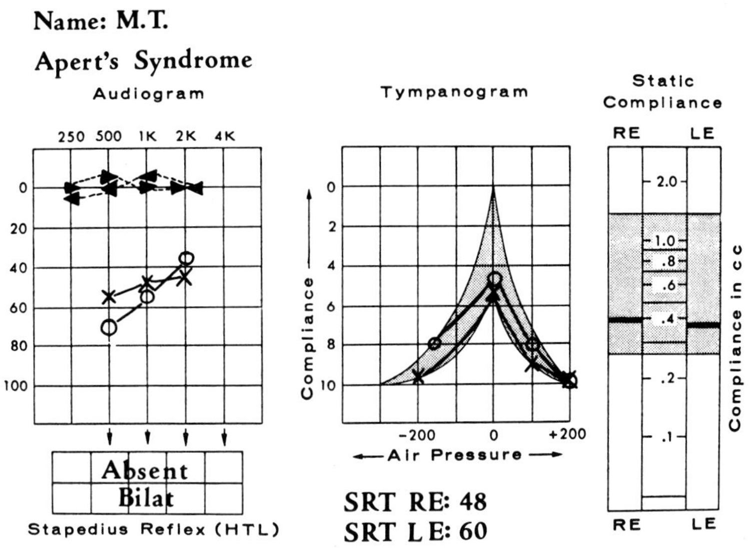

Figure 10-4 Impedance audiometric findings from an 11-year old with Apert's syndrome (acrocephalosyndactyly).

pneumatic otoscopy examination under the operating microscope showed normally mobile tympanic membranes. Static compliance was slightly lower than normal bilaterally and she had no acoustic reflexes. W.G. has not been operated on; however, we suspect that she has congenital stapedial footplate fixation and possible other middle ear ossicular anomalies (Fig. 10-5 and Fig. 10-6).

Treacher Collins Syndrome. (mandibular dysostosis). J.K. is a three and one-half-year old with moderate first arch manifestations of Treacher-Collins syndrome. He has typical downward sloping palpebral fissures, beaked nose, and micrognathia. Both ear canals are very narrow and tortuous, too tiny for the smallest pneumatic otoscope

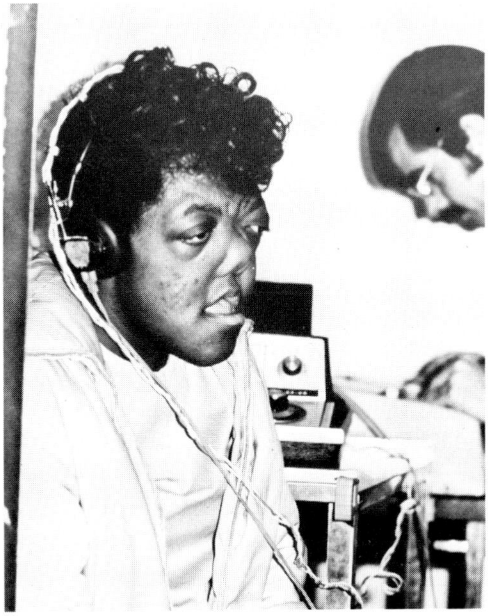

Figure 10-5 Apert's syndrome.

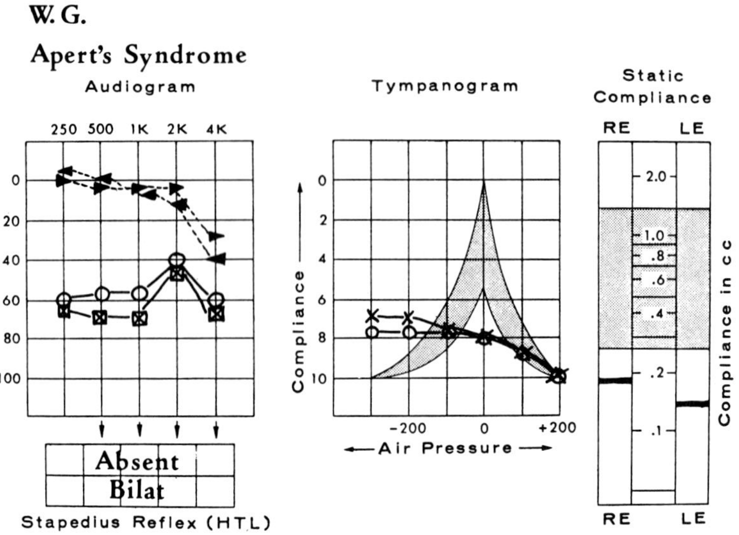

Figure 10–6 Impedance audiometry findings for the Apert's syndrome patient shown in Figure 5.

speculum. J.K. was diagnosed as having bilateral conductive hearing loss by age one year. He had bilateral SRTs of 45 dB and was fitted at two and one-half years with an earlevel air-conduction hearing aid which he wears continually. All ENT examiners report difficulty in viewing J.K.'s tympanic membranes. The impedance studies consistently demonstrated normal tympanograms and absent acoustic reflexes until approximately two months ago. At that time, the tympanograms were type B bilaterally, and a diagnosis of serous otitis media was made, which was medically treated. Hearing levels did not seem to change and the middle ear effusion did not clear with medication. Bilateral ventilation tubes were placed while J.K. was under general anesthesia, and thick serous fluid was removed bilaterally. The report of the operation indicated difficulty in verifying placement of the tubes, and though the right ear tube was felt to be definitely in place, some question remained about whether or not the left tube was successfully placed. Two weeks following the bilateral myringotomies with tubes, J.K. returned for evaluation. His mother reported doubt about improvement in the child's hearing. Otologic examination was inconclusive because the "ear canals were too small to verify tube placement." The hearing test showed no improvement in SRTs or pure-tone thresholds. The impedance Physical Volume Test showed a right ear volume of .9 cc and a left ear volume of .2 cc. This finding confirmed good placement of the tube in the right ear and a poor result with the tube in the left ear. The lack of hearing improvement continues to suggest the presence of a middle ear ossicular problem a common finding in mandibulofacial dysostosis. Although a physical volume of .9 cc is within general normal limit's, J.K.'s small ear canals have a normal volume of .2 cc. Thus a .9 cc volume is some four times his normal volume, representing the patency of the ventilation tube and his middle ear space (Fig. 10-7 and Fig. 10-8).

We have two patients with profound sensorineural deafness accompanying their craniofacial and skeletal problems who are enrolled as students in the state residential school for the deaf. Both patients are female, or normal intelligence, and communicate well with manual signs and fingerspelling. Both patients have radiologically confirmed middle ear ossicular anomalies overshadowed by their profound

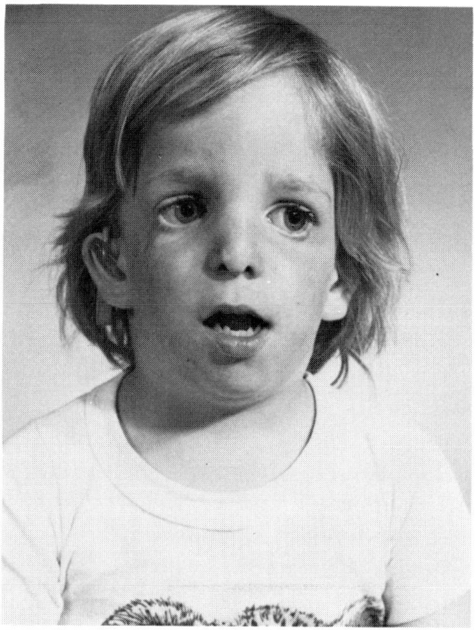

Figure 10-7 Youngster with mild penetrance of Treacher-Collins syndrome.

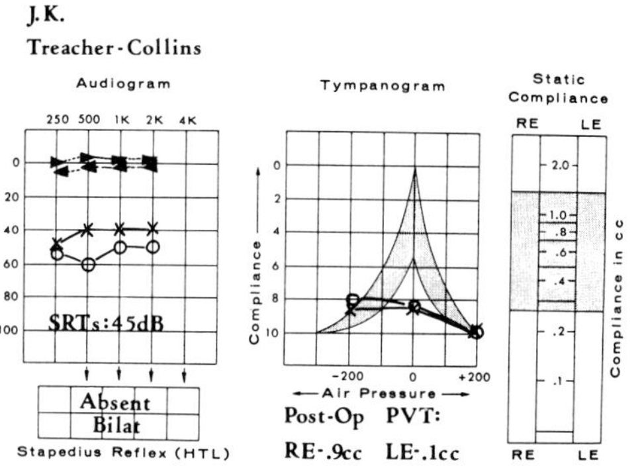

Figure 10-8 Impedance audiometry findings from a Treacher-Collins youngster shown in Figure 7.

sensorineural deafness. The key to their middle ear anomalies was type B (flat) tympanograms in light of normal eardrum appearance and normal mobility with pneumatic otoscopy.

Mobius Syndrome. The first young girl has bilateral facial weakness (nearly complete paralysis), submucous cleft palate with bifed uvula, obvious malformations of the external ears, and macrostomia or greatly exaggerated width of the mouth

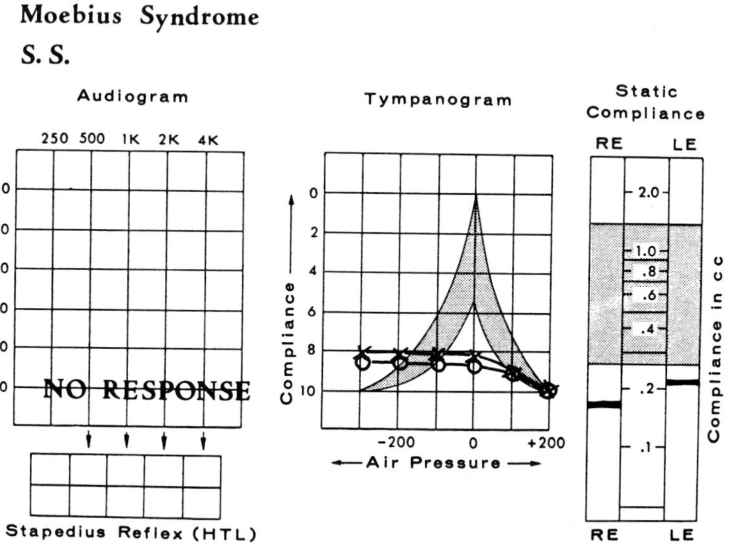

Figure 10-9 Impedance audiometry findings in Mobius syndrome.

resulting from failure of proper union of the maxillary and mandibular processes. In addition to no measureable hearing, radiographic tomographic studies reveal symmetric middle ear anomalies involving malleus and incus deformities and absence of the oval window bilaterally. The cochlea and vestibular system appear normal by x-ray, but the internal auditory canals are hypoplastic, measuring only 1.5 mm in diameter instead of the normal diameter of approximately 8.0 mm. The external ear canals and tympanic membranes are normal bilaterally on otoscopic examination and pneumatic massage. The impedance study indicated type B tympanograms, low static compliance, and absent acoustic reflexes (Fig. 10-9).

Klippel-Feil Syndrome. (brevicollis). The second female student with profound sensorineural hearing loss and middle ear anomalies has congenital absence of several cervical vertebrae with obvious shortening of the overall length of her cervical spine. Her neck appears short with slight webbing. She has a bifed uvula and submucous cleft palate. She is the seventh of eight children and was initially seen at age three and one-half because of absence of speech development. Her external ears appear slightly larger and somewhat low-set, with normal tympanic membranes and external ear canals. Radiographic tomography revealed bilateral fused ossicular masses. Again the impedance study was sensitive to the ossicular deformity producing type B tympanograms, low static compliance, and absent acoustic reflexes (Fig. 10-10 and Fig. 10-11).

EAR DISEASE IN NATIVE AMERICANS

Otitis media is currently the most serious health problem among the native American Indian and Eskimo population of North America. Much effort and money has been expended over the past years to gain control over the widespread problems of alcoholism and tuberculosis among American Indians. The success in these health programs, however, brought to light a new health problem—otologic disease and hearing impairment. This fact was cited in the President's Message on Indian Affairs, July 8th, 1970, when the four major health problems were listed in order as (1) otitis media, (2) mental health, (3) alcoholism, and (4) maternal and child care.

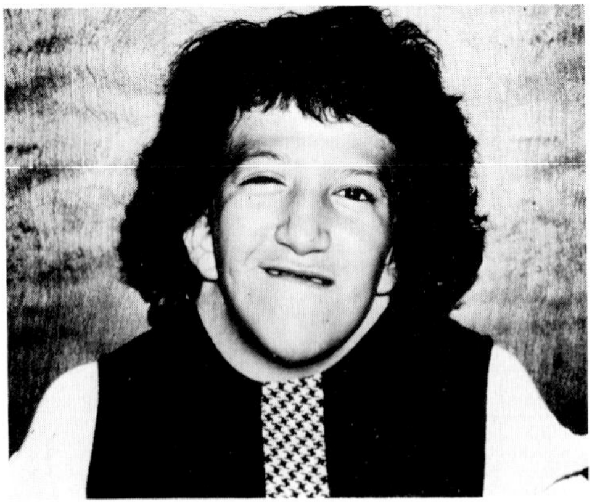

Figure 10-10 Profoundly deaf girl with Klippel-Feil syndrome and right-sided facial paralysis.

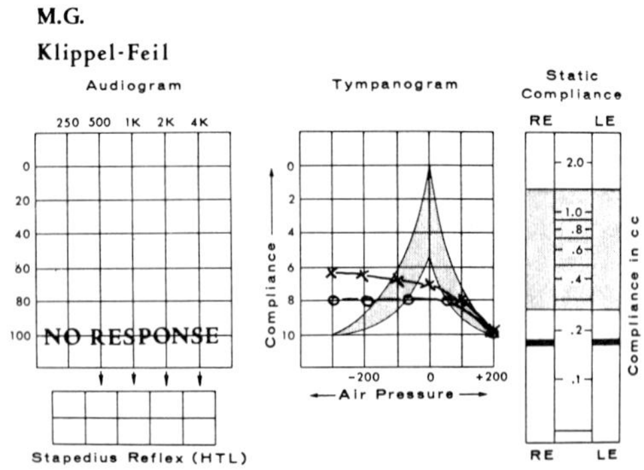

Figure 10-11 Impedance findings for the Klippel-Feil patient shown in Figure 10-10.

Health problems are readily evident among Native American populations because of their poor home conditions, harsh physical and psychologic environment, inadequate water facilities, crowded living conditions, unsanitary waste disposal, inadequate refrigeration, nonexistent insect control, and poor nutrition. With new federal financial support great strides in the health care for American Indians and native Alaskan's are being made. Cultural barriers, poverty, poor transportation, and lack of education about issues continue to make solutions to health problems more difficult. But progress is on the way, and in time, otitis media will be tumbled from its "number one" position in the list of serious health problems facing Indians and Eskimos (Johnson and Watrous, 1978).

The magnitude of the otitis media problem in this special population of Native Americans is immense. The Department of Health, Education and Welfare, Indian Health Service, is responsible for the health care of nearly 500,000 American Indians belonging to more than 250 tribes and 53,000 native Alaskans living in some 300 villages. While numerous gains gave been made over the past few years, the health status of Native Americans is still far below the standard for the rest of the nation. According to J.L. Stewart, of the Indian Health Service, data from the past seven years indicate that initial visits for otitis media have increased from a rate of 5,688 per 100,000 to 12,290 per 100,000. The Indian Health Service estimates a reservoir of over 22,000 unoperated patients potentially in need of otologic surgery; an additional 13,000 Native Americans are estimated to need hearing aids (Stewart, 1975).

Ear Disease in American Indians

Review of publications dealing with the incidence of ear disease in various American Indian populations also shows a high percentage of middle ear disorders. Johnson (1967) reported the incidence of chronic otitis media in the Navajo population to be twelve to fifteen times higher than found in Caucasian Americans.

Jaffe (1968) published a widely referenced article concerning the incidence of ear diseases of all types in the Navajo. Aural atresia prevalence was 58 in 60,000 cases; external otitis was uncommon, although foreign bodies in the form of "sheep ticks" were often found residing in the external ear canal; the pattern of onset of acute otitis media was common in infants, often leading to chronic suppurative otitis media; chronic suppurative otitis media was the most common Navajo otologic disease, with 4.2 percent of central perforations in 2000 patients; approximately 30 percent of these perforations had suppuration at examination; atelectatic middle ears were noted in 4.8 percent (96 per 2,000 cases); and no cholesteatomas were noted in over 200 tympanoplasties. Jaffe cites inbreeding among the Navajos as a major cause of frequently seen bifed uvula and aural atresias. One hundred years ago there were only 5000 Navajos while today's Navajo population is estimated at 125,000 to 150,000.

Other reports have been published on various American Indian tribes. Data on ear disease in some 385 South Dakota Indian children were presented by Gregg and colleagues in 1970 indicating that at least 24 percent of the group had significant ear disease history based on otolaryngologic and radiographic studies. Rossi (1972) used audiometry and tympanometry to evaluate ear disease in 504 New Mexican Pueblo Indian children. Two reports are available on ear problems in 3,043 Indians of Montana (Axelsson and Lewis, 1974; Lewis, 1975). As expected, otitis media, both acute and chronic, was the most commonly diagnosed disease, with an unexpected high incidence of sensorineural hearing loss (10.2 percent) in relatively young Indians. McCandless (1974) reported a correlation of 93 percent between impedance and otoscopy in the Wind River Reservation Indians of Wyoming. McCandless reported that conventional hearing screening missed nearly 40 percent of those children with significant otitis media. He felt that although otoscopy could be completed in less time than required for impedance testing, the impedance technique could be done in 2 to 3 minutes per child by trained technicians.

Hearing Impairment in Eskimos

In 1956, Hayman and Kester reported that the prevalence of active otitis media in Alaskan native children was as high as 17 percent. Ear disease in Eskimo children is such a common occurrence that most native Alaskan parents do not consider otorrhea to be a disease (Maynard, 1969). Brody (1965) reported a study in which 31 percent of an Eskimo village population had at least one episode of draining ears within the evaluation year, with two thirds of the group with ear disease indicating more than one episode of otorrhea. He stated that ear disorders in Eskimos are established by the age of two years, and those children who by age two did not have draining ears were unlikely to develop ear problems.

Several additional studies on Eskimo populations have been published confirming the extraordinarily high incidence of middle ear disease. Reed and Colleagues (1967) followed 378 Eskimo children during their first four years. In this group, 62 percent had one or more episodes of otorrhea—65 percent of this group had middle ear problems prior to age one, 89 percent by age two years. He reported that the *frequency* of episodes had more influence on the degree of hearing impairment than the age of onset of the initial otorrhea episode. Ling and Colleagues (1969) examined 525 children and adults in a single village and found active ear disease present in 30.8 percent of the group. Reed and Dunn (1970) found that 43 percent of 641 Eskimo children experienced 532 episodes of otitis media, with the highest incidence occurring in children less than two years of age. Kaplan (1973) reported that 38 percent of a group of Eskimo children had one or more bouts of otorrhea prior to age one, and 76 percent of these children commonly experienced otorrhea when they were subsequently evaluated at seven to ten years of age.

Although impedance screening is reportedly in wide use in Alaska, only a few reports have been published (Harker and Van Wagoner, 1974, 1976). In one study, more than 700 southeast Alaskan schoolaged children, with 35 of the children under the age of two years, were evaluated with pure tones, audiometry, otoscopy, and an "abbreviated" impedance technique. Pure-tone results could not be obtained in approximately 30 percent of the group because of their young age; however, impedance results were obtained in all but 1.3 percent of the group. Some 10 percent of the children passed the hearing screening but failed the impedance test. It was concluded that " . . . so far as to say in younger children, if only one test were available, impedance testing would be preferred."

Profoundly Deaf Children

Children attending schools for the deaf are not routinely evaluated by otolaryngologists. These deaf children seldom complain about their ears or of changes in their hearing sensitivity due to otologic pathologic factors. Bone conduction measurements are of limited usefulness in this special population with severe-to-profound sensorineural hearing impairment. Only a few published articles are available describing impedance measurement results from children attending schools for the deaf.

Two early reports were published about some 250 deaf children from the Minnesota School for the Deaf (Keating et al., 1972; Rose et al., 1972). These children, aged five to twenty-one years, were given otologic examination, hearing tests, tympanometry, and acoustic reflex tests. Tympanometry showed an incidence of abnormal findings greater than 10 percent for children of twelve years or younger, and less than 10 percent for children of all ages. The eight-year-old group had the highest percentage of abnormal tympanograms (54 percent). On the initial tympanogram test, seventy-nine ears had high negative pressure, yet only twenty-one of these ears were noted by otoscopy to be retracted. Otoscopic re-examination of seventy-two ears with middle ear pressure greater than −100 mm H_20 increased the otoscopic rating of "retraction" from twenty-one to fifty-one ears. The authors concluded that " . . . in an otologic examination, awareness of the possibility of negative middle ear pressure results in an increase in eardrums being rated retracted." Acoustic reflexes were examined in the 193 deaf children who had normal tympanometry. From this group of 193, acoustic reflexes were elicited in only thirty children in at least one frequency in at least one ear. Only seven of these thirty children had acoustic reflexes present bilaterally. The authors make a valiant but unsuccessful effort to relate the presence or absence of acoustic reflexes in deaf children to "good or poor" hearing aid utilization.

Porter (1972) purported to establish normative date for otoadmittance measurements in eighteen deaf children with severe-to-profound hearing loss. He did find statistically significant differences in conductance, susceptance, admittance, and impedance values between "normal-hearing" and "deaf" children's ears. The actual mean impedance value between the two groups was only 157 ohms, which is probably clinically insignificant. Unrelated to his experimental procedure, however, Porter reported results of impedance measurements in forty-two deaf students from the Kansas School for the Deaf. Abnormal admittance values consistent with middle ear pathologic findings were noted in 16.7 percent of the group, subsequently confirmed to have otitis media or middle ear effusion.

Brooks (1975) studied impedance in 306 children who were residents of two schools for the deaf in England during 1969. He pointed out two important conclusions: (1) The incidence of middle ear effusion is the same in deaf and normal-hearing children at five years of age, but the rate at which the disease diminishes in subsequent years is considerably slower in the deaf group; and (2) the residual level of middle ear disorders at age eleven and older is markedly higher in deaf children. Brooks reported that 7 percent of the deaf students older than eleven years had middle ear disease. Keating also found a high incidence of abnormal tympanogram's (25 percent) of deaf students aged twelve to thirteen years. Brooks concluded that although the incidence of middle ear problems in deaf children is at least equal to that noted in normal-hearing children, the likelihood of *detection* of the middle ear problem is considerably less.

Rossi and Sims (1977) reported the use of acoustic reflex measurements in the severely and profoundly deaf in an effort to evaluate the validity of audiometrically determined air-bone gaps. They conducted impedance studies of thirty-five deaf students showing that some 80 percent of the "air-bone gaps" produced by audiometry were, in fact, invalid. They recommend the use of impedance measurements of the acoustic reflex to resolve the ambiguity of responses due to probable tactile-vibratory stimulation with the audiometric bone oscillator from true conductive components. Riding and colleagues (1978) evaluated children in the Western Pennsylvania School for the Deaf with impedance and otoscopy and found 25 percent of the children in primary grades had some type of aural pathologic findings during the school year.

These studies show that impedance audiometry provides a useful means of evaluating the conductive mechanism in patients with profound deafness. The Brooks study brought out an important additional fact about the increase in hearing loss which accompanies middle ear problems. In deaf children this additional hearing loss may have a significant deleterious effect on hearing aid performance. If the child is mature enough to recognize the need to turn up the hearing aid gain, problems may be created with distortion and feedback; if the child is too young to note the change in hearing, poor performance with the hearing aid may also result. Impedance audiometry should, by all means, be a routine procedure for children attending schools for the deaf.

STAPEDIUS REFLEX IN MYASTHENIA GRAVIS

Myasthenia gravis is a neuromuscular disease characterized by abnormal fatigue of the muscles, particularly those innervated by the facial nerve. Symptoms usually develop early in the disease process with drooping of one or both upper eyelids (ptosis). Ptosis combined with facial diplegia (paralysis) result in a sad, sleepy expression which is characteristic of this condition.

The chief complaint of these patients is rapid muscle fatigue. For example, in attempting to comb the hair, it may become impossible to raise the arm above the head more than a few times. Some individuals also have difficulty chewing food owing to the rapid onset of fatigue in the muscles of deglutition. Because of the general weakness of these muscles, swallowing may be difficult and speech becomes an effort.

Blom and Zakrisson (1974) observed abnormal acoustic reflex decay in three patients with myasthenia gravis. Morioka and colleagues (1976) observed elevation of the acoustic reflex threshold in myasthenia gravis patients prior to medication with edrophonium chloride (Tensilon). After medication, lower intensity levels were required to elicit the reflex.

Warren and colleagues (1977) studied acoustic reflex decay to a 1-minute sound stimulus of 500 Hz in six patients with myasthenia gravis. In the six patients the magnitude of the stapedius muscle declined 30 to 75 percent, which was not demonstrated during the initial 10 seconds of stimulation. Thirty to forty-five seconds after intravenous injection of edrophonium chloride, no observable reflex decay was noted.

IMPEDANCE MEASUREMENTS WITH STUTTERERS

In 1973, McCall and Rabuzzi verified the reflex association between middle ear muscles and laryngeal muscles in cats. Although electromyographic evidence of middle ear muscle activity in association with vocalization in cats and man had been previously reported, McCall and Rabuzzi proved that reflex contraction of the stapedius and tensor tympani muscles was indeed activated by electric stimulation of the internal branch of the superior laryngeal nerve. Acoustic reflex discharges in the tympanic muscles were observed to occur also in association with reflex contraction of the cricothyroid muscle.

Based on the finding of the McCall and Rabuzzi study, Jerger conducted a small pilot project to compare middle ear muscle activity related to the onset of speech in stutterers and nonstutterers.— Although technically difficult to instrument, Jerger was able to show that the middle ear muscle activity, monitored with a specially designed acoustic impedance meter and a probe tone of 1400 Hz, occurred reflexively in nonstutterering speakers about 100 msec *prior* to the onset of vocalization. However, a group of three stutterers consistently showed altered middle ear muscle activity with the onset of their auditory muscle reflex occurring some 200 to 600 msec *following* the onset of vocalization.

A recent study of central auditory function in stutterers also revealed some interesting findings relative to middle ear muscle activity (Hall and Jerger, 1978). A series of tests designed to evaluate central auditory performance was administered to a group of ten stutterers and a carefully selected matched group of ten nonstutterers. As a group, the stutterers did indeed show evidence of central auditory deficiency, suggesting a subtle disorder at the brain stem level. Of particular interest was the finding that the amplitude function of acoustic reflex measurements, at threshold and in 5-dB increments to a maximum intensity of 110 dB HL at 2000 Hz, showed a consistently more gradual slope for the stutterers than for the nonstutterers.

ACKNOWLEDGEMENT

The author would like to acknowledge the efforts of a number of persons who supplied data or information used in preparation of this manuscript: Karen Bedwell, Elaine Carlson, Patricia Clees, Carol Cox, Marion Downs, James Jerger, Marilyn Krajicek, Richard Von Wagoner, Raymond Wood, and Janet Zarnoch. Portions of this chapter were presented at the International Symposium on Impedance Screening for Middle Ear Disease in Children, Nashville, 1977.

REFERENCES

Abahazi, D.A. and Greenberg, H. J.: Clinical acoustic reflex threshold measurements in infants. *J. Speech Hear. Dis.* 42:514, 1977.

Axelsson, A. and Lewis, C.: Aspects on delivery of ear, nose and throat care to Montana Indians. *Health Care and the Poor* 89:6; 551, 1974.

Bashore, S.R.: The use of tympanometry for screening developmentally disturbed children. *Audio. Hearing Educ.* 2:6; 35, 1976.

Berman, S.A., Balkany, T.J. and Simmons, M.A.: Otitis media in the neonatal intensive care unit. *Pediatrics* 62:2; 198, 1978.

Bess, F.H., Lewis, H.D. and Cieliczka, D.J.: Acoustic impedance measurements in cleft palate children. *J. Speech Hear. Dis.* 40, 13, 1975.

[1]J. Jerger, personal communication.

Bess, F.H., Schwartz, D.M. and Redfield, N.P.: Audiometric, impedance and otoscopic findings in children with cleft palates. *Arch Otolaryngol.* 102, 465, 1976.

Billings, B.L. and Lowry, L.D.: Tympanometry, impedance and aural reflex testing in a cleft palate population. *Cleft Palate J.* 11, 21, 1974.

Blom, S. and Zakrisson, J.E.: The stapedius reflex in the diagnosis of myasthenia gravis. *J. Neurol. Sci.* 21, 71, 1974.

Bluestone, C.D., Wittel, R.A. and Paradise, J.L.: Roentgenographic evaluation of eustachian tube function in infants with cleft and normal palates. *Cleft Palate J.* 9, 93, 1972.

Borus, J.: Acoustic impedance measurements with hard of hearing mentally retarded children. *J. Ment. Defic. Res.* 16, 196, 1972.

Brody, J.A., Overfield, T. and McAlister, R.: Draining ears and deafness among Eskimos. *Arch. Otolaryngol.* 81, 29, 1965.

Brooks, D.N.: Middle ear effusion in children with severe hearing loss. *Impedance Newsletter*, Vol. 4. New York, American Electromedics, 1975, 6-7.

Brooks, D.N., Wooley, H. and Kanjilal, G.C.: Hearing loss and middle ear disorders in patients with Down's Syndrome (Mongolism). *J. Ment. Defic. Res.* 16, 21, 1972.

Fulton, R.T. and Lamb, L.: Acoustic impedance and tympanometry with the retarded: a normative study. *Audiol.* 11, 199, 1972.

Fulton, R. and Lloyd, L.: Hearing impairment in a population of children with Down's Syndrome. *Am. J. Ment. Defic.* 73, 298, 1968.

Glovsky, L.: Audiological assessment of a mongoloid population. *Trng. Sch. Bull.* 33, 27, 1966.

Gregg, J. B., Steele, J. P., Clifford, S. and Werthman, H.E.: A multidisciplinary study of ear disease in South Dakota. *S. Dak. J. Med.* 23, 11, 1970.

Hall, J.W. and Jerger, J.F.: Central auditory function in stutterers. *J. Speech Hear. Res.* 215, 324, 1978.

Harker, L.A. and Van Wagoner, R.: Application of impedance audiometry as a screening instrument. *Acta Otolaryngol.* 77, 198, 1974.

Harker, L.A. and Van Wagoner, R.S.: Eustachian tube malfunction in Southeast Alaska. *Alaska Med.* 18:2; 13, 1976.

Hayman, C. and Kester, F.: Eye, ear, nose and throat infections in natives of Alaska. *Northwest Med.* 56, 423, 1956.

Howie, V.M., Ploussard, J.H. and Sloyer, J.L.: Natural history of otitis media. *Ann. Otol. Rhinol Laryngol.* (Suppl. #25) 85:18, 1976.

Jaffe, B.J.: The incidence of ear diseases in the Navajo Indians. *Laryngoscope* 58:2126, 1968.

Jaffe, B.F.: Heredity and congenital factors affecting newborn conductive hearing. *Conference Proceedings on Newborn Hearing Screening*, California State Department of Public Health, Berkeley, California, 1971; 87–100.

Jarvis, J.F.: Audiologic status of children with cleft palate: a review of 350 cases. *Audiol.* 15, 242, 1976.

Jerger, S., Jerger, J., Mauldin, L. and Segal, P.: Studies in impedance audiometry II: Children less than 6 years old. *Arch. Otolaryngol.* 99:1, 1974.

Johnson, R.L.: Chronic otitis media in school age Navajo Indians. *Laryngoscope* 77:1990, 1967.

Johnson, J.S. and Watrous, B.S.: An acoustic impedance screening program with an American Indian population. In Harford, E.R., Bess, F.H., Bluestone, C.D. and Klein, J.O. (Eds.): *Impedance Screening for Middle Ear Disease in Children* New York; Grune & Stratton, 1978, 257–270.

Jordan, O.: Mental retardation and hearing defects. *Scand. Audial* 1:1; 29, 1972.

Kaplan, G.J.: Long-term effects of otitis media: a ten year cohort study of Alaskan Eskimo Children. *Pediatrics* 52, 577, 1973.

Keating, L., Rose, D., Facer, G. et al.: Acoustic-impedance measurements in the deaf. In *Proceedings of Impedance Symposium*, Rochester, Minnesota, 1972, 177–181.

Keith, R.W.: Impedance audiometry with neonates. *Arch. Otolaryngol.* 97, 465, 1973.

Keith, R.W.: Middle ear function in neonates. *Arch. Otolaryngol.* 101, 376, 1975.

Keith, R.W., Murphy, K.P. and Martin, F.: Acoustic impedance measurement in the otological assessment of multiply handicapped children. *Clin. Otolaryngol.* 1:221, 1976.

Lamb, L. and Norris, T.: Acoustic impedance measurements. In Fulton, R. and Lloyd, L. (Eds.): *Audiometry for the Retarded.* Baltimore, Williams & Wilkins Co., 1969.

Lamb, L. and Norris, T.: Relative acoustic impedance measurements with mentally retarded children. *Am. J. Ment. Defic.* 75:1; 51, 1970.

Lewis, C.: The Montana otitis media project. *Hearing Instruments* 26:4; 21, 1975.

Ling, D., McCoy, R.H. and Levinson, E.D.: The incidence of middle ear disease and its educational implications among Baffin Island Eskimo Children. *Canad. J. Pub. Health* 60:385, 1969.

Lloyd, L. and Reid, M.J.: The incidence of hearing impairment in an institutionalized mentally retarded population. *Am. J. Ment. Defic.* 71, 746, 1966.

Maynard, J.E.: Otitis media in Alaskan Eskimo children: an epidemiological review with observations on control. *Alaska Med.* 93, 1969.

McCall, G.N. and Rabuzzi, D.D.: Reflex contraction of middle-ear muscles secondary to stimulation of laryngeal nerves. *J. Speech Hear. Res.* 16: 56, 1973.

McCandless, G.A. and Allred, P.L.: Tympanometry and emergence of the acoustic reflex in infants. In Harford, E.R., Bess, F.H., Bluestone, C.D. and Klein, J.O. (Eds.): *Impedance Screening for Middle Ear Disease in Children.* New York, Grune & Stratton, 1978, 57–67.

McCandless, G. and Thomas, G.: Impedance audiometry as a screening procedure for middle ear disease. *Trans. AAOO* 78, 98, 1974.

Morioka, W.T., Neff, P.A., Boisserane, T.E., Hartman, P.W. and Cantrell, R.W.: Audiotympanometric findings in myasthenia gravis. *Arch. Otolaryngol.* 102:211, 1976.

Northern, J. and Downs, M.: *Hearing In Children,* 2nd Ed. Baltimore; Williams & Wilkins Co., 1978.

Paradise, J.L. and Bluestone, C.D.: Early treatment of the universal otitis media of infants with cleft palate. *Pediatrics* 53:38, 1974.

Paradise, J.L., Smith, C.G. and Bluestone, C.D.: Tympanometric detection of middle ear effusion in infants and young children. *Pediatrics* 58:198-206, 1976.

Porter, T.A.: Normative otoadmittance values for three populations. *J. Aud. Res.* 12:1; 53, 1972.

Reed, D. and Dunn, W.: Epidemiologic studies of otitis media among Eskimo children. *Public Health Rep.* 85:8; 699, 1970.

Reed, D., Struve, S. and Maynard, J.E.: Otitis media and hearing deficiency among Eskimo children: a cohort study. *Am. J. Pub. Health* 57:9; 1675, 1967.

Reichert, T.J., Cantekin, E.I., Riding, K.H., Cohn, B.L. and Bluestone, C.D.: Diagnosis of middle ear effusions in young infants by otoscopy and tympanometry. In Harford, E.R., Bess, F.H., Bluestone, C.D. and Klein, J.O. (Eds.): *Impedance Screening for Middle Ear Disease in Children.* New York, Grune & Stratton, 1978, 257–270.

Riding, K.H., Reichert, T.J., Findlay, R.C. and Stool, S.E.: Tympanometric and otologic evaluation of students in a school for the deaf. In Harford, E.R., Bess, F.H., Bluestone, C.D. and Klein, J.O. (Eds.): *Impedance Screening for Middle Ear Disease in Children.* New York; Grune & Stratton, 1978, pp. 279–291.

Rittmanic, P.A.: The mentally retarded and mentally ill. In Rose, D. (Ed.): *Audiological Assessment.* Englewood Cliffs, New Jersey, Prentice-Hall, 1971, 369–401.

Rose, D., Keating, L., Facer, G. and Whicker, J.: Reflex measures in various types of ear pathology. In *Proceedings of Impedance Symposium,* Rochester, Minnesota, 1972, 261–268.

Rossi, D.F.: Hearing deficiency in Pueblo Indian children: results of a mass screening program. *Rocky Mt. Med. J.* 65, 1972.

Rossi, D.F. and Sims, D.G.: Acoustic reflex measurements in the severely and profoundly deaf. *Audiol. Hear. Educ.* 3:4; 6, 1977.

Sando, I. and Wood, R.P.: Congenital middle ear anomalies. *Otolaryngol. Clin. North Am.* (Symposium) 4:291, 1971.

Schwartz, D.M. and Schwartz, R.H.: Acoustic impedance and otoscopic findings in children with Down's Syndrome. Presented at the Society for Ear, Nose and Throat Advances in Children, October 1977, Chicago, Illinois.

Schwartz, D.M. and Schwartz, R.H.: A comparison of tympanometry and acoustic reflex measurements for detecting middle ear effusion in infants below seven months of age. In Harford, E.R., Bess, F.H., Bluestone, C.D. and Klein, J.O. (Eds.): *Impedence Screening for Middle Ear Disease in Children.* New York, Grune & Stratton, 1978, 91–96.

Shurin, P.A., Pelton, S.I., Klein, J.O.: Otitis media in the newborn infant. *Ann. Otol. Rhinol. Laryngol.* (Suppl. 25) 85: 216, 1976.

Snow, C.S. and McCandless, G.: Acoustic reflexes in spasticity and hypotonia. *Impedance Newsletter,* Vol. 4. New York; American Electromedics, 1975, 1–2.

Stewart, J.L.: The Indian Health Service hearing program: an overview. *Hearing Instruments* 26:4; 22, 1975.

Stool, S.E.: Diagnosis and treatment of ear disease in cleft palate children. In Bzoch, K. (Eds.): *Communicative Disorders Related to Cleft Lip and Palate.* Boston; Little, Brown & Co., 1971, 264, 273.

Warren, W.R., Gutmann, L., Cody, R.C., Flowers, P. and Segal, A.T.: Stapedius reflex decay in myasthenia gravis. *Arch. Neurol.* 34, 496, 1977.

Zarnoch, J.M. and Balkany, T.J.: Tympanometric screening of normal and intensive care unit newborns: validity and reliability. In Harford, E.R., Bess, F.H., Bluestone, C.D. and Klein, J.O. (Eds.): *Impedance Screening for Middle Ear Disease in Children.* New York; Grune & Stratton, 1978, 69–79.

Zarnoch, J.M. and Northern, J.L.: Acoustic Reflex Measures for the Prediction of Hearing Sensitivity in Deaf-Blind and Retarded Deaf-Blind Children. Paper presented before the Society for Ear, Nose and Throat Advances in Children (SENTAC), Fifth Annual Meeting, October 1977, Chicago, Illinois.

Chapter Eleven

THE USE OF IMPEDANCE MEASURES IN HEARING AID FITTING

GEARY A. McCANDLESS, Ph.D.
ROBERT W. KEITH, Ph.D.

INTRODUCTION

The goal of amplification is to achieve appreciation of acoustic energy at all frequencies in the speech spectrum while at the same time avoiding overamplification in the noncommunicative bandwidth. It is essential that sound be presented at a level which is comfortable over long periods of time and which does not produce physiologic or psychologic overload.

There has been much debate concerning the "best" way of obtaining optimal amplification for the hearing-impaired. Determining gain and frequency response from pure-tone sensitivity data or from comfortable listening levels appears to have value, as does fitting by prescription of electroacoustic characteristics, comparative hearing aid trials from stock aids, or selection by subjective impressions of clarity and quality. The failure of one technique to emerge as clearly superior after nearly forty years of trial suggests that while positive aspects can be found in most fitting methods, most lack the precision and proven validity one might wish.

To add objectivity and reliability to the hearing aid selection process, it is essential that physical measures with corresponding quantification by numbers be used as a means of assessing hearing aid function rather than descriptive words. While subjective evaluation of sound quality is important as a final step in the selection process, effects of varying electroacoustic characteristics must be expressed in terms that are less ambiguous than "harsh," "tinny," or "pleasant." These impressions, of course, must correlate at some point with specific measurable electroacoustic characteristics.

Impedance tests contribute to the fitting process by providing quantifiable measures that describe the status of the auditory system; they are influenced relatively little by subjective state and may be related to many aspects of auditory function, such as overload and perhaps even loudness. It seems reasonable, therefore, that impedance tests have good potential to improve upon current clinical practices of hearing aid selection and fitting.

As a matter of good clinical practice, all potential hearing aid candidates should receive an impedance test battery including tympanometry and ipsilateral and contralateral acoustic reflex thresholds at 250, 500, 1000, 2000, and 4000 Hz (Madell, 1976). Contralateral reflex decay and physical volume tests should also be included. Routine inclusion of these tests alerts the clinician to the pathologic factors in the tympanic membrane or middle ear system which may affect the fitting process. Also, acoustic reflex (AR) thresholds may help define the dynamic range and detect retrocochlear pathologic factors. Whether impedance findings suggest conductive, cochlear, or retrocochlear impairment, each type requires special consideration in the process of hearing aid fitting.

The presence of acoustically induced intra-aural muscle reflexes is mandatory for purposes of hearing aid fitting. When no viable reflex can be elicited, the procedures discussed in this chapter are inappropriate. Unfortunately, they are often of no assistance in cases where needed most, as with very young children, with mentally retarded subjects, or where a significant conductive component exists. Even the presence of a unilateral conductive pathologic factor makes the use of impedance tests for hearing aid fitting impossible, since the reflex is usually elevated or abolished bilaterally. The impedance technique is also limited in severe-to-profound sensorineural losses, since the reflex may sometimes be absent. Jerger and colleagues (1972) reported a significant number of absent reflexes in severe or profound hearing loss and found, for example, that reflexes could be obtained in only about 50 percent of subjects with losses greater than 85 dB HL. More encouraging, however, as related to hearing aid fitting, is that only 10 or 15 percent of subjects with sensorineural hearing loss less than 55 dB show absent reflexes. Since most hearing aid candidates have losses classified as mild or moderate, impedance testing can be utilized for at least 80 percent of potential hearing aid users.

USE OF ACOUSTIC REFLEX MEASURES IN SELECTING ELECTROACOUSTIC CHARACTERISTICS

Acoustic gain, frequency response, and saturation sound pressure level (SSPL) are accepted as basic electroacoustic measures important to hearing aid fitting. Factors such as transient distortion, compression, attack and recovery time, total bandwidth, harmonic distortion, smoothness of frequency response curve, and perhaps other characteristics are important considerations but will not be discussed here as we do not yet know how these factors affect hearing in the impaired ear. Before appropriate specific electroacoustic values can be incorporated into a hearing aid, measures of auditory function must first be made for each prospective user to determine his specific requirements. Optimum frequency response can be inferred by speech discrimination tests or by using some other predictive formula or technique (Victoreen, 1973; Berger, 1976).

The AR threshold has been of particular interest because of its potential use as an indicator of intensity overload. The interest in the acoustic reflex for this application emerged primarily because of the work by Metz (1946), who suggested that AR may indicate presence of loudness recruitment and that it represents an upper boundary of the dynamic range of hearing. Most studies employing measures to specify electroacoustic characteristics have, as a consequence, been related to loudness tolerance and SSPL as contrasted with measures of gain and frequency response (McCandless and Miller, 1972; McCandless, 1973, Olsen and Hipskind, 1973; Holmes and Woodford, 1976; Snow and McCandless, 1976; Rappaport and Tait, 1976; Dennenberg and Altshuler, 1976; and Keith, 1978.) Much less work has been reported relating the use of reflex measures to determine real ear gain or frequency response requirements for hearing aids (Dudich, Kieser, Keith, 1975; Tonisson, 1975; Rappaport and Tait, 1976; Snow and McCandless, 1976; and Preves and Orton, 1978).

Preliminary clinical experience clearly indicates AR measures to have practical value in hearing aid fittings. However, specific clinical tests have not yet been widely used at this time. We do not know exactly how reflex activity relates to subjective loudness for long periods of time, nor whether gain and frequency response determinations from reflex measures result in increased hearing aid acceptance and use. However, reflex thresholds have been demonstrated to be reliable and stable. Therefore, if they can be related consistently to subjective values of loudness, overload, or other aspects of auditory function, they can be used in the fitting process. Some of the previously reported work and suggested techniques will be discussed here.

USE OF THE ACOUSTIC REFLEX TO DETERMINE SSPL

The Acoustic Reflex as an Indicator of Loudness and Overload.

There are three main reasons for limiting the output of a hearing aid or otherwise reducing the total exposure time of intense sounds to the ear: (1) to prevent subjective loudness discomfort; (2) to prevent physiologic overload and possible distortion; and (3) to prevent physical trauma to the ear.

While there seems to be a general consensus that the output of a hearing aid must not exceed certain psychologic, physiologic, or physical limits, precisely what these limits should be and how they relate to various aspects of loudness discomfort have not been well defined (Rintelman and Bess, 1977). The uncertainties and variance of loudness discomfort levels (LDL) have been graphically described as "non-standard measures subject to uncertain interpretation" (Millin, 1975). Despite the apparent disagreement as to exact LDL thresholds and diversity of measurement technique, it can safely be said that subjective, physiologic, and physical overload occurs in the same general intensity range of about 85 to 110 dB SPL in normal ears, and that these measures are influenced by a variety of factors such as total time the stimulus is present, the bandwidth and waveform of the test stimulus (Margolis and Popelka, 1975), the level of background noise, and even the instructional method used to assess overload function (Morgan, Wilson, Dirks, 1974). If acoustic reflex measures are to be used to assess overload and to specify SSPL, it is essential that relationships of the reflex to loudness discomfort levels, temporary and permanent threshold shifts, and high-intensity distortion be examined.

EFFECTS OF ACOUSTIC REFLEXES ON LOUDNESS

The finding by Metz (1952) and later by Jepsen (1963) and Jerger (1970) that the

AR threshold occurs at reduced sensation levels in cochlear pathologic conditions implies the reflex is elicited when the activating stimulus exceeds some constant critical loudness (Jerger, Burney, Mauldin, 1974). This concept has been challenged by others (Hood and Poole, 1966; Ross, 1968; Margolis and Popelka, 1975; and Morgan and Dirks, 1975), who suggest that loudness is not the determinant of reflex thresholds; rather, elicitation of the reflex is more closely related to physical characteristics of the activating stimulus such as waveform and bandwidth. There is evidence that energy to the cochlea is reduced through action of the middle ear muscles at high-intensity levels for frequencies below 2000 Hz (Simmons, 1959; Borg, 1972). The attenuating effects of the AR have been estimated to be from as little as 5 to 10 dB (Bekesy and Rosenblith, 1961), to as much as 40 dB (Wiggers, 1937). Recent studies suggest the actual reduction is more typically 8 to 10 dB (Morgan and Dirks, 1975) and that the effects of the muscles are limited to the intensities of 90 dB SPL and higher.

If, as some believe, the reflex acts to reduce the energy of stimuli below 2000 Hz, we might expect to hear loudness change as the acoustic reflex threshold (ART) is crossed, or that the rate of loudness would decrease with increasing intensity. There is actually little evidence to show that dramatic changes in the magnitude estimates of loudness occur at AR thresholds. Loudness estimates apparently are quite linear to levels above the AR threshold (Stevens, 1955). It seems reasonable that minute contractions of middle ear muscles may not result in subjective changes of loudness (Morgan and Dirks, 1975). More logically, loudness alteration might not be expected until the magnitude of contraction is sufficient to alter significantly the impedance of the ear, and even then would be limited only to the lower frequency range.

ACOUSTIC REFLEXES AND LOUDNESS DISCOMFORT

Both researchers and clinicians have examined the AR as a possible means of identifying loudness discomfort. The objective is to use this measure as one criterion of overload, especially with patients who are unable to make loudness discomfort judgments because of age or pathologic conditions. If a constant relationship can be demonstrated between LDL and AR thresholds, it can be reasoned that the reflex might be used as the determinant of acoustic overload and in specifying SSPL. Reported research has been confusing in this relationship and as yet has not been entirely clarified.

Although loudness magnitude increases somewhat linearly up to levels producing sensations of pain, at some point below this level, subjective annoyance or discomfort occurs. Sensations of annoyance, discomfort, or alteration of quality to steady-state stimuli clearly appear in the intensity range approximating the AR threshold. Whether these sensations more closely approximate the AR threshold (McCandless, 1973) or the point of maximal reflex contraction (Olsen and Hipskind, 1973) has not been finally determined. The reason for this may be the wide divergence of methodology used in obtaining objective measures of loudness discomfort. Almost certainly, sensations of physical discomfort or pain are not caused by contraction of middle ear muscles, since the reflex is activated many times during each day even while talking. It is more likely that whatever mechanism causes the middle ear muscle contraction also ascribes to that stimulus some attribute of annoyance or irritability. Measures of tolerance or discomfort have been variously referred to as threshold of discomfort (TD), annoyance level, loudness discomfort level (LDL), uncomfortable loudness level (ULL or UCL), tolerance level or threshold, level of maximum audibility, and so on. Unfortunately, not only do these terms have slightly different connotations, but there are many differing techniques used to make these measures.

A loudness discomfort threshold is defined by some as the point at which a sound first becomes annoying, while others obtain estimates of loudness resulting in physical pain (Holmes and Woodford, 1976). Inconsistencies in measurement technique result in poor agreement as to what constitutes a real LDL, how it should properly be measured, and how it relates to SSPL settings. The confusion over discomfort measures is well illustrated by Berger (1976). "The typical text book on audiology pays little attention to the UCL determination, evidently under the assumption that most everyone involved with the audiometric testing readily understands the concept and the measurement protocol. Since the UCL is critical to appropriate SSPL, choice for setting in the hearing aid, the lack of specifics about it in the literature is unfortunate."

The problem in comparing AR thresholds to LDL has not been so much with the AR measure as with variability of subjective responses in the LDL tests. Table 11-1 illustrates good consistency of AR thresholds in normal subjects done in different laboratories and using a variety of impedance instruments. By contrast, this table also shows the greater variance of the LDL measurements and the ranges for pure-tone stimuli typically varying from as low as 84 to as high as 106 dB SPL. Patients with hearing loss also show considerable variance of LDL values owing to manifestations of the pathologic condition itself.

As previously mentioned, instructional differences greatly influence the loudness discomfort level, often shifting the values as much as 20 dB. Relationships of LDL to AR thresholds were mentioned by Hood and Poole in 1966. Although they did not investigate the reflex directly, they reported no particular relationship between the AR reflex threshold and the loudness discomfort levels in the affected ears. Their criterion for LDL was defined only as the point the subject "first expressed a feeling of loudness discomfort," but instructions were not described in detail. Later, Niemeyer (1971) stated that the LDL indicates that overload of the sensory cells is commencing. He further stated that AR thresholds are 10 to 20 dB lower than the threshold discomfort in ears with noise-induced trauma. Correspondence of his LDL measures may have been influenced largely by instructions; but since he did not specify the techniques or instructions used in the study, this correlation cannot be ascertained.

In 1972, McCandless and Miller found a high average correlation between the AR and LDL thresholds for pure-tone stimuli. In this study the LDL was described specifically as the point of *beginning* discomfort. Care was taken to instruct subjects to report impressions of a point where sound *first* begins to become uncomfortable. Results of the study showed some individual variability, but 90 percent of the subjects reported AR and discomfort thresholds to agree within ± 5 dB.

TABLE 11-1. Comparison of loudness discomfort and acoustic reflex thresholds*

		LDL	ART	r
Olsen and Hipskind	1000 Hz	87	91	re: HL
Duditch et al.	1000 Hz	84	93	re: SPL
Miller	500-2000 Hz	100	99	re: SPL
McLeod	1000 Hz	98	95	re: SPL
Berger	1000 Hz	106	92	re: SPL

*Data for normal ears for pure-tone stimuli from five different studies
Adapted in part from Ritter, 1977

Morgan and colleagues (1974) found a ± 3.5 dB average difference between LDL and reflex thresholds for pure tones using instructions phrased to determine not only when discomfort had occurred, but also when sound was "too loud" or "annoying," or when it was "above the level to which they would choose to listen for any period of time." Using broad-band stimuli, Morgan reported the AR threshold to be as much as 30 dB lower than the loudness discomfort level.

Other investigators—Berger (1976, 1979), Dennenberg and Altschuler (1976), Keith (1977), and Ritter and colleagues (1979)—have questioned the presumed relationship between the loudness experience and acoustic reflex and also the use of the reflex in the hearing aid selection procedures. According to these authors, while there is a high average correlation between loudness discomfort and acoustic reflex thresholds, these two measures do not necessarily appear at corresponding levels in individual subjects with sufficient consistency to infer loudness discomfort from acoustic reflex measures.

Recognizing the dependence of LDL measures on instruction to the subjects, Miller (1972) studied the effects of slight instructional changes on the LDL and related these measures to the AR threshold. He found as much as a 20-dB individual variance in LDL measures, but reported the difference between AR and LDL thresholds to average less than 2 dB for frequencies 250 to 4000 Hz when using a point where the sound first *starts* to become uncomfortable as the measure of discomfort. When instructions were changed only slightly to represent a point at which pure tones *clearly* became unpleasant, similar to those used by Morgan and colleagues (1974), Berger (1976), and Dennenberg and Altschuler (1976), the average discomfort threshold was elevated by 7 dB. Miller also found changes in instructions which reflected the point at which the stimulus becomes intolerable or physically uncomfortable to raise the measured LDL for pure tones from 100 to 122 dB SPL. The dramatic influence of instruction on the discomfort threshold levels explains in part where relationships between discomfort and reflex thresholds have been inconsistent. Most importantly it emphasizes the need to specify instructions used in relating LDL to the AR threshold especially for purposes of determining SSPL in hearing aids, and even suggests the AR threshold to be the most stable measure in recommending SSPL.

In summary, confusion remains regarding the relationship of acoustic reflex thresholds to loudness discomfort levels. It should be remembered, however, that the primary source of variance is not the reflex threshold but the LDL threshold. Until investigators more carefully define and standardize LDL tests, discrepancies between the two measures will persist.

ACOUSTIC REFLEX—PHYSIOLOGIC OVERLOAD AND DISTORTION

It seems generally accepted that if speech or other stimuli are raised above the AR threshold or beyond a point of beginning discomfort, a person is still able to discriminate most speech sounds even though there may be mechanical distortion produced by the conducting mechanism or cochlea. In fact, undistorted speech remains fairly clear in normal ears and in most ears with mild cochlear pathologic findings to levels above 100 dB SPL. This is illustrated by discrimination-intensity function tests in which speech clarity remains fairly good at high-intensity levels. However, evidence is accumulating which suggests that significant distortion occurs above this level. It is interesting to note that normal ears and many with cochlear pathogic findings show a slight reduction in speech discrimination rollover at high sensation levels of 5 to 20 percent (Jerger et al, 1968). This suggests that sufficient distortion occurs in the ear at high intensities to affect speech clarity to some degree. If distorted or degraded speech is used as the stimulus, the effects of high-level distortion are more obvious; that is, a greater discrimination reduction or rollover is produced. Evidence of distortion at levels above the AR threshold or discomfort level can be demonstrated clinically in some patients. Qualitative changes in a pure-tone stimuli or speech stimuli are described as sound becoming tinny or raspy as intensity is increased to levels above 95 dB SPL.

Few studies have actually analyzed speech discrimination at high-intensity levels with intra-aural muscle activity in mind. The middle ear has been reported to have a linear input-output function up to 130 dB SPL; whereas, considerable distortion may originate in the cochlea at levels beginning at 80 to 90 dB SPL, a level closely corresponding to the AR threshold (Borg and Zakrisson, 1973). Nonlinearity in the cochlear microphonics of animals also appears at about this level. At slightly higher levels subharmonics can be recorded in the cochlear microphonics of animals, the intensity of which can reach the magnitude of the fundamental frequency (Dallos and Linnell, 1964). The upward spread of masking also influences high-intensity discrimination. The spread of masking at low sensational levels is limited to a very narrow frequency range.

There is evidence that the middle ear muscles may reduce rather than produce distortion at high intensities. This evidence is based primarily upon the observation that when the middle ear muscles are paralyzed, distortion is greatly increased and reduction of speech discrimination occurs (Borg and Zakrisson, 1973; McCandless and Goering, 1974; and McCandless and Schumacher, 1979). Reductions in speech discrimination scores of 30 to 70 percent may result in ears with stapedial paralysis at intensity levels beginning very close to where the reflex would normally occur. Borg and Zakrisson (1973) have suggested that normal stapedius function extends the dynamic range of the ear by 15 to 20 dB.

In summary, there is both direct and indirect evidence that auditory distortion occurs at levels near or slightly above the acoustic reflex threshold. The reflex, therefore, might serve as a good indicator of beginning nonlinearity or distortion, even though it may not actually be the cause of these effects. Distortion at high-intensity levels is subjectively subtle and has minimal effect on discrimination of undistorted speech but may have a more significant effect in the impaired ear. Were it not for the action of the intra-aural muscles which extend the dynamic range, even greater distortion might occur. While reflex thresholds generally occur above the range of common environmental sounds, neither the normal nor the impaired ear can avoid producing distortion at high intensities, whether intense sound comes directly from the environment or is introduced via a hearing aid. Since it is likely that distortion increases rapidly above acoustic reflex thresholds, it seems reasonable to consider the AR threshold for sustained stimuli as a potential guide for the SSPL.

ACOUSTIC REFLEX AND ACOUSTIC TRAUMA

A third reason for limiting output of a hearing aid is to minimize the potential risk of additional hearing loss from overexposure to intense sound. The notion that individuals with end organ hearing loss are less susceptible to further damage by noise seems to have little basis in fact. Subjects whose AR reflex is absent owing to the severity of hearing loss but who have functioning hair cells might even be considered to be at higher risk for acoustic trauma through amplification because they have no protective acoustic reflex function. It is actually quite difficult to document increased hearing loss by excessive noise through amplification. This is because of difficulty in quantifying total sound pressures actually reaching the ear through a hearing aid. Moreover, the potential for noise-induced hearing loss is greatly influenced by the acoustic spectrum and total exposure time of the sound. Many hearing aids are capable of presenting sound in excess of 130 dB SPL, so the potential of noise damage due to amplification must be considered with each fitting.

The possibility of noise trauma due to excessive sound pressure in adults seems to be minimized because users typically lower the volume to tolerable—and consequently safer—levels when in noisy situations. Also, few users are exposed to continuous high-level environmental noise. The greatest potential for damage appears to be in infants and children or others not capable of adjusting volume controls or unable to complain adequately when loud sounds become uncomfortable. There have been several clinical reports of trauma in children due to over amplification by hearing aids (Harford and Markle, 1955; MacRae and Farrant, 1965; Ross and Lerman, 1967; Jerger and Lewis, 1975; and Rintelman and Bess, 1977). Kasten and Braunlin (1970) reported the traumatic effects of a hearing aid on a child with a moderate loss who showed a substantial drop in hearing after wearing an aid for fourteen months. This child's aid had only 20 to 30 dB of real-ear gain and an SSPL of 120 dB, illustrating how little gain and SSPL may be potentially damaging.

It is interesting to note that long-term exposure is potentially damaging at levels approximating the acoustic reflex threshold (about 90 dBA for an 8-hour exposure). However, it should not be inferred that all noise exceeding the reflex threshold is dangerous. Recommended safe levels of the Occupational Safety and Health Administration (OSHA) indicate a 5-dB increase in the safe listening level when exposure time is cut in half, i.e., 95 dB for 4 hours, 100 dB for 2 hours, with an upper limit of 115 dB for 15 minutes or less. The intermittent nature of sound found in most environments may not exceed the damage risk criterion levels for noise established by the U.S. Department of Labor and OSHA (OSHA, 1974). If the environmental noise is sufficient to stimulate the reflex into tonic contractions one might infer that this level is potentially damaging over long periods of time for sustained high-level stimuli. Adaptation of the middle ear muscles might occur, reducing their protective action after a few minutes of constant stimulation. Also, the middle ear muscles have little attenuating effect of frequencies above 2000 Hz, so damage at these higher frequencies might result in any case.

The evidence to date would suggest that for purposes of protection from intense sounds introduced by amplification, setting the SSPL to levels corresponding with the beginning reflex thresholds for brief sounds would not be appropriate. It is the total exposure time that is of most concern, and while there has been some research regarding the contraction of the muscles as related to noise trauma, there is little evidence that sound that triggers occasional bursts of reflex activity would be potentially damaging if it does not exceed known damage risk criterion. Therefore, for purposes of setting SSPL, an appropriate level would be below the level at which typical environmental sounds produce constant contraction of the middle ear muscles.

TEMPORARY THRESHOLD SHIFT

Even if the total exposure time of intense sounds falls below a level expected to produce permanent and irreversible damage, reports by users of subjective "muffling" or "dullness" of sound after wearing the aids for a period of time are quite common. This suggests that temporary threshold shift (TTS), altered loudness, or pitch or timber changes has occurred (Ward, 1973). While TTS may not be an infallible predictor of susceptibility to permanent threshold shift except at high frequencies, sounds sufficient to cause TTS through hearing aids should be considered potentially damaging as well as capable of producing unwanted distortion in the cochlea. Although subjects with hearing loss demonstrate less TTS than those with normal ears, it is apparently because they have "less to lose" (Ward, 1973). When the amount of TTS is added to the amount of hearing loss, the total drop in threshold due to fatiguing noise is about the same as in normal ears. Cochlear losses, therefore, enjoy little if any exposure level advantage over the normal ear, and in this context they have more to lose (Selters, 1964). The implication, of course, is that sound pressures that are potentially damaging or fatiguing to the normal ear may have the same effect in the ear with sensory hearing loss—at least in those with mild-to-moderate loss, since their thresholds of overload are at or near normal levels (Hood and Poole, 1966).

Although the influence of middle ear muscle activity on TTS has not been extensively studied, the correspondence of the AR threshold levels reported to produce TTS and permanent damage over time are amazingly close. For example, Hood and Poole (1966) reported dramatic TTS shifts from pure-tone stimuli occurring above 90 dB SL. Selters (1964) showed a rapid elevation of TTS in normal ears beginning at 90 dB SL. If one wishes to set hearing aid gain and SSPL at levels at which TTS would not occur, the reflex threshold activity when wearing amplification may be a useful measure for this purpose.

CLINICAL PROCEDURE FOR SETTING SSPL USING THE ACOUSTIC REFLEX

One technique of determining SSPL values for hearing aid candidates is to limit the output of the aid at or slightly above the acoustic reflex threshold for pure tones as illustrated in Figure 11–1. Reflex thresholds are determined for frequencies 500, 1000,

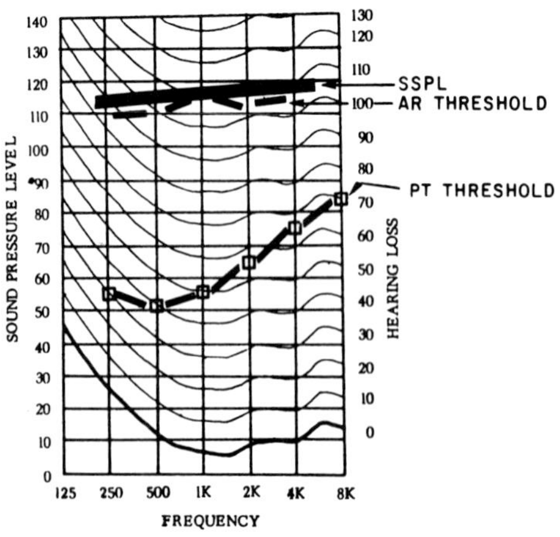

Figure 11-1 Method of determining appropriate SSPL level, based on acoustic reflex thresholds for pure tones. Pure tone and acoustic reflex thresholds are displayed in SPL. Appropriate SSPL level is at or slightly above best-fit line of AR thresholds at frequencies 500-4000 Hz.

2000, and 4000 Hz. SSPL is set at or slightly above a best-fit line for these frequencies. To set SSPL at the point of beginning reflex activity elicited by a speech stimulus would result in input settings that might unnecessarily limit upper usable auditory ranges.

Using speech stimuli, the output of the aid should be set 5 to 8 dB higher than the acoustic reflex thresholds, since verbal stimuli produce lower reflex thresholds than do pure tones. (McCandless and Miller, 1972; Olson and Hipskind, 1973; Dudich, Keiser, Keith, 1975; and McLeod, 1977). Figure 11–2 illustrates this concept. The acoustic reflex for speech is recorded as intensity is increased. Not until the reflex is nearly 10 dB above the level of beginning muscle activity does it become subjectively uncomfortable. Setting SSPL to levels below those that would eliminate all reflex activity does not seem to be a method of choice, based on the many studies related to loudness and loudness discomfort. Transient sounds lasting a few milliseconds are not recorded as annoying, whereas sounds of long duration causing sustained middle ear contraction are invariably judged to be uncomfortable.

In summary, the output of an aid should be limited to levels just below these at which speech and normal environmental sound cause sustained muscle contraction, but should allow for occasional reflex activity caused by peaks of energy. Using pure-tone stimuli, one might elect to set SSPL between 300 and 3000 Hz at levels that barely produce constant reflex contractions but never at levels exceeding about 10 dB above this point.

ACOUSTIC REFLEX MEASURES IN SETTING ACOUSTIC GAIN

Subjects with cochlear impairment typically utilize hearing aid gain corresponding to about one half their hearing loss owing to recruitment and narrowing of dynamic range (Lybarger, 1963; McCandless, 1973; and Berger, 1976). Setting gain is a more critical issue for children than for adults, since the latter are able to adjust volume controls to a desirable listening level for each situation.

The viewpoint that the AR is not mediated by loudness of the signal poses a theoretic argument against the use of the reflex method of establishing hearing aid gain. Gain most often conforms to a comfort level setting or MCL. However, the MCL

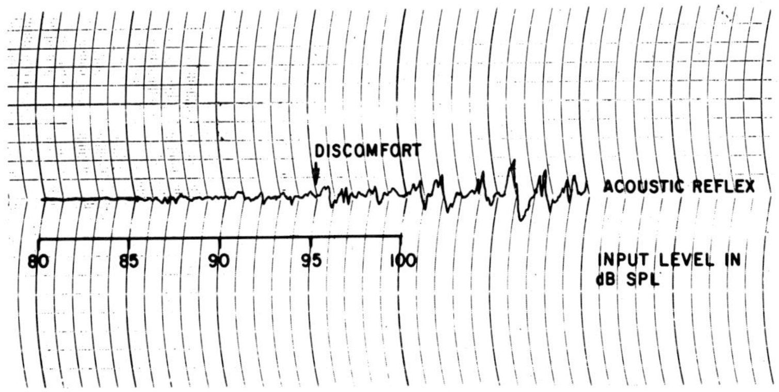

Figure 11-2 Acoustic reflexes to running speech stimulus are shown. Note that sensation of discomfort does not occur at reflex threshold for speech but at about 10 dB above point of beginning reflexes.

for speech is elevated by a background of noise while the AR stays constant. In quiet, the AR and most comfortable loudness (MCL) for speech are correlated so the AR procedure has been proved successful in setting gain for many children (Keith, 1978).

The influence of the reflex on speech discrimination is also an important issue when relating gain to the reflex. Rappaport and Tait (1976) examined this relationship by measuring speech discrimination in noise at the reflex threshold and at levels 10 dB above and 10 dB below the AR threshold. Although considerable variation was found between measures, the highest speech discrimination occurred at the point of beginning reflex activity.

Keith (1978) examined the AR as it related to the MCL. Using a 70 dB speech signal, he found that hearing aid gain adjusted to the AR threshold resulted in 62.5 percent of the hearing aid users reporting speech to be at MCL and 37.5 percent reported it was too loud. He indicated that setting the aid at or just below the AR threshold levels yielded settings inappropriate for most subjects. He then modified his procedure by dividing subjects into two groups. Those whose AR threshold was less than 90 dB were adjusted exactly to the AR threshold, and subjects with reflexes above 90 dB HTL adjusted their aids to just below the AR threshold. Using this procedure he found 75 percent of the hearing aid users were amplified to their MCL.

Measuring Real Gain

It is sometimes helpful not only to set gain on a hearing aid but actually to measure the use gain at a specific volume setting. Tonisson (1975) described a technique for determining real ear or functional gain based on measurements of aided and unaided reflex thresholds, as illustrated in Figure 11-3. He used narrow-band stimuli presented free field to elicit the reflexes with and without a hearing aid. Real-ear gain was defined as the difference in dB between the aided and unaided thresholds. Results showed general correspondence between the measures, but considerable individual variation was found between real ear gain vs gain measured in a 2 cc

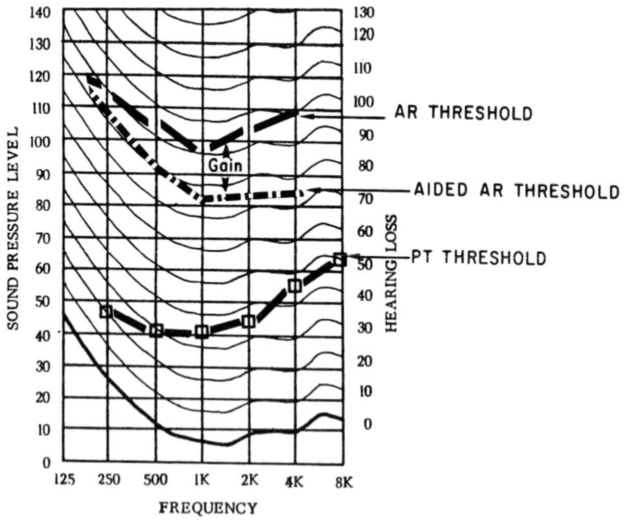

Figure 11-3 Functional or real-ear gain based on acoustic reflex thresholds are shown. The amount of shift in reflex threshold from unaided to aided condition reflects functional gain at each frequency tested.

coupler. Tonnison indicated that the AR method of determining gain offers advantages over coupler measures in that real-ear values reflect not only influences of hearing aids but also effects of ear mold, pinna, and ear canal.

In 1978, Preves and Orton replicated Tonnison's work using pulsed tones as stimuli. They too reported some differences in insertion vs coupler gain using reflex measures. In most cases insertion gain was slightly greater than functional gain; the mean differences ranged from .3 dB at 250 Hz to 4.6 dB at 5000 Hz. These values are not great, however, suggesting reasonable validity for use of the reflex gain procedures.

In summary, as reflex techniques for determining optimum and real-ear gain are developed, they can add objectivity to existing clinical procedures. More importantly, they offer a method of setting gain in children based on more objective criteria than procedures that set the volume control on some arbitrary basis.

Several investigators have reported clinical procedures for using the reflex to adjust gain in hearing aids (Horning, 1975; Tato and Rainville, 1976; Snow and McCandless, 1976; Bragg, 1977; and Keith, 1978). The procedure usually followed is to place the hearing aid on one ear of the subject and the impedance probe in the opposite ear, as shown in Figure 11-4. The speaker may be at 0°, 90° or other azimuth depending on the preference of the examiner. Sound field speech at 60 to 70 dB SPL or other stimuli are presented as free field, and the volume control is adjusted upward until the reflex is first seen on the compliance meter or recorder. Gain must be set at levels at which conversational speech and most environmental sounds do not produce a constant reflex contraction. Figure 11-5 shows the aided reflex activity to a speech stimuli as the volume control is gradually turned up. Sensations of discomfort are seen when the reflex contraction becomes sustained. The volume should be set at a lower level to prevent this tonic contraction.

EAR CANAL VOLUME AND HEARING AIDS

The use of the acoustic impedance meter to measure ear canal volume between the probe tip cuff and the tympanic membrane has special significance for hearing aid fittings, selection, and utilization (Northern, 1978). In the presence of an intact eardrum and a hermetically sealed probe tip cuff in the ear canal, the average enclosed canal cavity is approximately 1.2 cc for an adult. In infants, the physical ear canal volume value may be as small as 0.5 cc. It seems likely that these same ear canal volumes exist when the ear canal is tightly sealed with a nonvented ear mold.

Clinicians are aware, of course, that hearing aid specifications are reported in dB

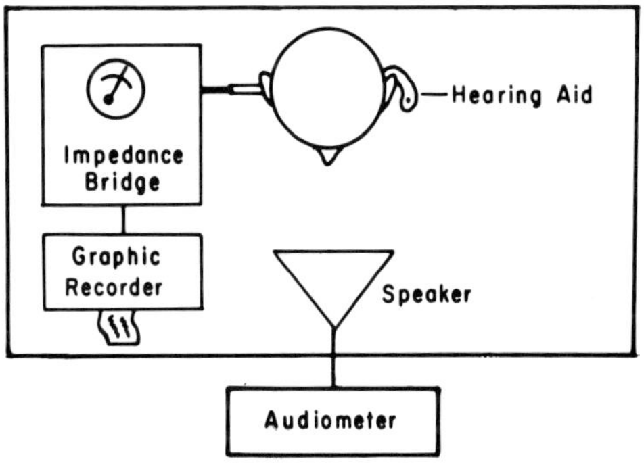

Figure 11-4 Block diagram of arrangement of subject and equipment for measuring acoustic reflexes while wearing hearing aid. AR can be monitored on compliance meter but is best done using a graphic recorder.

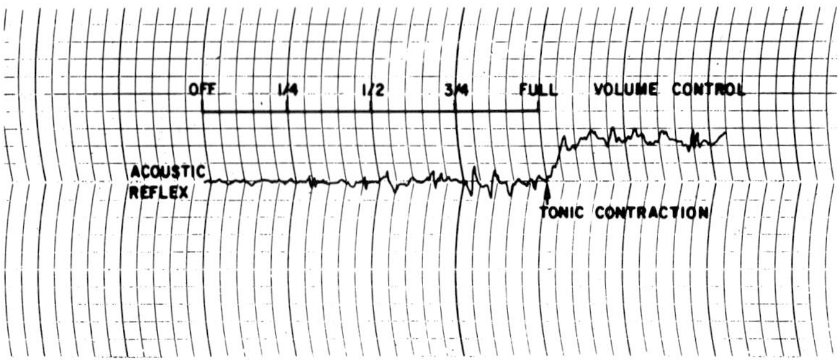

Figure 11-5 Aided acoustic reflex is shown to increase in amplitude as volume control of hearing aid is raised to maximum. At higher levels, AR is seen to be in tonic contraction, but superimposed compliance changes corresponding to peak energy in speech stimulus can still be seen.

relative to a 2.0 cc cavity. However, hearing aid specifications relative to a 2.0 cc cavity will be significantly altered when the hearing aid is coupled tightly to an ear canal that is less than 2.0 cc in volume. In fact, *each time the cavity volume is reduced by half, the entrapped sound pressure is increased by 6 dB.* It can be expected that hearing aid sound pressures measured on a 2.0 cc cavity will be delivered to an adult 1.0 cc ear canal with 6 dB more intensity than shown on the standard hearing aid frequency response curve (Cole, 1975). Small children with ear canal volumes of .5 cc may actually receive 12 dB more amplification than indicated on the hearing aid specification report.

Clinicians who select hearing aids based on the aid's reported 2.0 cc specifications must be aware that over amplification may result from coupling the aid and full ear mold to a 1.0 cc or smaller ear canal. According to Sachs and Burkhard (1972) the 2.0 cc coupler underestimates aided sound pressure level relative to the human ear canal by as much as 15 dB in the higher frequencies. The acoustic impedance meter can provide important information to establish ear canal volume prior to selection of the hearing aid.

THE ACOUSTIC REFLEX IN SELECTING OPTIMUM FREQUENCY RESPONSE

Relatively little research or clinical findings has been reported utilizing reflex measures in predicting optimum frequency response. Using the procedure described previously by Tonnison (1975), the reflex thresholds are obtained for pure tones in a free-field setting. Gain at discrete frequencies can be measured and the aided frequency response computed. Figure 11-6 shows the aided and unaided reflex thresholds for a frequency-modulated tone presented free field to a two-and-one-half-year-old child. His audiometric and reflex thresholds are shown in SPL. Aid A shifts the reflex thresholds 15 dB at 500 Hz, 15 dB at 1000 and 2000 Hz, and 20 dB at 4000 Hz. Aid B lowered the AR threshold 15 dB at 500 Hz, 15 dB at 1000 Hz, 25 dB at 2000 Hz, and 25 dB at 4000 Hz. Aid B clearly has more functional gain at the higher frequencies and is more appropriate for this particular child. Using the reflex technique, the clinician can simultaneously measure average real gain and frequency response. The data can be used predictively to determine optimum gain and frequency response to compare the function of various clinical aids or can be used with a master hearing aid.

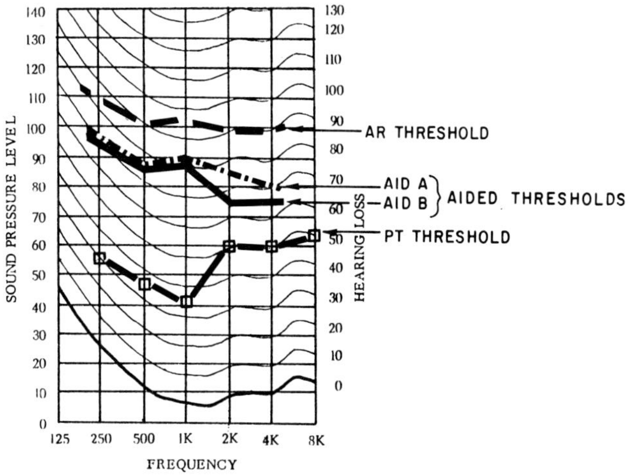

Figure 11-6 Comparison of frequency response of two hearing aids based on aided reflex threshold measures. Differences in frequency response between various aids are reflected in aided AR thresholds. Note that in this case, aid B has more functional gain at 2000 and 4000 Hz than aid A.

SUMMARY

Use of a variety of traditional hearing aid selection procedures has failed to establish a single method that is clearly superior and that results in an optimal hearing aid fitting that is free of subjective judgment. These procedures are especially deficient when they are used with very young children or with other individuals who are unable to provide listener reaction to the aided signal. Use of the acoustic reflex as a guide to the establishment of optimal gain, SSPL, and frequency response may provide the objectivity that is desired.

Use of the acoustic reflex to determine SSPL is done for three reasons: (1) to prevent subjective loudness discomfort; (2) to prevent physiologic overload and possible distortion; and (3) to prevent acoustic trauma to the ear. A suggested clinical procedure for establishing SSPL is to limit the output of the hearing aid to levels at or slightly above the acoustic reflex for pure tones when the hearing aid volume control is set to approximately three-fourths gain.

For those who question the potential value in using the AR to indicate intensity overload, an appropriate question might be, "How many hearing aid wearers will tolerate their aids to be worn at levels which produce sustained contraction?" To the present time the authors have found none. To establish an appropriate hearing aid gain, present sound-field speech at 60 to 70 dB SPL and adjust the volume control until the acoustic reflex is just visible to occasional peaks of acoustic energy. To select optimum frequency response, measure the hearing aid's real-ear gain by determining the difference between aided and unaided AR thresholds to sound-field, narrow-band, or pulse-tone stimuli.

While the techniques discussed in this chapter need to be validated through further research and clinical trials, it appears that acoustic reflex measurements in hearing aid fitting have useful application with some patients and deserve further investigation and refinement.

REFERENCES

Bekesy, G.V. and Rosenblith, W.A.: The mechanical properties of the ear. In Stevens, S. (Ed.): *Handbook of Experimental Psychology*. New York, John Wiley Co., 1951.

Berger, K.W.: Prescription of hearing aids: a rational. *J. Am. Audiol. Soc.* 2: 71, 1976.

Berger, K.W.: The use of uncomfortable loudness level in hearing aid fitting. *Maico Audiolog.* 15: 2, 1976.

Borg, E.: Acoustic middle ear reflexes: a sensory control system. *Acta Otolaryngol. (Suppl.)* XXX, p. 304, 1972.

Borg, E. and Zakrisson, J.E.: Stapedius reflex and speech feature. *J. Acoust. Soc. Am.* 54: 525, 1973.

Bragg, V.C.: Toward a more objective hearing aid fitting procedure. *Hearing Instruments* : 6, 1977.

Cole, W.A.: Hearing aid gain: a functional approach *Hearing Instruments*. 26, 10: 22-24, 1975.

Dallos, P.J. and Linnell, C.O.: Subharmonic components in cochlear-microphonic potentials. *J. Acoust. Soc. Am.* 40:1; 4, 1966.

Dennenberg, L.J. and Altshuler, M.W.: The clinical relationship between acoustic reflexes and loudness perception. *J. Am. Audiol. Soc.* 2:3, 79, 1976.

Dudich, T.M., Keiser, M. and Keith, R.W.: Some relationships between loudness and the acoustic reflex. *Impedance Newsletter*, Vol. 4. Acton, Mass., American Electromedics, 1975, 12–15.

Harford, E. and Markle, D.M.: The atypical effect of a hearing aid on one patient with congenital deafness. *Laryngoscope* 65:970, 1955.

Holmes, D. and Woodford, C.: Acoustic reflex thresholds and loudness discomfort level relationships in deaf children. *J. Acoust. Soc. Am.* 59: 1; 83, 1976.

Hood, J.D. and Poole, J.P.: Tolerable limit of loudness: its clinical and physiological significance *J. Acoust. Soc. Am.* 40:47, 1966.

Horning, J.: Tympanometry and hearing aid selection. *National Hearing Aid Journal* April, 8/50, 1975.

Jepson, O.: Middle ear reflexes in man. In Jerger, J. (Ed.). *Modern Developments in Audiology*. New York, Academic Press, 1963, 193–239.

Jerger, J., Speaks, C. and Trammell, J.L.: A new approach to speech audiometry. *J. Speech Hear. Dis.* 33:4; 318, 1968.

Jerger, J.: Clinical experience with impedance audiometry. *Arch. Otolaryngol.* 92:311, 1970.

Jerger, J., Burney, P., Mauldin, L. et al.: Predicting hearing loss from the acoustic reflex. *J. Speech Hear. Dis.* 39:1, 1974.

Jerger, J., Jerger, S. and Maulding, L.: Studies in impedance audiometry: normal and sensorineural ears. *Arch. Otolaryngol.* 96:513, 1972.

Jerger, J. and Lewis N.: Binaural hearing aids: are they dangerous for children? *Arch. Otolaryngol.* 101:480, 1975.

Kasten, R.N. and Braunlin, R.J.: Traumatic hearing aid usage: a case study. Paper presented at the annual convention of American Speech and Hearing Association, New York, 1970.

Keith, R.W.: An acoustic reflex technique of establishing hearing aid settings. Paper presented at the Annual Convention of the American Speech and Hearing Association, Houston, November 1976.

Keith, R.W.: An acoustic reflex technique of establishing hearing aid settings. *J. Am. Aud. Soc.* 1979. In press.

Lybarger, S.: Simplified fitting systems for hearing aids. Radioear Corp., Cannonsburg, Pennsylvania.

Macrae, J.H. and Farrant, R.H.: The effect of hearing aid use on the residual hearing of children with sensorineural deafness. *Ann. Otol.* 74:409, 1965.

Madell, J.R.: Hearing aid evaluation procedures with children. In Ruben, M. (Ed.): *Hearing Aids: Current developments and Concepts*. Baltimore, University Park Press, 1976, 103–109.

Margolis, R.H. and Popelka, G.R.: Loudness and the acoustic reflex. *J. Acoust. Soc. Am.* 58:6; 1330, 1975.

McCandless, G. and Miller, D.: Loudness discomfort and hearing aids. *National Hearing Aid Journal* June 7/28/32, 1972.

McCandless, G.: Hearing aids and loudness discomfort. Paper presented at Otocongress 3, Copenhagen, 1973.

McCandless, G.A. and Goering D.: Changes in loudness after stapedectomy. *Arch Otolaryngol.* 100: 344, 1974.

McCandless, G.A. and Schumacher, M.: Speech discrimination function in facial paralysis. *Arch. Otolaryngol.* 1979. In press.

McLeod, H.: The relationship between the acoustic reflex and loudness discomfort in normal and sensorineural ears. Unpublished Ph.D. dissertation, Bowling Green State University, Bowling Green, Ohio, 1977.

Metz, O.: The acoustic impedance measured in normal and pathological ears. *Acta Otolaryngol.* (Suppl. #63) 1946.

Metz, O.: Threshold of reflex contractions of muscles of the middle ear and recruitment of loudness. *Arch. Otolaryngol.* 55:536, 1952.

Miller, D.: The effects of instruction and practice on the level and stability of the loudness discomfort threshold. Unpublished Ph.D. dissertation, University of Utah, Salt Lake City, Utah, 1972.

Millin, J.P.: Practical and philosophical considerations. In Pollack, M.C. (Ed.): *Amplification in the Hearing Impaired*. New York, Grune & Stratton, 1975, 115–142.

Morgan, D.E. and Dirks, D.D.: Influence of middle-ear muscle contration on pure tone suprathreshold loudness judgments. *J. Acoust. Soc. Am.* 57:2; 411, 1975.
Morgan, D.E., Wilson, R.H. and Dirks, D.O.: Loudness discomfort level: selected methods and stimuli. *J. Acoust. Soc. Am.* 56:2; 577, 1974.
Niemeyer, W.: Relations between the discomfort level and the reflex threshold of the middle ear muscles. *Audiol.* 10:172, 1971.
Northern, J.L.: Hearing aids and acoustical impedance measurements. *Monographs in Contemporary Audiology* 1:2, Maico Hearing Instruments, 1978.
Olson, A.E., Hipskind, N.M.: The relation between levels of pure tones and speech which elicit the acoustic reflex and loudness discomfort. *J. Aud. Res.* 13:71, 1973.
Preves, D.A. and Orton, J.F.: Use of acoustic impedance measures in hearing aid fitting. *Hearing Instruments* June 22, 1978.
Rappaport, B.Z. and Tait, C.A.: Acoustic reflex threshold measurement in hearing aid selection. *Arch. Otolaryngol.* 102: 3; 129, 1976.
Rintleman, W.F. and Bess, F.H.: High-level amplification and potential hearing loss in children. In Bess, F.H. (Ed.): *Childhood Deafness: Causation, Assessment and Management.* New York, Grune & Stratton, 1977, 267–293.
Ritter, R.: The effect of instructional patterns on the relationship between loudness discomfort levels and acoustic reflex thresholds. Unpublished Ph.D. dissertation, University of Denver, Denver, Colorado, 1978.
Ritter, R. Johnson, R. and Northern, J.: The controversial relationship between loudness discomfort levels and acoustic reflex thresholds. *J. Am. Soc. Audiol.* 4:4; 123, 1979.
Ross, M. and Lerman, J.: Hearing aid usage and its effect upon residual hearing. *Arch. Otolaryngol.* 86: 639, 1967.
Ross, S.: On the relation between the acoustic reflex and loudness. *J. Acoust. Soc. Am.* 43:768, 1968.
Sachs, R.M., Burkhard, M.D.: Insert earphone pressure response in real ears and couplers. Abstract, *J. Acoust. Soc. Am.* 52, 1(Part 1):183, 1972.
Selters, W.: Adaptation and fatigue. *J. Acoust. Soc. Am.* 36:2202, 1964.
Simmons, B.F.: Middle ear muscle activity at moderate sound levels. *Ann. Otol. Rhinol. Laryngol.* 68:1126, 1959.
Snow, T. and McCandless, G.: The use of impedance measures in hearing aid selection. *National Hearing Aid Journal* January 7/32–33, 1976.
Stevens, S.S.: The measurement of loudness. *J. Acoust. Soc. Am.* 27:5; 815, 1955.
Tato, J.M. and Rainville, M.J.: Utilization du reflexe stapedien pour l'adaption des protheses. (The use of stapedius reflex in the fitting of hearing aids.) *Audiol.* 15:428, 1976.
Tonisson, W.: Measuring in-the-ear gain of hearing aids by the acoustic reflex method. *J. Speech Hear. Res.* 18:5, 1975.
Victoreen, J.A.: *Basic Principles of Otometry.* Springfield, Charles C. Thomas, 1973.
Ward, W.D.: Adaptation and fatigue. In Jerger, J. (Ed.): *Modern Developments in Audiology.* 1973, 301–339.
Wiggers, H.C.: The functions of the intra-aural muscles. *Am. J. Physiol.* 120:771, 1937.

Chapter Twelve

APPLICATIONS OF IMPEDANCE AUDIOMETRY TO ANIMAL RESEARCH

LARRY MAULDIN, B.A.
JAMES JERGER, Ph.D.

Historically, experimental animals have provided investigators with much information regarding acoustic impedance measures. Various animal species have been employed in the study of absolute impedance, middle ear transfer function, acoustic reflex thresholds, and the dynamics and effects of acoustic reflex activity in normal ears. These results have been applied in the study of impedance measures in humans. The clinical applications of impedance measures in the evaluation of humans with various auditory pathologic conditions have been well defined in previous chapters. Until recently, however, impedance audiometry has not been utilized in studying pathologic states in animals.

TYMPANOMETRY

Tympanometry in animals has been employed in the evaluation of the development of middle ear impedance in neonatal animals, the monitoring of middle ear air pressure, and the assessment of various surgically created middle ear impairments. In each of these applications, tympanometry provided valid and reliable information.

The use of tympanometry to evaluate the development of middle ear impedance in the neonatal hamster was described by Relkin and colleagues (1978). These investigators used a carefully calibrated tympanometer to assess middle ear admittances for signals spanning the range from 800 to 1800 Hz. Hamsters were classed in age groups of 6, 12, 16, 20, 25, 30, 35, 51, and 69 days. Relkin and associates found that prior to 16 days of age the admittance could not be measured reliably. From day 16 to day 35 middle ear admittance increased rapidly. Admittances measured at days 51 and 69 showed only a slight further increase. In addition, admittances measured after day 16 showed an orderly frequency effect. The

800 Hz signal always yielded the lowest admittance, while the 1800 Hz signal always resulted in the highest admittance.

In 1974 Eliachar and colleagues and Miller and Holmquist presented results from experimental animals showing that the tympanogram provides a valid estimate of middle ear pressure. Cannulae were surgically implanted to allow the experimenters to control and monitor the middle ear air pressure in guinea pigs (Eliachar et al.) and rhesus monkeys (Miller and Holmquist). Both studies indicated that the external canal air pressure which produces maximum compliance (minimum impedance) corresponds closely to the actual middle ear air pressure. More recently, Cantekin and coworkers (1977) used tympanograms to monitor the air pressure and status of the middle ears of rhesus monkeys serving as animal models for the study of Eustachian tube function.

Effects of experimental middle ear surgery on impedance measures in the squirrel monkey were described by Jerger and colleagues (1978a). Both acoustic reflexes and tympanograms were recorded before and after experimental surgery to produce middle ear disorders. Lesions studied included middle ear mass, ossicular discontinuity, middle ear mass plus ossicular fixation, and mastoid mass obliteration. Each monkey was tested on at least six occasions, three times before surgery and three times after surgery. In each test session, tympanograms were recorded at each 200-Hz increment for probe tone frequencies from 200 to 3000 Hz.

Jerger and colleagues were able to record tympanograms reliably in the squirrel monkeys. Preoperative tympanograms on the monkeys showed probe tone frequency effects that were remarkably similar to the effects observed in humans. As the probe tone frequency was successively raised above the frequency that gave a deep, single-peak tympanogram, a "W" shaped tympanogram appeared, grew more pronounced, and then declined to a shallow, single-peak tympanogram. Although this progression of pattern changes is the same in both humans and squirrel monkeys, the absolute frequency at which analogous patterns are seen is quite different. A particular tympanometric pattern in squirrel monkeys will appear at a probe tone frequency that is approximately 1000 Hz higher than the probe tone frequency that produced its counterpart in humans. Figure 12–1 illustrates these described effects in a human and a squirrel monkey. The probe tone frequencies yielding deep, single-peak tympanograms are 200 and 1200 Hz for the human and monkey, respectively. At 1200 Hz, a "W" pattern is obvious in the human tympanogram, while for the monkey, the "W" shape is not readily apparent until 2400 Hz. Similar effects were observed in all the monkeys during preoperative testing.

Postoperatively, the tympanometric patterns resulting from the experimental surgical procedures were similar to those observed in humans with the same middle ear pathologic findings. Tympanograms in ears with middle ear mass lesions showed a flattening and decrease in depth, while surgery to create ossicular discontinuity produced abnormally deep tympanograms that showed a "W" pattern at a lower probe tone frequency than had been the case preoperatively. In all the monkeys the tympanometric measures accurately reflected the nature of the experimental middle ear disorder.

Two conclusions may be drawn from the studies reporting tympanometric measures in animals. First, tympanometry is a valid technique for assessing middle ear air pressure and the functional status of the middle ear. Changes in tympanometric patterns with middle ear disorders are analogous in animals and humans. The second conclusion, extremely important for clinical application of tympanometric measures

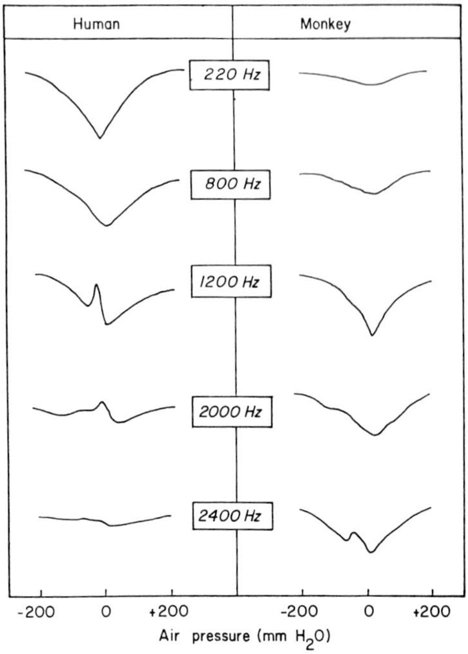

Figure 12-1 Typical human and monkey tympanograms at various probe tone frequencies. Similar patterns are seen in human and monkey tympanograms as probe tone frequency increases. A specific pattern in the monkey is obtained at a higher probe tone frequency than analogous pattern in human.

in animals, is that the frequency of the probe tone used to record tympanograms has a great influence on the tympanometric pattern observed. Relkin and colleagues (1978) were unable to detect admittances for probe tone frequencies below 800 Hz in hamsters; Jerger and colleagues (1978a) found that tympanograms below 1200 Hz were shallow and somewhat rounded in shape in squirrel monkeys. The probe tone frequency that yields a deep, single-peak tympanogram in one species of experimental animal may be quite different from the frequency that yields the same pattern in another species. Therefore, the instrumentation employed in impedance measurement in animals should be sufficiently flexible to allow the use of a wide range of probe tone frequencies. The appropriate probe tone frequency or range of probe tone frequencies may then be determined for the experimental animals being used.

ACOUSTIC REFLEX

Acoustic reflex thresholds are routinely employed in humans as indicators of amount of conductive hearing loss or as a means of predicting degree of sensorineural hearing loss. In unilateral conductive hearing loss, the amount of conductive loss is estimated from the elevation of acoustic reflex thresholds when sound is delivered to the affected ear (Jerger et al., (1974a). Degree of sensorineural hearing loss is predicted from the comparison of acoustic reflex thresholds for pure-tone signals and noise signals (Jerger et al., 1974b). Until recently these applications of acoustic reflex measures have not been attempted in animals.

Acoustic reflexes have been described in squirrel monkeys subjected to experimental middle ear surgery (Jerger et al., 1978a) and in squirrel monkeys with experimentally induced sensorineural hearing loss (Jerger et al., 1978b). In both studies, acoustic reflex thresholds were determined for pure-tone signals at 500, 1000, 2000, and 4000 Hz, as well as for broad-band random noise. Acoustic reflex thresholds were obtained in at least three separate sessions before and three sessions after the experimental treatment.

Reflexes in normal monkeys revealed a pattern similar to that observed in humans. The reflex threshold to broad-band noise was considerably better than the averaged threshold for 500, 1000, and 2000 Hz signals. This relationship, the noise-tone difference (NTD), is employed to predict degree of sensorineural hearing loss in humans (Jerger et al., 1974b) and was similarly employed in the squirrel monkey.

Middle Ear Surgery

In the monkeys subjected to experimental middle ear surgery, the preoperative NTDs suggested normal hearing in both ears in each monkey. Following the unilateral middle ear surgery, two effects were observed. First, when the impedance measuring probe was in the surgically altered ear, reflex activity, in general, either was not observed or was present at elevated threshold levels. Jerger and colleagues attributed this to the change in the "resting" impedance of the middle ear system.

The second effect of middle ear surgery was apparent when the impedance measuring probe was in the normal ear and the acoustic signal was delivered to the ear with a middle ear disorder. On the first postoperative test session, all monkeys showed substantially elevated reflex thresholds. In the permanent middle ear disorders, reflex thresholds remained elevated throughout postoperative testing. In the temporary middle ear disorders, reflex thresholds progressively improved during the postoperative testing. In all monkeys, NTDs indicated normal sensorineural levels postoperatively.

The reflex thresholds with sound in the ear operated on provided quantitative information on middle ear transmission losses resulting from the experimental surgery. These losses must be compensated for on a decibel-for-decibel basis. By comparing postoperative reflex thresholds with the average preoperative reflex thresholds, Jerger and colleagues were able to estimate the degree of conductive hearing loss present at any test session.

Sensorineural Hearing Loss: Ototoxic Drugs

Changes in the NTD following direct irrigation of the inner ear with gentamicin solution were described by Jerger and colleagues (1978b) as being quite variable. These changes, however, predicted degrees of sensorineural hearing loss which correlated well with post-mortem histopathologic studies. Figure 12–2 shows pre- and postoperative reflex thresholds on four monkeys. Postoperatively, reflexes were not observed for any of the signals with sound in the ear treated with gentamicin. All tympanograms were normal on each postoperative test. In addition, reflex thresholds were at normal levels when sound was delivered to the unoperated ear. Thus, having ruled out the possibility of middle ear disorder, a prediction of profound sensorineural loss in the operated ear was made on all four monkeys. Histologic studies, also shown in Figure 12–2, revealed extensive morphologic damage in each animal and supported the prediction of profound loss.

In two monkeys, postoperative reflex activity was observed. Figure 12–3 shows that in one monkey (# 4092) a small change in the NTD resulted in the prediction of a

#4865	STIM	PRE	POST	DIFF
	BBN	81.3	—	—
	500	121.0	—	—
	1000	108.3	—	—
	2000	94.7	—	—
	NTD	26.7	—	—
	PREDICTION		PROFOUND LOSS	

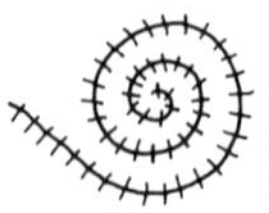

#3649	STIM	PRE	POST	DIFF
	BBN	87.3	—	—
	500	111.3	—	—
	1000	98.7	—	—
	2000	89.0	—	—
	NTD	12.4	—	—
	PREDICTION		PROFOUND LOSS	

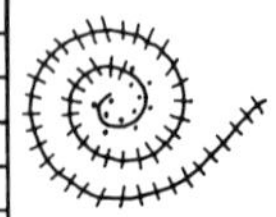

#5386	STIM	PRE	POST	DIFF
	BBN	79.7	—	—
	500	119.3	—	—
	1000	110.0	—	—
	2000	102.7	—	—
	NTD	31.0	—	—
	PREDICTION		PROFOUND LOSS	

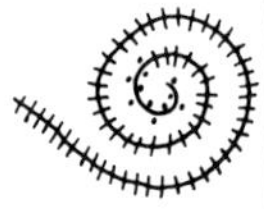

#4297	STIM	PRE	POST	DIFF
	BBN	89.0	—	—
	500	118.0	—	—
	1000	98.7	—	—
	2000	87.3	—	—
	NTD	12.3	—	—
	PREDICTION		PROFOUND LOSS	

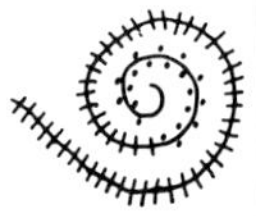

Figure 12–2 Preoperative and postoperative reflex thresholds (in decibels sound pressure level) on treated ears of four monkeys receiving unilateral direct irrigation of inner ear with gentamicin. Postoperative absence of reflexes in all monkeys suggests profound sensorineural loss. Diagrammatic cochlear representations show extent of damage revealed histologically. Slashed lines indicate severe destruction; dotted lines, moderate destruction; BBN, broad-band noise; NTD, noise-tone difference.

mild sensorineural loss, while a larger NTD change in the second monkey (#3725) resulted in the prediction of a moderate sensorineural loss. The first monkey showed only a limited extent of damage in the basal region of the cochlea on histologic studies. The second showed more severe damage that extended further apically. In these animals histologic studies correlated well with the predicted losses.

Sensorineural Hearing Loss: Noise Exposure

Jerger and colleagues (1978b) also described changes in the NTD following noise exposure. Figure 12–4 shows results obtained on one monkey undergoing unilateral

#4092	STIM	PRE	POST	DIFF
	BBN	85.7	94.0	-8.3
	500	106.3	101.3	5.0
	1000	100.3	100.3	0.0
	2000	89.0	97.3	-8.3
	NTD	12.8	5.6	7.2
	PREDICTION		MILD LOSS	

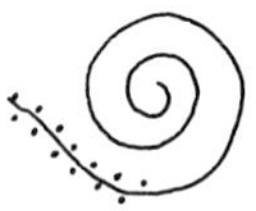

#3725	STIM	PRE	POST	DIFF
	BBN	89.0	100.7	-11.7
	500	113.0	108.0	5.0
	1000	103.7	108.7	-5.0
	2000	94.0	99.0	-5.0
	NTD	14.6	4.5	10.1
	PREDICTION		MODERATE LOSS	

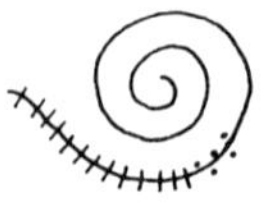

Figure 12–3 Preoperative and postoperative reflex thresholds (in decibels sound pressure level) and threshold differences (before-after) on treated ears of two monkeys receiving unilateral direct irrigation of inner ear with gentamicin. Diagrammatic cochlear representations show extent of damage revealed histologically. Note correlation between extent and severity of damage and predicted hearing loss. Slashed lines indicate severe destruction; dotted lines, moderate destruction; smooth lines, no destruction; BBN, broad-band noise; NTD, noise-tone difference.

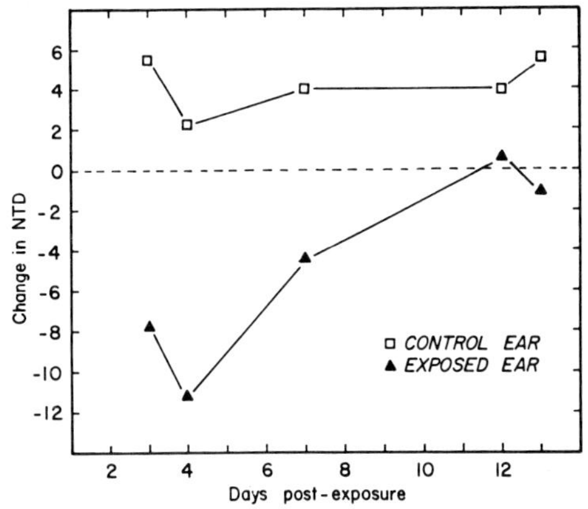

Figure 12-4 Effects of noise exposure on noise-tone difference (NTD). Changes in NTD (post-exposure NTD–pre-exposure NTD) are plotted for monkey recovering from unilateral noise exposure. Note systematic return of NTD to its pre-exposure level on exposed ear.

noise exposure. The figure compares the average pre-exposure NTD with the NTD measured on each post-exposure test session for both the control ear and the ear exposed to broad-band noise at 115 dB SPL for 2 hours. While the control ear showed a relatively constant NTD, the exposed ear yielded a large decrease in the NTD on the first two post-exposure test sessions. This change in the NTD suggested that the noise exposure produced a moderate-to-severe sensorineural loss. Thereafter the NTD began to increase, indicating recovery from the noise exposure. By the twelfth day after the exposure, a return of hearing to normal levels is predicted. Similar patterns of changes in the NTD were observed on two other monkeys undergoing noise exposure. Noise exposure resulted in reduction of the NTD with subsequent return of the NTD to normal levels during the post-exposure period. The NTD seems to provide an accurate reflection of both the degree of noise-induced hearing loss and the time course of recovery.

COMBINED USE OF TYMPANOMETRY AND ACOUSTIC REFLEXES

As is the case in humans, the use of either tympanograms or acoustic reflexes as a sole measure of middle ear function in animals will provide only limited information. Acoustic reflexes accurately reflect the degree of dysfunction in middle ear disorders. However, they offer little information about the nature of the disorder; this information is provided by the tympanometric measures. Neither acoustic reflexes nor tympanograms, in isolation, can provide an overall description of the disorder. However, when used in combination, the two measures offer a powerful technique for evaluating the status of experimental animals.

Jerger and colleagues (1978a) evaluated the agreement between impressions of middle ear status determined independently from impedance findings and from histologic studies. Of the seven monkeys evaluated, only one monkey showed poor agreement between impedance and histologic factors. In the remaining monkeys, overall agreement between impedance and histologic factors was fair in two monkeys and good in four monkeys. The general conclusion was that agreement between impedance findings and histologic findings was quite satisfactory.

In the evaluation of sensorineural losses in experimental animals, the noise-tone difference accurately reflects changes in cochlear sensitivity. Increasing sensorineural loss produces progressively smaller NTDs. In the case of profound sensorineural loss, acoustic reflex activity is not observed. However, middle ear disorders can also result in the failure to observe reflex activity. In such cases, erroneous predictions of profound sensorineural hearing loss would be made. Tympanograms provide a means of detecting many of the middle ear disorders that may arise in animals. Thus, even when the measure of interest is the acoustic reflex, both reflexes and tympanograms should be recorded to control for the possible artifactual effects of middle ear disorder.

APPLICATIONS OF IMPEDANCE MEASURES IN ANIMALS

Impedance measures, tympanograms, and acoustic reflexes, offer a sensitive, easily administered means of assessing middle ear function and cochlear sensitivity in animals. Immediately apparent applications are the monitoring of middle ear function of animals serving as experimental models for the study of middle ear disorders and the predictions of sensorineural hearing levels in ototoxic drug and noise exposure experiments. Of no less value, however, is the application of impedance measures as screening and/or monitoring tests of middle ear function and cochlear sensitivity in animals used in any type of auditory experimentation. Unsuspected and undetected middle ear disorders in experimental animals can render entire experiments useless. The quickly administered impedance measures offer a technique for detecting many of these disorders in their early stages, before the experimental data must be considered completely invalid. In some experiments where estimates of threshold sensitivity are needed, predictions based on the noise-tone difference (NTD) may be sufficient to supplant time-consuming behavioral training techniques. In combination, tympanograms and acoustic reflexes provide a stable baseline assessment of middle ear function and cochlear sensitivity against which any changes may be compared.

In recent years, the use of impedance measures as a screening procedure in children has gained widespread popularity among pediatricians. At present, we are aware of at least one innovative practitioner of veterinary medicine who is attempting to employ impedance measures in a similar manner in a clinical veterinary practice. Perhaps the next decade will witness the growth of applications of impedance measures in animals similar to that observed in humans over the last decade.

REFERENCES

Cantekin, E., Bluestone, C., Saez, C., Doyle, W. and Phillips, D.: Normal and abnormal middle ear ventilation. *Ann. Otol. Rhinol. Laryngol. (Suppl.)* 41:1, 1977.

Eliachar, I., Sando, I. and Northern, J.: Measurement of middle ear pressure in guinea pigs. *Arch. Otolaryngol.* 99:172, 1974.

Jerger, J., Anthony, L., Jerger, S. and Mauldin, L.: Studies in impedance and audiometry: III. Middle ear disorders. *Arch. Otolaryngol.* 99:165, 1974a.

Jerger, J., Burney, P., Mauldin, L. and Crump, B.: Predicting hearing loss from the acoustic reflex. *J. Speech Hear. Disord.* 39:11, 1974b.

Jerger, J., Mauldin, L. and Igarashi, M. Impedance audiometry in the squirrel monkey. Effect of middle ear surgery. *Arch. Otolaryngol.*104:214, 1978a.

Jerger, J., Mauldin, L. and Igarashi, M.: Impedance audiometry in the squirrel monkey. Sensorineural losses. *Arch. Otolaryngol.* 104:559, 1978b.

Miller, J. and Holmquist, J.: An animal model for study of Eustachian tube and middle ear function. *Scand. Audiol.* 3:63, 1974.

Relkin, E., Saunders, J. and Konkle, D.: A tympanometric evaluation of the development of middle ear admittance in neonatal hamsters. Paper presented at the ninety-fifth meeting of the Acoustical Society of America, Providence, Rhode Island, 1978.

Index